Brain Protection in Cardiac Surgery

Robert S. Bonser • Domenico Pagano
Axel Haverich
(Editors)

Brain Protection in Cardiac Surgery

Springer

Prof. Robert S. Bonser MD, FRCP, FRCS, FESC, FACC
Professor and Consultant Cardiac Surgeon
Department of Cardiothoracic Surgery,
Queen Elizabeth Hospital,
University Hospital Birmingham NHS Trust,
Edgbaston, Birmingham, UK

Mr. Domenico Pagano
Cardiothoracic Surgery
Beaumont Road 208
B30 1NX Birmingham
Bournville
United Kingdom

Prof. Axel Haverich
Medizinische Hochschule
Hannover (MHH) Klinik für Herz-, Thorax-,
Transplantations- und
Gefäßchirurgie
Carl-Neuberg-Str. 1
30625 Hannover
Germany

ISBN: 978-1-4471-6833-1 ISBN: 978-1-84996-293-3 (eBook)

DOI: 10.1007/978-1-84996-293-3

A catalogue record for this book is available from the British Library

Softcover re-print of the Hardcover 1st edition 2011

Printed on acid-free paper

Springer Science+Business Media (www.springer.com)

Foreword

"You are old, Father William," the young man said,
And your hair has become very white;
And yet you incessantly stand on your head –
Do you think, at your age, it is right?"
"In my youth," Father William replied to his son,
I feared it might injure the brain;
But, now that I'm perfectly sure I have none,
Why, I do it again and again."[1]

These verses from the poem *Father William*[1] were composed by Lewis Carroll, the author of *Alice's Adventures in Wonderland.* They suggest that brain damage might be induced by serial insults – albeit in this case, by standing on one's head!

The recognition that cardiac surgical operations might be associated with brain injury was reported by Fox et al. in 1954,[2] the very year in which Gibbon reported the first successful clinical use of the heart-lung machine in cardiac surgery.[3] Succeeding years saw numerous studies confirming the association between cardiac surgery and cerebral injury.

Although much research effort has been expended over the years, brain damage in cardiac surgical patients remains a significant and challenging problem, not least because of the increased susceptibility of our progressively ageing patients. Progress has been made, but perhaps not as much as in other areas of cardiac surgical morbidity and mortality. There are several reasons for this, not least the fact that the brain has proved to be a difficult organ to study. Much of the research has focused on either functional or structural cerebral damage. Studies which have attempted to increase the understanding of the potential importance and relative incidence of these two components of the overall cerebral pathology have been relatively few. It has to be said that a strong consensus providing a clear indication of the principal pathophysiology (or pathophysiologies) has yet to emerge.

This book focuses on a thorough review of where we are currently in our understanding of brain injury in cardiac surgery and the strategies currently employed to lessen its incidence and severity in our patients. The editors have gathered together an impressive group of established experts and researchers in this field. The chapters are broad in the overall coverage of the subject, and commendably, they are also very forward-looking in their suggestions for future research and development, emphasizing the potentially important contributions from new developments in basic science, pharmacology, imaging modalities, etc.

I congratulate the editors and authors for this informed and stimulating book, which deserves to find a place on the desk of all of us who, rightly, believe that the understanding and ultimate prevention of serious brain injury in cardiac surgery patients remains a mountain yet to be conquered.

London Professor Ken Taylor

References

1. *Father William* verses are reprinted from *The Hunting of the Snark and Other Poems and Verses.* Lewis Carroll. New York: Harper & Brothers; 1903.
2. Fox HM, Risso ND, Gifford S. Psychological observations of patients undergoing mitral surgery. *Psychosomat Med.* 1954;16;186–208.
3. Gibbon JH. Application of a mechanical heart and lung apparatus to cardiac surgery. *Minnesota Med.* 1954; 37:171–185.

Preface

We welcome the reader to the *Monographs in Cardiac Surgery* series. These monographs have the objective to fully summarize the information available to date regarding particular facets of cardiac surgery – indications, operative techniques, pre-operative care, post-operative outcomes – so that the reader can have a full and up-to-date understanding of the history, current understanding, and future direction in a given area. As such, the series should be of interest to cardiac surgeons in practice or training, anesthesiologists, intensive care physicians, and potential researchers.

Brain injury remains one of the most dreaded complications of cardiac surgery. The range of injury is broad; while a stroke may be easily defined and diagnosed, more subtle injuries most definitely occur. There remains debate as to how these are diagnosed and there is a lack of standard definitions allowing inter-study comparison. If we are to have confidence in strategies that may reduce brain injury, we need to have confidence in the end-points used to define that injury. We need to better understand the phenomena associated with neuropsychometric testing; we need to fully elucidate the relationship between structural brain injury, embolism counting, and surrogate biomarkers; and we need an improved understanding of the clinical significance of abnormalities detected on post-operative magnetic resonance imaging.

In this, the first of the series, we have tried to construct a detailed background of studies of neurological morbidity and neuroprotection from a range of experts in the field of neuroprotection, providing a detailed reference for clinicians in the field. We have attempted to inter-connect the different strands of injury – be it the pathology, the imaging, the clinical and cognitive examination, potential biomarkers – and have then provided summary reports of treatment strategies that may reduce such injury. One of our objectives was to provide a reference background to stimulate research. As we look to the future, the design of studies attempting to reduce such injury becomes increasingly important and we hope that the fundamental background information provided in these chapters will fuel interest, initiate novel prevention and therapeutic strategies, and inform the investigator how to develop and design their research study.

Robert S. Bonser
Domenico Pagano
Axel Haverich

Series Preface

This series is directed toward surgeons, physicians, and healthcare workers involved in the care of patients requiring cardiac, cardiothoracic, and cardiovascular surgery. The scientific developments in this field continue to be prodigious and are published in an ever-increasing journal base. We hope that the series will also provide an important resource to research workers in the quest to accelerate the translation of basic research findings into clinical study and practice. The knowledge base in our disciplines is changing rapidly and there is an important requirement to consolidate the wide-ranging information on which clinicians must base their practice.

In the series, eminent experts, serving as editors or authors, offer their accounts of innovations within our areas of practice. In some, a thorough review of the available literature is undertaken to provide a balanced reference tool for investigators to pose future research questions and understand the studies that have been previously performed to best design subsequent studies and analyses. In others, state-of-the-art, technical advances are described, affording surgeons a platform to refine their practice, providing information on thresholds of when to recommend interventions and guidance on which intervention might be appropriate.

Each and every anesthetic and surgical procedure carries a risk of mortality and complications. Much has been done in to define and quantitate risk and to establish which factors may predict adverse outcome. Although such definition and quantitation may allow us to improve our counseling of patients regarding the risks of procedures, it does not necessarily allow us to categorically decide whether patients should undergo an intervention or whether they are best served by continued medical treatment or alternative modes of therapy. One of the focuses of the series will not only be the reports of which patients are at risk of which complications but also concentrate on what avenues are available to reduce risk.

The series focuses on all aspects of cardiovascular patient care.

Some volumes will focus on specific conditions or operative procedures while others will focus on aspects of patient care, improvements in patient management, and reduction of complications. Developments in the field are continuous and, therefore, clinicians need to understand which developments in basic research can be translated into improved patient care and how these can be investigated in clinical studies and trials. This series will continue to accelerate this process providing a detailed reference on which to base innovation and answer important clinical questions in our disciplines.

We have consciously emphasized the importance of future research direction within the series and, as co-editors, we pledge to support our professional colleagues and the series readers as they share advances within our field of practice.

Robert S. Bonser
Domenico Pagano
Axel Haverich

Contents

Contributors

Yasir Abu-Omar MBChB, DPhil, MRCS Specialist Registrar
Department of Cardiothoracic Surgery, Papworth Hospital, Papworth Everard, UK

Robin Peter Alston MBChB, MD, FRCA Consultant
Department of Anaesthesia, Critical Care and Pain Medicine,
Royal Infirmary of Edinburgh, Edinburgh, Scotland, UK

Miguel F. Arango MD Anesthesiologist
Department of Anesthesiology, London Health Sciences Centre,
London, Ontario, Canada

Joseph E. Arrowsmith MB, BS, MD, FRCP, FRCA Consultant
Department of Anaesthesia and Intensive Care, Papworth Hospital,
Papworth Everard, Cambridgeshire, UK

Robert A. Baker PhD, BMedSci(Hons), Dip Perf, CCP (Aus)
Director Cardiac Surgery Research and Perfusion
Department of Cardiac and Thoracic Surgery, Flinders Medical Centre and Flinders University, Adelaide, South Australia, Australia

William A. Baumgartner MD Director of Cardiac Surgery Research Laboratory and The Vincent L. Gott Professor
Department of Cardiac Surgery, The Johns Hopkins Hospital,
Baltimore, Maryland, USA

Martin Bendszus MD Director
Department of Neuroradiology, University of Heidelberg, Heidelberg, Germany

Sunil K. Bhudia MD, FRCS(CTh) Specialist Registrar
West Midlands Cardiothoracic Rotation, Edgware, Middlesex, UK

Robert S. Bonser MD, FRCP, FRCS, FESC, FACC
Professor and Consultant Cardiac Surgeon
Department of Cardiothoracic Surgery, Queen Elizabeth Hospital,
University Hospital Birmingham NHS Trust, Edgbaston, Birmingham, UK

Michael A. Borger MD, PhD Staff Surgeon
Department of Cardiac Surgery, Leipzig Heart Center, Saxony, Leipzig, Germany

André Y. Denault MD Anesthesiologist
Department of Anesthesiology, Montreal Heart Institute and Université de Montréal, Montréal, Quebec, Canada

Alain Deschamps MD, PhD, FRCPC Anesthesiologist
Department of Anesthesiology, Montreal Heart Institute, Montreal, Quebec, Canada

Gabriele Di Luozzo MD Cardiothoracic Surgeon
Department of Cardiothoracic Surgery, Mount Sinai School of Medicine, New York, USA

George Djaiani MD, DEAA, FRCA, FRCPC
Associate Professor of Anesthesia
Department of Anesthesia and Pain Management, Toronto General Hospital, UHN, University of Toronto, Toronto, Ontario, Canada

Vamsidhar B. Dronavalli MBBS, MRCS
Research Fellow and Honorary Registrar
Department of Cardiothoracic Surgery, Queen Elizabeth Hospital, University Hospital Birmingham NHS Trust, Edgbaston, Birmingham, UK

Maruthi S. S. R. Ganugapenta MBBS, MD(Anaesthesia), FCARCSI Clinical Fellow
Department of Anaesthesia and Intensive Care, Papworth Hospital, Papworth Everard, Cambridgshire, UK

Rebecca F. Gottesman MD, PhD Assistant Professor
Department of Neurology, Johns Hopkins University School of Medicine, Baltimore, Maryland, USA

Maura A. Grega MSN, CCRP Research Nurse and Program Coordinator
Department of Surgery, Johns Hopkins University, Baltimore, Maryland, USA

Randall B. Griepp MD Cardiothoracic Surgeon and Director of Aortic Surgery
Department of Cardiothoracic Surgery, Mount Sinai School of Medicine, New York, USA

Alina M. Grigore MD, MHS Associate Professor of Anesthesiology
Department of Anesthesiology, Mayo Clinic Hospital, Phoenix, Arizona, USA

John W. Hammon MD Professor of Surgery
Department of Cardiothoracic Surgery, Wake Forest University School of Medicine, Winston-Salem, North Carolina, USA

Deborah K. Harrington MD, MRCS Registrar Cardiothoracic Surgery
Department of Cardiothoracic Surgery, Queen Elizabeth Hospital, University Hospital Birmingham NHS Trust, Edgbaston, Birmingham, UK

Marjan Jahangiri MBBS, FRCS, FRCS CTh, MS
Professor of Cardiac Surgery
Department of Cardiothoracic Surgery, St. George's, University of London, London, UK

Richard A. Jonas MD Chief
Children's National Medical Center, Washington, DC, USA

Timothy J. Jones MD, FRCAS (CTh) Paediatric Cardiac Surgeon
Cardiac Unit, Birmingham Children's Hospital, Birmingham, UK

Min Lou MD, PhD Assistant Professor
Department of Neurology, The 2nd Affiliated Hospital of Zhejiang University, Hangzhou, Zhejiang, China

Guy M. McKhann MD Professor of Neurology
Department of Neurology, Johns Hopkins University, Baltimore, Maryland, USA

Reza Motallebzadeh MA, MB, BChir, MRCS, MD
Specialist Registrar and Wellcome Trust Clinical Research Fellow
Department of Surgery, Addenbrooke's Hospital, Cambridge, Cambridgeshire, UK

John M. Murkin MD, FRCPC Director
Cardiac Anesthesiology Research, Department of Anesthesiology and Perioperative Medicine, University of Western Ontario, London, ON, Canada

Harish Ramakrishna MD, FASE Senior Associate Consultant, Section Chief
Cardiothoracic Anesthesiology, Department of Anesthesiology, Mayo Clinic Arizona, Phoenix, Arizona, USA

Basel Ramlawi MD, MMSc Chief Resident
Division of Cardiac Surgery, University of Western Ontario and London Health Sciences Center, London, Ontario, Canada

Aaron M. Ranasinghe MD, MRCS Clinical Lecturer
Department of Cardiovascular Medicine, University of Birmingham, Birmingham, UK

Magdy Selim MD, PhD Associate Professor
Neurology, Harvard Medical School, Beth Israel Deaconess Medical Center, Boston, Massachusetts, USA

Frank W. Sellke MD Chief
Cardiothoracic Surgery Research, Department of Surgery, Beth Israel Deaconess Medical Center, Harvard Medical School, Boston, Massachusetts, USA

Ola A. Selnes PhD Professor
Department of Neurology, Johns Hopkins University School of Medicine, Baltimore, Maryland, USA

Colin Smith MB ChB, MD, FRCPath Senior Lecturer
Department of Pathology, University of Edinburgh, Edinburgh, Scotland, UK

David A. Stump PhD Professor
Department of Anesthesiology and Cardiothoracic Surgery, Wake Forest University School of Medicine, Winston-Salem, North Carolina, USA

David P. Taggart MD (Hons), PhD, FRCS Professor
Cardiovascular Surgery, Nuffield Department of Surgery, University of Oxford, Headington, Oxford, UK

Eric S. Weiss MD, MPH Resident
General Surgery, Department of Surgery, The Johns Hopkins University School of Medicine, Baltimore, Maryland, USA

Molecular and Biochemical Basis of Brain Injury Following Heart Surgery – Interventions for the Future

1

Eric S. Weiss and William A. Baumgartner

1.1 Introduction

Cardiac surgical procedures such as coronary artery bypass grafting (CABG), valvular replacement and heart transplantation, as well as many others are life-saving procedures for hundreds of thousands of US patients each year. However, despite this clinical utility, many patients who undergo cardiac surgery suffer neurological injury as a result. In addition to the morbidity and mortality caused by neurological injury, these complications are associated with increases in hospital length of stays, costs, and admissions to rehabilitation facilities.

By far, the most feared neurological complication of cardiac surgery is stroke, with an incidence of between 1% and 6%.[1,2] However, subtle decreases in neurocognition and impairments in level of consciousness occur frequently in the early postoperative period and can be equally distressing for patients and their families. Impaired consciousness can lead to additional neurological sequelae including encephalopathy, delirium, and depression.[3]

It is believed that atherosclerotic emboli from the aorta and hypoperfusion in watershed brain territories are the principal causes of stroke following cardiac surgery. The pathogenesis of cognitive impairment is likely multifactorial and generally depends on whether the impairment occurs early or late after cardiac surgery. Early deficits are likely related to microemboli, hypotension, general anesthesia, and inflammatory state initiated by cardiopulmonary bypass (CPB) while late deficits are likely related to increasing age, preoperative neurocognitive conditions, and vascular disease common for this group of patients.[4]

The development at our institution of a basic laboratory approach to understand the molecular and biochemical basis of neurologic injury following many types of cardiac surgical procedures is an important stepping stone to the development of effective neuroprotective strategies. Neurological complications of cardiac surgery are a national and international heath concern and the development of preventative strategies can have benefits not only for those patients with neurologic complications from cardiac surgery, but potentially for those patients suffering brain injury from a number of factors such as stroke, traumatic brain injury and anoxic brain injury. In this chapter, we will review the known molecular mechanisms of brain injury following cardiac surgery, detail preventative strategies that have arisen from an understanding of those mechanisms, and describe new approaches for neuroprotection. We are confident that a molecular understanding of brain injury will lead to improvements in the health and well-being of patients who undergo cardiac surgery.

1.2 Current Neuroprotective Strategies

There are several neuroprotective strategies currently employed to prevent neurologic injury following cardiac surgery. These focus on prevention of hyperthermia (>37°C) during rewarming as well as the avoidance of rapid rewarming, use of arterial line filters, avoidance of hyperglycemia, minimization of

E.S. Weiss (✉)
Department of Surgery, The Johns Hopkins University School of Medicine, Baltimore, Maryland, USA
e-mail: eweiss3@jhmi.edu

R.S. Bonser et al. (eds.), *Brain Protection in Cardiac Surgery*,
DOI: 10.1007/978-1-84996-293-3_1, © Springer-Verlag London Limited 2011

direct aortic manipulation, the use of alpha stat pH techniques in CPB, decreased levels of hemodilution, and avoidance of cardiotomy suction to minimize the risk of fat emboli.[3] Although these techniques have resulted in a diminution of stroke and neurocognitive dysfunction, when these events do occur, they can result in devastating complications for patients and families. In a series from the Johns Hopkins Hospital examining 2,711 patients who received cardiac surgery over a 4-year period, the incidence of stroke was 2.7% and those who suffered stroke had a 22% perioperative mortality rate.[5] Furthermore, 6.9% of patients developed encephalopathy, which was associated with a mortality rate of 7.5%. These numbers were in contrast to the low mortality rate of 1.4% for those patients not suffering from any cognitive impairment. Thus, while our current neuroprotective strategies are likely helpful, they are not sufficient to fully protect patients from neurological complications following cardiac surgery. Understanding the molecular and biochemical basis for brain injury may lead to novel therapies.

1.3 Hypothermic Circulatory Arrest, a Model for Understanding Brain Injury in Cardiac Surgery

Clinical neurological complications such as delirium and encephalopathy are often subtle on exam and can consequently be difficult to model and study. Even stroke has a large variability in severity among patients. It is often advantageous to examine severe forms of injury to identify important mediators and pathogenic mechanisms. When effective treatments are developed for the severe form of pathology, investigators can be encouraged about potential applications for more mild presentations. Our laboratory efforts have consequently focused on understanding the brain injury that occurs after hypothermic circulatory arrest (HCA), a commonly utilized technique in cardiac surgery, which unfortunately also can result in deleterious neurological complications. Over the next several sections, we will discuss the molecular basis of brain injury following HCA.

1.3.1 Clinical Aspects of HCA

In 1950, Bigelow demonstrated the value of whole body hypothermia and total circulatory arrest for cardiac operations.[6] Subsequently, the technique of HCA was first adopted into clinical practice for complex repairs of congenital cardiac malformations. Providing a bloodless operative field, unobstructed by cannulae or clamps, HCA remains the current cornerstone for procedures involving the aortic arch and descending thoracic aorta, as well as for repairs of congenital heart defects. Despite its utility in clinical medicine, HCA is not without adverse neurological sequelae. While it is generally accepted that safe durations of HCA range from 45 to 60 min, many patients who undergo HCA suffer neurologic complications such as ischemic infarction, seizures, and delayed neuropsychomotor development.[7–9]

1.3.2 Excitotoxicity in HCA

Postmortem histology after HCA shows a pattern of selective neuronal death. The neurons most affected are those in the basal ganglia, cerebellum, and hippocampus. These affected brain regions are protected against injury by glutamate receptor antagonists, suggesting that excitotoxicity is the mechanism of cell death in this model.[10]

Glutamate, the most abundant free amino acid in the central nervous system (CNS), serves as a neurotransmitter that mediates signaling in excitatory pathways. Excessive accumulation of glutamate contributes to neuronal ischemic injury by overactivating neuronal receptors, precipitating a cascade of intracellular events that leads to neuronal death, a phenomenon termed glutamate excitotoxicity by Olney in 1978.[11] There is now overwhelming support for the hypothesis that excessive extracellular concentrations of excitatory amino acids mediate their toxicity through glutamate receptor channels, especially the N-methyl-D-aspartate (NMDA) receptor gated ion channel (Fig. 1.1).

Excessive intracellular Ca^{2+}, induced by NMDA activation, overstimulates normal physiological processes, activating a series of enzymes such as kinases, proteases, phosphatases, and endonucleases which

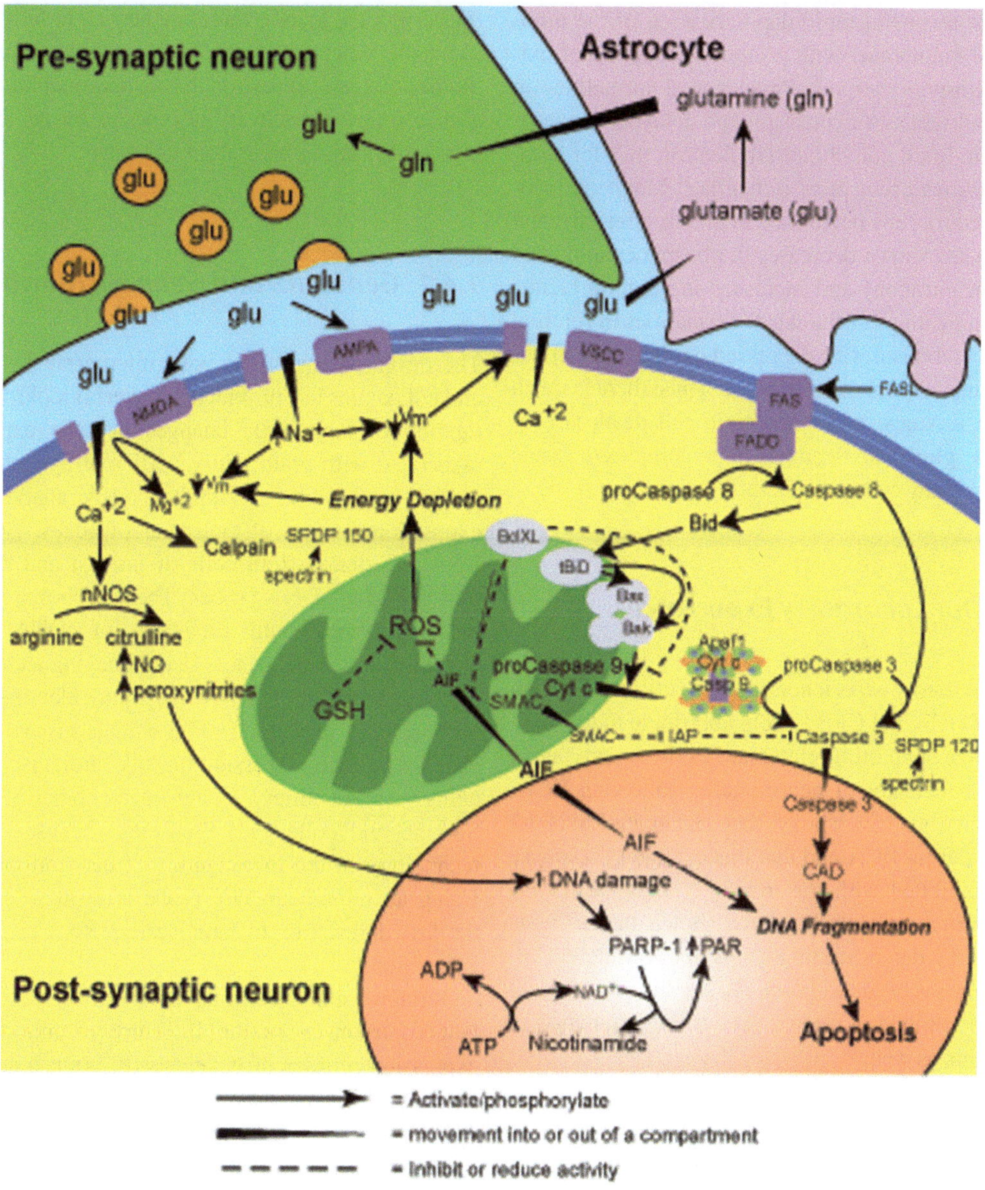

Fig. 1.1 Glutamate excitotoxicity pathway. Some of the known pathways by which glutamate excitotoxicity leads to cellular death

ultimately lead to damaged neurons.[12,13] It is felt that elevations in cytosolic Ca^{2+} induces nitric oxide synthase (NOS) to produce nitric oxide (NO), which in large quantities is cytotoxic.[14–17]

NO and its derivatives can damage cells via a variety of mechanisms. First, NO interacts with superoxide (O^{2-}) to form peroxynitrite (ONOO-), which can oxidize nitrate tyrosine residues. In addition, NO can interact with oxygen to form N_2O_3, which can nitrosylate cysteine residues. NO and its derivatives can further activate poly (ADP-ribose) polymerase (PARP), which depletes NAD and leads to cell death. Additional studies have shown that NO can damage DNA directly.[18–20]

In addition to elevating intracellular NO levels, high cytosolic Ca^{2+} levels may trigger the release of cytochrome c from the mitochondria, activating cysteine proteases called caspases that act as the direct effectors of programmed cell death or apoptosis.[21] Additionally, there is mounting evidence that disturbance of mitochondrial function itself may be central in the process of delayed cell death (apoptosis) after ischemia[22] (Fig. 1.1). Exposure of rat cerebellar granule cells to glutamate results in rapid depolarization of the mitochondrial membrane, with prompt uncoupling of oxidative phosphorylation.[23] Persistent abnormalities in mitochondrial DNA expression and delayed decreases in specific brain mitochondrial electron transfer complex activities occur after ischemia.[24] Magnetic resonance spectroscopy performed in infants after perinatal asphyxia has shown decreases in phosphocreatine and ATP concentrations and increases in cerebral lactate levels[25] indicating continuing abnormalities in cerebral energy metabolism with depressed oxidative phosphorylation in neuronal mitochondria. Thus, there is much evidence to suggest that apoptotic cell death is triggered by glutamate leading to a complex cascade involving many cellular effectors.

1.3.3 Our Laboratory Experience

In our laboratory experience, we have utilized a canine model of HCA and CPB to help contribute to the body of evidence supporting glutamate excitotoxicity as an important mediator of neurotoxicity following HCA. Specifically, we have shown that glutamate levels are elevated during HCA and that this excitatory response can be inhibited with the use of NMDA or AMPA receptor antagonists.[10] We have shown that NOS is important by demonstrating levels of citrulline in CSF of canine subjects undergoing HCA.[14,16,17] Use of NOS inhibitors resulted in improved neurologic function in the animals as well.[26]

1.4 New Directions in Identifying Molecular Mechanisms of Brain Injury and Cardiac Surgery

Thus, independent experiments in several laboratories have validated the role of glutamate excitotoxicity in models of HCA. However, while we know much about the effectors of brain injury with HCA, we know comparatively little about the regulation of those effectors at the transcriptional level. As a substantial portion of neurons die in a delayed fashion from apoptosis, it is reasonable to expect that alterations in gene expression may underlie many of the deleterious changes associated with neuronal injury from HCA. Focus at this transcriptional level is therefore needed to fully understand the process by which neurons die from HCA. Studies of gene expression during neuronal injury may also lead to the discovery of other pathways involved in neuronal injury heretofore unknown.

1.4.1 Genomics and Gene Microarrays

The development of the gene microarray by Brown and colleagues has provided a powerful tool for investigation of large-scale changes in gene expression associated with brain injury.[27] Microarray technology makes it possible to simultaneously analyze gene expression for tens of thousands of genes. Typically, RNA is isolated from cells of interest and reversed transcribed to cDNA probes. These probes are placed on a microarray with thousands of cDNA strands cloned from known genes. Using imaging technology, active genes from the RNA sample are identified. This approach has been used to investigate disease-related changes in gene expression for myocardial ischemia,[28] aging,[29] brain injury,[30] and many other diseases. Soriano and colleagues pioneered the use of array technology in the investigation of cerebral ischemia. Using an oligonucleotide probe array they provided the first description of large-scale mRNA differential expression.[31]

Ramlawi and colleagues have provided an important contribution to the literature examining gene expression profiles of patients with brain injury after cardiopulmonary bypass.[32] The investigators evaluated 42 patients who underwent CPB for either coronary bypass grafting or valvular procedures or both. Patients were administered neurocognitive tests preoperatively and at 3 days after their operation. A total of 17 patients were found to have neurocognitive decline (defined by a decrease of 25% from baseline) Serum of all patients were evaluated for differential gene expression using an affymetrix gene microarray. Patients with neurocognitive decline were found to have alterations in genes involved in inflammation, cell adhesion and antigen presentation. This study determined that patients who sustain neurocognitive decline following cardiac surgery have different gene expression profiles from those who do not develop decline and also identified important potential genes in for brain injury following CPB.

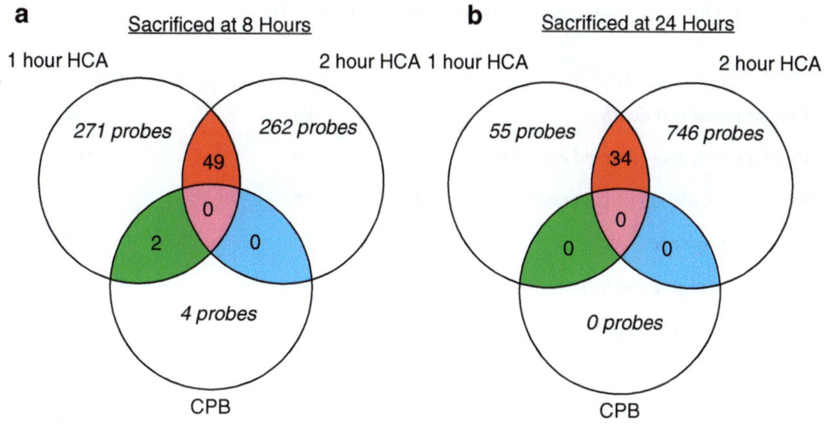

Fig. 1.2 Venn diagrams depicting the number of differentially expressed genes (as defined by absolute fold change of 1.5 and false discovery rate of <10%) for experimental groups sacrificed at either 8 h (**a**) or 24 h (**b**) after either HCA or CPB treatment

1.4.2 The Canine Genome

In our own laboratory, we have utilized gene microarrays to identify important mediators of brain injury in our canine model of CPB and HCA. The first complete sequence of the canine genome for the breed boxer was published in December of 2005.[33] The landmark project served as the culmination of many advances in the field of canine genomics which have provided new insights into canine diseases and the phylogeny of breeds. Now that the canine genome has been sequenced, we can perform microarray analyses in our model. Through a genomic approach, we hope to discover how the brain transcriptome responds to hypothermic circulatory arrest and CPB. We have applied microarray technology to study gene expression for canine subjects that have undergone HCA for either 1 or 2 h or CPB alone. We have found several changes in gene expression in all three groups (Fig. 1.2). Furthermore, similar to data by Ramlawi, we have found that alterations in genes involved in apoptosis and inflammation predominate in the canine model of brain injury following HCA (Table 1.1).

1.5 Valproic Acid – A Novel Neuroprotectant During HCA

Valproic acid (VPA) is a short chain fatty acid commonly used to treat mood and seizure disorders in humans.[34] Interest in VPA as a neuroprotectant stemmed from a recent body of scientific evidence demonstrating that VPA has neuroprotective effects in vitro.[35–37] A widely proposed mechanism explaining these effects is that VPA acts as a histone deacetylase (HDAC) enzyme inhibitor. The HDAC enzymes represent a broad class of proteins responsible for catalyzing the hydrolysis of acetyl groups on certain amino acids of histone proteins. Deacetylated histones bind susceptible regions of DNA with high affinity, leading to chromatin condensation and reduction in transcription factor activity.[35] Histone deacetylase inhibitors, such as valproic acid, have been shown to cause hyperacetylation of histones, which in turn release from DNA and allow the transcription of proteins that protect against oxidative stress.

Because of the importance of transcription in neuroprotection, our group applied valproic acid in a blinded manner to our canine model of HCA.[38]

In these experiments, five dogs received bolus infusion (750 mg) of VPA prior to HCA along with a continuous infusion of sodium valproate, 2.25 g (75 mg/kg) during HCA. When compared to control animals, dogs receiving VPA demonstrated significantly improved neurologic scores at 24, 48, and 72 h after HCA (Fig. 1.3) In addition, histological analysis revealed less pathologic damage in the VPA treated animals. Importantly, the entorrhinal cortex, an area involved with learning and memory, was significantly protected in dogs treated with valproic acid. In order to validate these results, we measured the levels of N-acetyl-aspartate (NAA) quantification in three key areas of the brain at both 24 and 72 h following injury. NAA loss is a well-known marker of brain injury. As injury severity increases, NAA levels decline, indicating worsening injury. After treating dogs with valproic acid, the cortex, hippocampus, and cerebellum

Table 1.1 Differential gene expression in a canine model of HCA

Biological process	Significantly regulated genes	Annotated genes in dataset	*p*-value
Programmed cell death	***93***	***766***	***4.90E–05***
Regulation of programmed cell death	66	510	9.90E–05
Negative regulation of programmed cell death	36	224	5.80E–05
Immune response	***85***	***619***	***9.30E–07***
Activation of immune response	13	64	1.60E–03
Adaptive immune response	17	78	1.40E–04
Lymphocyte-mediated immunity	14	72	1.70E–03
Humoral immune response	15	72	5.60E–04
Immunoglobulin-mediated immune response	12	52	7.80E–04
Complement activation	10	37	5.40E–04
Innate immune response	18	111	3.50E–03
Wound healing	24	120	2.90E–05
Inflammatory response	39	245	3.60E–05
Cytokine secretion	6	22	6.80E–03
Protein kinase cascade	***53***	***377***	***5.60E–05***
Ik B/N FkB cascade	22	130	7.40E–04
Circulatory system process	***26***	***156***	***3.30E–04***
Blood circulation	23	140	8.80E–04
Heart contraction	10	49	5.30E–03
Hemostasis	21	97	2.70E–05
Cell component organization and biogenesis	***239***	***2,418***	***3.80E–04***
Actin cytoskeletal organization and biogenesis	30	202	9.00E–04
Ribonucleoprotein complex biogenesis and assembly	31	203	4.60E–04

demonstrated preservation of near-normal N-acetyl-aspartate levels.[38]

The finding that VPA has dramatic effects on neuronal survival of animals in our model leads us to speculate that differential expression of protective genes may be an important mechanism underlying this functional protection. We are in the process of examining the brains of VPA-treated animals with microarrays, and have begun a phase I safety study examining the effects of VPA administration in clinical cardiac surgery. We feel that VPA administration may be a promising therapeutic option to help limit brain injury in HCA and other types of cardiac surgery.

1.6 Future Directions – Proteomics and the Development of Biomarkers for Brain Injury in Cardiac Surgery

1.6.1 Proteomics

Proteomics is the study of the protein composition of cell or body tissue and encompasses posttranslational changes that occur following protein genesis. With recent technological advances, the entire protein profile of a cell can be obtained and examined. In this way, differentially produced proteins can be isolated, identified, and described for the disease of question.

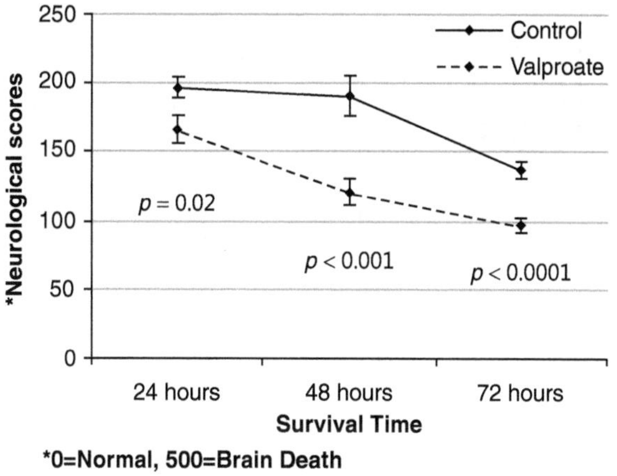

Fig. 1.3 Clinical neurologic scores for control versus valproate dogs at 24, 48, and 72 h after hypothermic circulatory arrest (Adapted from Williams et al.[38] Copyright Elsevier 2006)

Investigators at Duke University have provided an important description of proteomic changes that occur in the brain following hypothermic circulatory arrest.[39] Using two-dimensional gel electrophoresis and protein mass spectroscopy, they have investigated the protein profile of neonatal 10 piglets that were subjected to deep hypothermic circulatory arrest. The findings of this study were that 10 proteins were differentially expressed, including apolipoprotein A1 and neuron specific enolase, both proteins that have been shown to be important in other models of brain injury.

Because proteomics studies, such as this one, investigate the functional components of the cell (unlike genomics which studies potential protein products), the data obtained from proteomic strategies is very powerful for predicting phenotypic changes. Proteomics has perhaps its most useful application in the development of biomarkers for diagnosis and prognosis.

1.6.2 The Need for Biochemical Markers to Monitor Brain Injury

Brain injury resulting from various etiologies is a significant international health concern. Unlike other organ-based diseases where biomarkers exist for diagnosis and guidance of treatment, no such definitive tests exist for brain injury. Accurate and specific biomarkers have important applications in diagnosis, prognosis, and clinical research of all forms of brain injury.[40] Their development will facilitate the identification and treatment of brain injury after cardiac surgery.

1.6.3 α[Alpha]II-Spectrin Breakdown Products: A Novel Brain Injury Biomarker

Biomarkers should be present in an accessible biological material, predict the magnitude of injury, and be highly sensitive and specific for a disease in question. Work by Dr. Ronald Hayes' laboratory at the University of Florida and Banyan Biomarkers Inc., has focused on the use of proteolysis of α[alpha]II-spectrin as a prototypical biochemical marker.[40,41] α[alpha]II-spectrin is the major structural component of the cortical membrane cytoskeleton and is particularly abundant in axons and presynaptic terminals.[42,43] Importantly, α[alpha]II-spectrin is a major substrate for cysteine proteases (calpain and caspase-3) involved in necrotic and apoptotic cell death.[44] There is considerable evidence that α[alpha]II-spectrin is processed to signature cleavage products, spectrin breakdown products (SBDP), of molecular weight 150 kDa (SBDP150) and 145 kDa (SBDP145) by calpain. It is additionally cleaved to both a transient fragment of molecular weight 150 kDa (SBDP150i) and a major cleavage product of molecular weight 120 kDa (SBDP120) by caspase-3 (Fig. 1.4). Evidence for this pattern of breakdown has been described in in vitro neuronal cell culture models of mechanical stretch injury,[45] excitotoxicity,[45] and glucose oxygen deprivation.[46] More importantly, experimental evidence in mice suggests that the presence of SBDPs correlates with permanent neurodegeneration in a model of hippocampal traumatic injury.[47]

1.6.4 Advantages of SBDP150 and SBDP120 over Other Current Markers

The use of α[alpha]II-spectrin breakdown products as biomarkers for CNS injury are associated with several advantages over other biomarkers. Specifically, they are readily present in high levels in neurons and and

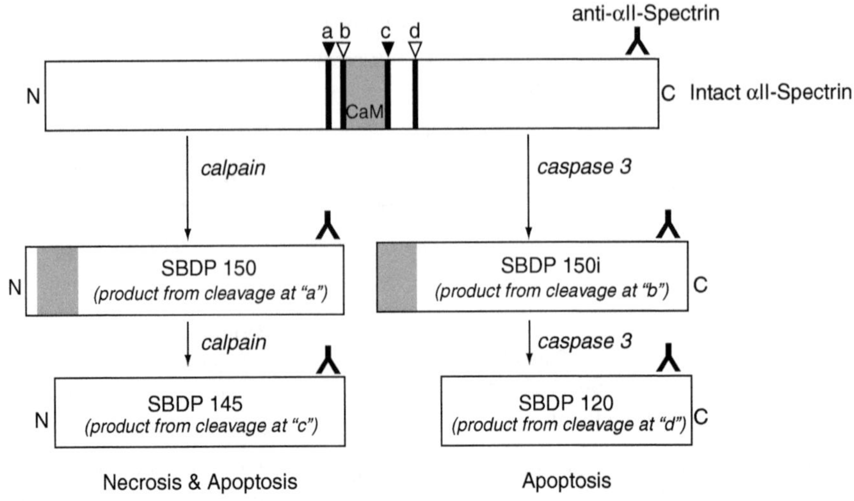

Fig. 1.4 In excitotoxity neuronal injury models, such as HCA, alpha II spectrin is vulnerable to specific calpain and caspase-mediated cleavage, generating fragments SBDP150 and SBDP120. This schematic presents the breakdown pathways for α[alpha]II spectrin and illustrates that necrotic cell death is calpain mediated whereas apoptosis is caspase mediated (From Weiss et al.[53])

low levels in other CNS cells such as glia.[44] α[alpha] II-spectrin is not present in erythrocytes and therefore measurements of αII-spectrin degradation are not confounded by blood contamination.[48] Finally, assessment of levels of necrosis and apoptosis in the CNS is valuable because these two major pathways of cell death are important in ischemic CNS injury such as occurs with cardiac surgery.

In our laboratory, we feel that α[alpha]II-spectrin breakdown products represent a novel way to assess CNS injury following cardiac surgery. We have thus examined the presence of these proteins in our canine model of HCA. Although we only have preliminary data at this point, we have found elevated levels of spectrin breakdown products in the cerebral spinal fluid of animals undergoing HCA. We feel that the use of these biomarkers may represent a novel method to not only gauge prognosis, but also predict outcomes prior to HCA.

1.7 Early and Late Cognitive Dysfunction May Result from Different Etiologies

Many of the molecular mechanisms underlying brain injury that we have previously discussed deal with acute changes in neurologic function occurring early after cardiac surgery. For a certain subset of patients, late neurocognitive dysfunction can also occur and be equally troublesome. Whereas early dysfunction likely results from microemboli, hypotension, and inflammation, we believe that the etiology for late neurocogintive dysfunction is largely related to the preoperative neurological state of the patient as well as the cardiovascular risk factors that they possess.[4]

There has been much support for this hypothesis. A study from our own institution examined cognitive performance 3 years following coronary bypass grafting and compared that to a control group with coronary artery disease who did not have surgery.[49] The groups were well matched for cardiovascular risk factors. There was a similar incidence of neurocognitive decline in each group. From these results, the investigators concluded that the principal risk factors for neurocognitive decline are related to increasing age and comorbidities rather than the use of cardiopulmonary bypass; 6 years following continues to support this concept.[50] This notion has been confirmed by several other studies investigating series of patients undergoing cardiac surgery.[51,52] The concept that early and late neurocognitive decline operate by different mechanisms underscores the importance of identifying molecular mechanisms of brain injury to determine important mechanistic factors for both types of injury.

1.8 Clinical Relevance for Study of Molecular Mechanisms

Neurologic injury is a significant risk factor for patients undergoing all types of cardiac surgery. Although stroke, with an incidence of 1–6%, is the most serious complication, cognitive impairment (25–65%) and impaired level of consciousness (10%) can be significantly troublesome for patients and lead to further complications.[1] Furthermore, for patients requiring HCA, infarctions, seizures, subtle losses of memory, problems with cognition, and delayed neuropsychomotor development are common and potentially devastating complications. Study of the molecular mechanisms associated with brain injury following cardiac surgery is crucial to improve the understanding of these injuries and develop targeted treatment strategies. The strides that are made in genomics and proteomics will have benefit not only for our cardiac surgical patients but for all patients suffering brain injury from stroke, traumatic brain injury, anoxic brain injury, or a number of other factors.

References

1. Roach GW, Kanchuger M, Mangano CM, et al. Adverse cerebral outcomes after coronary bypass surgery. Multicenter Study of Perioperative Ischemia Research Group and the Ischemia Research and Education Foundation Investigators. *N Engl J Med*. 1996;335:1857-1863.
2. Redmond JM, Greene PS, Goldsborough MA, et al. Neurologic injury in cardiac surgical patients with a history of stroke. *Ann Thorac Surg*. 1996;61:42-47.
3. Baumgartner WA. Neuroprotection in cardiac surgery. *Ann Thorac Surg*. 2005;79:S2254-S2256.
4. Baumgartner WA. Neurocognitive changes after coronary bypass surgery. *Circulation*. 2007;116:1879-1881.
5. McKhann GM, Grega MA, Borowicz LM Jr, et al. Encephalopathy and stroke after coronary artery bypass grafting: incidence, consequences, and prediction. *Arch Neurol*. 2002;59:1422-1428.
6. Bigelow WG, Lindsay WK, Greenwood WF. Hypothermia; its possible role in cardiac surgery: an investigation of factors governing survival in dogs at low body temperatures. *Ann Surg*. 1950;132:849-866.
7. Bellinger DC, Jonas RA, Rappaport LA, et al. Developmental and neurologic status of children after heart surgery with hypothermic circulatory arrest or low-flow cardiopulmonary bypass. *N Engl J Med*. 1995;332:549-555.
8. Drew CE, Anderson IM. Profound hypothermia in cardiac surgery: report of three cases. *Lancet*. 1959;1:748-750.
9. Hickey PR. Neurologic sequelae associated with deep hypothermic circulatory arrest. *Ann Thorac Surg*. 1998;65:S65-S69. discussion S9–70, S4–6.
10. Redmond JM, Gillinov AM, Zehr KJ, et al. Glutamate excitotoxicity: a mechanism of neurologic injury associated with hypothermic circulatory arrest. *J Thorac Cardiovasc Surg*. 1994;107:776-786. discussion 86–87.
11. Olney J. Neurotoxicity of excitatory amino acids. In: McGeer EGOJ, McGeer PL, eds. *Kainic Acid as a Tool in Neurobiology*. New York: Raven; 1978:95.
12. Rothman SM, Olney JW. Glutamate and the pathophysiology of hypoxic–ischemic brain damage. *Ann Neurol*. 1986;19:105-111.
13. Won SJ, Kim DY, Gwag BJ. Cellular and molecular pathways of ischemic neuronal death. *J Biochem Mol Biol*. 2002;35:67-86.
14. Brock MV, Blue ME, Lowenstein CJ, et al. Induction of neuronal nitric oxide after hypothermic circulatory arrest. *Ann Thorac Surg*. 1996;62:1313-1320.
15. Montoliu C, Llansola M, Monfort P, et al. Role of nitric oxide and cyclic GMP in glutamate-induced neuronal death. *Neurotox Res*. 2001;3:179-188.
16. Tseng EE, Brock MV, Kwon CC, et al. Increased intracerebral excitatory amino acids and nitric oxide after hypothermic circulatory arrest. *Ann Thorac Surg*. 1999;67:371-376.
17. Tseng EE, Brock MV, Lange MS, et al. Nitric oxide mediates neurologic injury after hypothermic circulatory arrest. *Ann Thorac Surg*. 1999;67:65-71.
18. Endres M, Wang ZQ, Namura S, Waeber C, Moskowitz MA. Ischemic brain injury is mediated by the activation of poly(ADP-ribose)polymerase. *J Cereb Blood Flow Metab*. 1997;17:1143-1151.
19. Mandir AS, Poitras MF, Berliner AR, et al. NMDA but not non-NMDA excitotoxicity is mediated by Poly(ADP-ribose) polymerase. *J Neurosci*. 2000;20:8005-8011.
20. Pieper AA, Blackshaw S, Clements EE, et al. Poly(ADP-ribosyl)ation basally activated by DNA strand breaks reflects glutamate-nitric oxide neurotransmission. *Proc Natl Acad Sci USA*. 2000;97:1845-1850.
21. Zhang Y, Bhavnani BR. Glutamate-induced apoptosis in neuronal cells is mediated via caspase-dependent and independent mechanisms involving calpain and caspase-3 proteases as well as apoptosis inducing factor (AIF) and this process is inhibited by equine estrogens. *BMC Neurosci*. 2006;7:49.
22. Kroemer G, Galluzzi L, Brenner C. Mitochondrial membrane permeabilization in cell death. *Physiol Rev*. 2007;87:99-163.
23. Teshima Y, Akao M, Li RA, et al. Mitochondrial ATP-sensitive potassium channel activation protects cerebellar granule neurons from apoptosis induced by oxidative stress. *Stroke*. 2003;34:1796-1802.
24. Christensen T, Diemer NH. Reduction of mitochondrial electron transport complex activity is restricted to the ischemic focus after transient focal cerebral ischemia in rats: a histochemical volumetric analysis. *Neurochem Res*. 2003; 28:1805-1812.
25. Penrice J, Lorek A, Cady EB, et al. Proton magnetic resonance spectroscopy of the brain during acute hypoxia-ischemia and delayed cerebral energy failure in the newborn piglet. *Pediatr Res*. 1997;41:795-802.
26. Tseng EE, Brock MV, Lange MS, et al. Neuronal nitric oxide synthase inhibition reduces neuronal apoptosis after hypothermic circulatory arrest. *Ann Thorac Surg*. 1997;64:1639-1647.
27. Brown PO, Botstein D. Exploring the new world of the genome with DNA microarrays. *Nat Genet*. 1999;21:33-37.
28. Stanton LW, Garrard LJ, Damm D, et al. Altered patterns of gene expression in response to myocardial infarction. *Circ Res*. 2000;86:939-945.

29. Lee CK, Allison DB, Brand J, Weindruch R, Prolla TA. Transcriptional profiles associated with aging and middle age-onset caloric restriction in mouse hearts. *Proc Natl Acad Sci USA*. 2002;99:14988-14993.
30. Matzilevich DA, Rall JM, Moore AN, Grill RJ, Dash PK. High-density microarray analysis of hippocampal gene expression following experimental brain injury. *J Neurosci Res*. 2002;67:646-663.
31. Soriano MA, Tessier M, Certa U, Gill R. Parallel gene expression monitoring using oligonucleotide probe arrays of multiple transcripts with an animal model of focal ischemia. *J Cereb Blood Flow Metab*. 2000;20:1045-1055.
32. Ramlawi B, Otu H, Rudolph JL, et al. Genomic expression pathways associated with brain injury after cardiopulmonary bypass. *J Thorac Cardiovasc Surg*. 2007;134:996-1005.
33. Lindblad-Toh K, Wade CM, Mikkelsen TS, et al. Genome sequence, comparative analysis and haplotype structure of the domestic dog. *Nature*. 2005;438:803-819.
34. McNamara J. Drugs effective in the therapy of the epilepsies. In: Hardman JGLL, ed. *The Pharmacological Basis of Therapeutics*. New York: McGraw-Hill; 1996:461-486.
35. Jeong MR, Hashimoto R, Senatorov VV, et al. Valproic acid, a mood stabilizer and anticonvulsant, protects rat cerebral cortical neurons from spontaneous cell death: a role of histone deacetylase inhibition. *FEBS Lett*. 2003;542:74-78.
36. Ren M, Leng Y, Jeong M, Leeds PR, Chuang DM. Valproic acid reduces brain damage induced by transient focal cerebral ischemia in rats: potential roles of histone deacetylase inhibition and heat shock protein induction. *J Neurochem*. 2004;89:1358-1367.
37. Ryu H, Lee J, Olofsson BA, et al. Histone deacetylase inhibitors prevent oxidative neuronal death independent of expanded polyglutamine repeats via an Sp1-dependent pathway. *Proc Natl Acad Sci USA*. 2003;100:4281-4286.
38. Williams JA, Barreiro CJ, Nwakanma LU, et al. Valproic acid prevents brain injury in a canine model of hypothermic circulatory arrest: a promising new approach to neuroprotection during cardiac surgery. *Ann Thorac Surg*. 2006;81:2235-2241. discussion 41–42.
39. Sheikh AM, Barrett C, Villamizar N, et al. Proteomics of cerebral injury in a neonatal model of cardiopulmonary bypass with deep hypothermic circulatory arrest. *J Thorac Cardiovasc Surg*. 2006;132:820-828.
40. Wang KK, Ottens AK, Liu MC, et al. Proteomic identification of biomarkers of traumatic brain injury. *Expert Rev Proteomics*. 2005;2:603-614.
41. Liu MC, Akle V, Zheng W, et al. Comparing calpain- and caspase-3-mediated degradation patterns in traumatic brain injury by differential proteome analysis. *Biochem J*. 2006;394:715-725.
42. Goodman SR, Zimmer WE, Clark MB, Zagon IS, Barker JE, Bloom ML. Brain spectrin: of mice and men. *Brain Res Bull*. 1995;36:593-606.
43. Riederer BM, Zagon IS, Goodman SR. Brain spectrin(240/235) and brain spectrin(240/235E): two distinct spectrin subtypes with different locations within mammalian neural cells. *J Cell Biol*. 1986;102:2088-2097.
44. Wang KK, Posmantur R, Nath R, et al. Simultaneous degradation of alphaII- and betaII-spectrin by caspase 3 (CPP32) in apoptotic cells. *J Biol Chem*. 1998;273:22490-22497.
45. Pike BR, Zhao X, Newcomb JK, Glenn CC, Anderson DK, Hayes RL. Stretch injury causes calpain and caspase-3 activation and necrotic and apoptotic cell death in septo-hippocampal cell cultures. *J Neurotrauma*. 2000;17:283-298.
46. Nath R, Probert A Jr, McGinnis KM, Wang KK. Evidence for activation of caspase-3-like protease in excitotoxin- and hypoxia/hypoglycemia-injured neurons. *J Neurochem*. 1998;71:186-195.
47. Hall ED, Sullivan PG, Gibson TR, Pavel KM, Thompson BM, Scheff SW. Spatial and temporal characteristics of neurodegeneration after controlled cortical impact in mice: more than a focal brain injury. *J Neurotrauma*. 2005;22:252-265.
48. Pike BR, Flint J, Dutta S, Johnson E, Wang KK, Hayes RL. Accumulation of non-erythroid alpha II-spectrin and calpain-cleaved alpha II-spectrin breakdown products in cerebrospinal fluid after traumatic brain injury in rats. *J Neurochem*. 2001;78:1297-1306.
49. Selnes OA, Grega MA, Borowicz LM Jr, et al. Cognitive outcomes three years after coronary artery bypass surgery: a comparison of on-pump coronary artery bypass graft surgery and nonsurgical controls. *Ann Thorac Surg*. 2005;79:1201-1209.
50. Selnes OA, Grega MA, Bailey MM, et al. Cognition 6 years after surgical or medical therapy for coronary artery disease. *Ann Neurol*. 2008;63:581-590.
51. Mullges W, Babin-Ebell J, Reents W, Toyka KV. Cognitive performance after coronary artery bypass grafting: a follow-up study. *Neurology*. 2002;59:741-743.
52. Wahrborg P, Booth JE, Clayton T, et al. Neuropsychological outcome after percutaneous coronary intervention or coronary artery bypass grafting: results from the Stent or Surgery (SoS) Trial. *Circulation*. 2004;110:3411-3417.
53. Weiss ES, Wang KKW, Allen JG, et al. Alpha II-spectrin breakdown products serve as novel markers of brain injury severity in a canine model of hypothermic circulatory arrest. *Ann Thorac Surg*. 2009;88(2):543-550.

Cardiopulmonary Bypass Circuit and the Brain

2

Michael A. Borger, George Djaiani, and Robert A. Baker

Credit for the development of modern day cardiopulmonary bypass (CPB) is usually given to John Gibbons, who produced a functional heart–lung machine at the Mayo Clinic in the early 1950s.[1] The development of the CPB circuit and the field of perfusion in general have been instrumental in the advancement of cardiac surgery over the last 5 decades. However, important neurologic complications were described shortly after the widespread adoption of CPB.[2,3] Such central nervous system complications range from subclinical cognitive dysfunction to delirium, to focal stroke, to coma and/or death. An ever-increasing number of clinical and basic research investigations have focused on the impact of CPB on neurologic complications since the 1980s.[4–12]

Central nervous system complications of CPB are generally attributed to the following factors: (1) cerebral embolization – macro- and microembolization of gaseous and particulate matter; (2) hypoperfusion – secondary to emboli, hypotension, low-flow sates, or shunting; and/or (3) inflammatory response – cytokines release and activation of the kallikrein-kinin and complement systems.

Neuropsychological impairment has been a major focus of research on neurologic complications of CPB.[6–12] Several studies have demonstrated a correlation between cerebral microemboli during CPB and postoperative cognitive impairment,[11,13,14] although other factors probably play a contributory role.[15] The relatively high incidence of post-CPB cognitive impairment makes this an attractive endpoint for prospective interventional studies, since much smaller patient sample sizes are required than for the much more uncommon endpoints of stroke or death. However, three recent studies have demonstrated that patients undergoing CPB may have a prevalence of postoperative cognitive impairment that is no different from age- and disease-matched control patients who either undergo off-pump coronary bypass surgery, percutaneous coronary interventions, or no cardiac interventions at all.[16–18] These results have questioned the significance of previously published findings of a significant increase in cognitive impairment in patients undergoing cardiac surgery in long-term follow-up studies.[12]

Although the definition, prevalence, and clinical significance of post-CPB neuropsychological impairment is open to discussion, there exists general agreement regarding central nervous system complications in general that: (1) clinically overt and occasionally devastating complications (i.e., stroke or coma) occur in approximately 1–3% of patients[4,19–21]; (2) post-CPB delirium/encephalopathy occurs in 5–10% of patients[4,22,23]; and (3) reduction of non-physiologic events during CPB (i.e., embolization, hypoperfusion, inflammatory response) is a worthy goal that may reduce the frequency of such neurologic complications.[11,24,25]

Of the causative factors described above (i.e., emboli, hypoperfusion, and inflammation), a large number of studies on CPB equipment have focused on the reduction of cerebral embolization as the primary goal. Such an effort is understandable given that emboli are known to occur in the vast majority of patients undergoing CPB, an association has been demonstrated between emboli and postoperative neurologic/neuropsychologic impairment, and emboli are readily quantifiable and therefore amenable to investigational studies.[5,13,14,26,27]

The modern day CPB circuit, in addition to being a testament to cooperation between biomedical engineers and clinicians, is a highly complex and effective tool

M.A. Borger (✉)
Department of Cardiac Surgery, Leipzig Heart Center, Leipzig, Saxony, Germany
e-mail: michael.borger@med.uni-leipzig.de

R.S. Bonser et al. (eds.), *Brain Protection in Cardiac Surgery*,
DOI: 10.1007/978-1-84996-293-3_2, © Springer-Verlag London Limited 2011

that allows the field of cardiac surgery to improve the quality of life and survival of hundreds of thousands of patients worldwide every year. We will examine the CPB circuit according to its various components in the current chapter, with a brief review of their known effects on neurologic complications. Issues regarding CPB management (e.g., alpha/pH stat, temperature, pharmacologic neuroprotection) will be discussed elsewhere in this monograph.

2.1 Oxygenators

One of the earliest and most important advancements in the development of the modern CPB circuit was the replacement of the bubble oxygenator with the membrane oxygenator. Bubble oxygenators required direct contact between the blood and oxygen for gas exchange. A major limitation with these devices was their inability to remove bubbles before they could embolize to the brain. In addition, blood trauma was also an important issue. Although defoaming agents were used, clinically apparent cerebral embolization continued to occur at a not infrequent rate.[3,27]

Early membrane oxygenators were technically challenging to use and were subject to leakage. The development of microporous hollow fiber membrane oxygenators that were reliable and more efficient led to the progressive displacement of bubble oxygenators from the market. The superior emboli-handling characteristics of the membrane oxygenators were confirmed by Blauth et al. who examined 34 patients undergoing CPB.[28] Patients operated on with a membrane oxygenator had significantly less central nervous system emboli as quantified by retinal fluorescein angiography. Other investigators demonstrated that membrane oxygenators caused less complement and inflammatory marker activation than bubble oxygenators,[29,30] further tilting the scales toward membrane oxygenators. Very few cardiac surgery centers in the world continue to use bubble oxygenators as a result of these important studies.[31]

2.2 Filters

The implementation of arterial line filters was another early and important development in minimizing cerebral injury during CPB. In 1976, Loop and co-investigators used ultrasonic insonation of the arterial line proximal and distal to a 20-μm woven nylon mesh arterial filter and demonstrated a 90% reduction in recorded emboli distal to the filter.[32] In one of the earliest studies to use transcranial Doppler monitoring of the middle cerebral artery during cardiac surgery, Payadachee et al. demonstrated that arterial filters resulted in a significant reduction in detectable cerebral emboli.[33] Furthermore, these investigators found a lower emboli count when a 25-μm filter was used in comparison to a 40-μm filter. A number of subsequent studies with similar conclusions led a consensus group to recommend arterial line filters during CPB as class I, level A evidence.[34]

Leukocyte-depleting filters were originally developed for allogeneic blood transfusion and have been investigated as a method of decreasing inflammatory activation during CPB. Although one study demonstrated a beneficial effect of such filters on the number of cerebral emboli during CPB and postoperative neuropsychologic outcomes,[35] other studies have failed to demonstrate any benefit.[36] Warren et al. concluded in a recent systematic review that there is currently insufficient evidence to support the routine use of leucocyte-depleting filters during CPB.[37]

Another potential "filter" that can be used in the CPB circuit is the dynamic bubble trap. Although this device is not a filter per se, it has a similar mode of action by directing gaseous microbubbles into the middle of the CPB tubing flow. The device has a collection tube placed in the middle of the downstream tubing, which subsequently removes the microbubbles from the circulation. Schoenburg et al. demonstrated in a randomized trial that the dynamic bubble trap results in an approximately 70% reduction of gaseous microemboli in the middle cerebral emboli of patients undergoing coronary bypass surgery.[38] Another filter-like mechanism uses ultrasound waves to redirect gaseous and particulate emboli away from the cerebral vessels in the patient's ascending aorta and arch.[39] This device is currently under early clinical investigation. Whilst the utilization of such devices is intrinsically interesting, the technology has not been developed into mainstream clinical practice.

2.3 Tubing and Coating

A variety of biocompatible surface-modified CPB circuits are clinically available, using differing technologies to provide a modified surface that is purported to be more biocompatible than traditional poly-vinyl chloride tubing. Various molecules have been incorporated into the circuits, including heparin, poly-2-methoxyethylacrylate, trillium- and synthetic protein-bonded circuits. Such circuits offer the possible advantage of decreasing the inflammatory response activated during CPB. It is hypothesized that this may translate into decreased neurologic injury. However, most studies of these circuits have focused on inflammatory, myocardial, or pulmonary outcomes rather than neurologic outcomes.

The biocompatible circuits that have undergone the most rigorous investigation to date are heparin-bonded circuits. Heyer et al. randomized 61 coronary bypass patients to receive heparin- versus non-heparin-bonded circuits and demonstrated better Trail-Making Test A scores 6 weeks after surgery in the heparin-bonded group.[40] Similarly, Baufreton et al. found a nonsignificant improvement in neuropsychological scores in patients randomized to receive a heparin-bonded circuit.[41] A larger study of 300 low-risk patients undergoing CABG surgery were randomized to either of the two different heparin-coated circuits or a control group.[42] Although the authors found that the use of a heparin-coated circuit was associated with lower transfusion requirements and decreased incidence of atrial fibrillation, there was no difference between the groups with respect to memory impairment. Such studies, plus others that have demonstrated decreased inflammatory activation, have led the consensus panel to conclude that "the use of biocompatible surface-modified circuits might be useful-effective at attenuating the systemic inflammatory response to CPB and improving outcomes" (class IIa, level B).[34]

2.4 Pumps

There are two basic types of pumps that are used for CPB: roller and centrifugal pumps. Roller pumps have been used since the introduction of CPB, have demonstrated extensive reliability, and have the theoretical advantage of being able to produce pulsatile perfusion. Centrifugal pumps have been used for over 30 years and offer the advantage of decreased blood trauma.[43] These pumps are therefore often used for patients who are expected to have long support times (e.g., complex operations, ECMO). Centrifugal pumps may also result in a decreased inflammatory response, but this point is controversial.

Scott et al. randomized 103 patients to receive either centrifugal or roller pumps during coronary bypass surgery.[44] Although these investigators found a lower incidence of neuropsychological dysfunction early (5 days) after CPB with a centrifugal device (33% versus 51%), the difference failed to reach statistical significance. Parolari et al. retrospectively examined 4,000 patients undergoing coronary and/or valvular surgery over a 5-year period and found a lower rate of stroke or coma in patients who were operated on with a centrifugal pump.[45] Despite these findings, there are currently no recommendations identifying the type of pump to be used during CPB, which may be beneficial in reducing adverse cerebral outcomes.

2.5 Venous Reservoirs

A large variety of venous reservoirs exist and they can be generally classified as hard shell ("open") or soft shell ("closed"). No clinical studies to date have shown a difference in cerebral embolization or other neurological outcomes between these two types of reservoirs. However, Mitchell et al. using an ex vivo model, demonstrated that operating the CPB circuit with low volume levels in various hard shell venous reservoirs was associated with an increased risk of subsequent air embolization, even when operating at or above the manufacturers' recommended minimum volume levels.[46] A recent survey of perfusion equipment revealed that hard shell venous reservoirs are used in over 80% of cardiac surgery centers.[31]

2.6 Cardiotomy Suction/Cell Saver

Cardiotomy suction has been identified as an important source of cerebral emboli during CPB. Although cardiotomy suction is an effective method of retrieving shed blood and minimizing blood loss during CPB, it also results in reinfusion of air, lipid, and cellular fragments from the pericardial well. Such embolic material has the ability to traverse the cardiotomy suction and arterial line filters. Lipid and gaseous emboli, in particular, have the ability to cross such filters either via distortion of their shape or by dispersing proximal to the filter and coalescing distal to it.[25]

Liu et al. were one of the first to demonstrate an association between cardiotomy suction and the number of microemboli, as measured by a Coulter counter in the CPB circuit.[47] Brooker and co-investigators confirmed that such emboli lead to significant cerebral injury in a canine model of CPB.[48] The use of cardiotomy suction was associated with a 15-fold increase in the number of SCADs (small capillary and arteriolar dilatations) during postmortem cerebral histologic examination, when compared to dogs that underwent CPB without cardiotomy suction. SCADs are dilatations of small arterial vessels that are thought to represent "footprints" of premortem lipid emboli and are known to increase in number with longer durations of CPB.[5,49]

Kincaid and co-investigators built on these findings to determine if substitution of cardiotomy suction with a cell saver device can reduce cerebral microembolization.[50] A canine model of CPB was used to demonstrate that the use of a cell saver resulted in a greater than 50% reduction in postmortem cerebral SCAD density, and that a continuous action cell saver was more effective than an intermittent action device. Interestingly, these investigators did not demonstrate any differences in cerebral SCAD density between three different types of arterial line filters.[50]

Such findings led to the development of the recommendation "that direct reinfusion of shed mediastinal blood into the CPB circuit should be avoided when possible (class I, level B)."[34] Another evidence-based appraisal of current practices suggested that cell saver processing of shed blood can be used, but that there is insufficient evidence to suggest efficacy.[51]

Two randomized clinical trials have recently been completed, after the abovementioned consensus statements were published, comparing standard cardiotomy suction to cell saver processing of shed blood during coronary bypass surgery. Rubens et al. randomized 268 patients and found no difference in the number of intraoperative cerebral emboli or the incidence of postoperative neuropsychological impairment between the two groups.[52] By contrast, Djaiani et al. randomized 226 elderly patients and found a lower incidence of cognitive dysfunction 6 weeks postoperatively in the cell saver group (6% versus 15%, $p=0.04$), whilst similarly finding no difference in intraoperative cerebral emboli counts.[53] There were many differences in the design of these two trials that may have contributed to the conflicting results. Most importantly, two different cell saver systems with diverse processing capabilities and two different approaches to blood management were utilized. The Djaiani group used a continuous flow cell saver, whilst the Rubens group used an intermittent flow cell saver. In addition, shed mediastinal blood was retransfused into the patient up to 4 h postoperatively in the Rubens study but was completely discarded in the Djaiani study. Finally, the average patient age was older in the Djaiani study and different statistical techniques were used to assess neuropsychological outcomes in the two studies.

2.7 Cannulas

A multitude of different arterial cannulas exist for CPB. While some cannulas have been demonstrated to have lower blood flow exit velocities and to produce less turbulent flow ex vivo, clinical studies have failed to demonstrate a reduction in cerebral emboli for these cannulas.[54]

An arterial cannula with a deployable intra-aortic filter has undergone extensive clinical investigation.[55–57] Although this cannula has been demonstrated to capture particulate emboli in 97% of patients, no definite neurologic advantage has been demonstrated in such patients.[57]

The technique of arterial cannulation may also play a role in cerebral embolization during CPB. Borger et al. randomized 34 patients to undergo standard cannulation of the ascending aorta or cannulation of the aortic arch with placement of the tip of the cannula beyond the left subclavian artery.[58] These investigators demonstrated a 40% reduction in the number of cerebral emboli in patients randomized to the arch cannulation group ($p=0.04$), presumably because of diversion of emboli away from the cerebral vessels and toward the lower body.

2.8 Other Factors

Venous return to the CPB circuit can be performed using standard gravity-assisted or vacuum-assisted venous drainage (VAVD). Vacuum assist was developed in the last few years as a method of ensuring adequate CPB flow rates when using small venous cannulas, particularly during minimal invasive valve surgery. Willcox et al. introduced air into an experimental CPB circuit and found that VAVD resulted in increased emboli generation distal to the arterial filter when compared to conventional gravity drainage.[59] Jones et al. examined different CPB circuits and found that VAVD did not result in significant increases in the number of emboli, as long as vacuum suction was kept at −40 mm Hg or less.[60] Carrier et al. in a retrospective review of over 1,500 patients undergoing cardiac surgery over a 4-year period found that VAVD was not associated with an increased risk of postoperative stroke.[61] Such studies would suggest that VAVD is probably safe, as long as air entrainment and large negative suction pressures are avoided.

Reduced volume "mini-circuits" have been suggested as a method of reducing hemodilution and inflammatory activation during CPB. Whilst such effects may have an indirect neurologic benefit for the patient, other studies have demonstrated safety issues in relation to these circuits such as a limited capacity to manage circulating gaseous emboli and a subsequently increased risk of cerebral embolization.[62]

Modified ultrafiltration (MUF) is another method of minimizing patient hemodilution by performing ultrafiltration during CPB support and hemofiltration of the circuit after weaning from CPB. While some experimental studies have suggested a neurologic benefit for MUF, other studies have demonstrated no benefit.[63] Supportive clinical data of a neurologic benefit is lacking to date.

2.9 Iatrogenic Contributions to Emboli

Certain events that occur during most cardiac operations (referred to as "surgical events") have been demonstrated to be associated with generation of cerebral emboli.[64] Such events include the initiation/cessation of CPB, aortic crossclamping/declamping, the application of the side-biting clamp, and the insertion/removal of the cardioplegia vent. Multiple clamp applications to the ascending aorta, as may be required during construction of proximal coronary bypass anastomoses, has been identified as a particularly important source of cerebral embolization.[65] Hammon et al. in a prospective randomized clinical trial, demonstrated that the use of a partial occluding clamp was associated with a higher rate of neuropsychological deficit 6 months after coronary bypass surgery than a single crossclamping technique (57% versus 30% respectively, $p=0.005$).[66] Such findings should lead surgeons to avoid partial occluding clamps during coronary bypass surgery whenever possible, but routine partial clamping still exists in a significant proportion of cardiac surgery centers.

In addition to "surgical events," a variety of perfusion-related activities (referred to as "perfusionist events") have also been linked to the development of cerebral microemboli. Taylor et al. demonstrated that cerebral emboli are seven times more likely to occur during injection of drugs or sampling of blood, predominantly because of the injection of gaseous emboli into the CPB circuit during such procedures.[67] In addition, Borger et al. demonstrated that patients with an increased number of such perfusionist events have worse postoperative neuropsychological performance.[14] Several simple maneuvers by both the surgeon and the perfusionist can be performed in the operating room to minimize the generation of gaseous microemboli. For example, Rodriguez et al. demonstrated that simply removing air from the venous line prior to initiation of CPB can markedly reduce the number of cerebral emboli.[68]

Another potential method of minimizing cerebral emboli during CPB is with insufflation of the operative field with carbon dioxide. Carbon dioxide is many times heavier and more soluble than oxygen and may therefore result in less cerebral emboli in patients undergoing open chamber procedures (e.g., valve repair or replacement, ascending aorta surgery). Svenarud et al. randomized 20 patients undergoing valvular surgery to receive carbon dioxide insufflation of the surgical field or standard management, and noted a 78% reduction in the number of emboli in the ascending aorta (as assessed by TEE) in the carbon dioxide insufflation group.[69] Martens et al. recently randomized 80 patients undergoing valvular surgery to receive CO_2 insufflation or control treatment and found improved auditory-evoked potentials (shorter P300 wave peak latencies) 5 days postoperatively in the carbon dioxide group.[70] However, Martens et al. failed to demonstrate any differences in neuropsychological outcomes. While flooding of the surgical field with CO_2 may decrease cerebral gaseous emboli amount and duration during open chamber procedures, it may also result in increased systemic pCO_2 levels when administered over an extended period. It is therefore recommended to flood the perioperative field for only a few minutes prior to releasing the aortic crossclamp.

2.10 Conclusion

The development of the CPB circuit was critical to the advancement of cardiac surgery and the explosion in the number of procedures in the second half of the twentieth century. Neurological complications, however, were noted early after the first use of CPB and have been a focus of investigational research ever since. Several key components of the CPB circuit have undergone extensive modification as a result of these studies. Although more recent evidence questions the severity of postoperative cognitive dysfunction and the role of CPB in its development, serious neurological complications such as stroke and seizures continue to occur after cardiac surgery, particularly in high risk patients. Further studies to determine the optimal CPB components should focus on such high risk patients.

References

1. Gibbon JH Jr. The application of a mechanical heart and lung apparatus to cardiac surgery. *Minn Med.* 1954;37: 171-185.
2. Caguin F, Carter MG. Fat embolization with cardiotomy with the use of cardiopulmonary bypass. *J Thorac Cardiovasc Surg.* 1963;46:665-672.
3. Gilman S. Cerebral disorders after open-heart operations. *N Engl J Med.* 1965;272:489-498.
4. Roach GW, Kanchuger M, Mora M, et al. Adverse cerebral outcomes after coronary bypass surgery. *N Engl J Med.* 1996;335:1857-1863.
5. Moody DM, Bell MA, Challa VR, Johnston WE, Prough DS. Brain microemboli during cardiac surgery or aortography. *Ann Neurol.* 1990;28:477-486.
6. Shaw PJ, Bates D, Cartlidge NE, et al. Neurologic and neuropsychological morbidity following major surgery: Comparison of coronary artery bypass and peripheral vascular surgery. *Stroke.* 1987;18:700-707.
7. Wong BI, McLean RF, Naylor CD, et al. Central nervous system dysfunction after warm or hypothermic cardiopulmonary bypass. *Lancet.* 1992;339:1383-1384.
8. Shaw PJ, Bates D, Cartlidge NE, Heaviside D, Julian DG, Shaw DA. Early neurological complications of coronary artery bypass surgery. *BMJ.* 1985;291:1384-1387.
9. Savageau JA, Stanton B, Jenkins CD, Klein MD. Neuropsychological dysfunction following elective cardiac operation. I. Early assessment. *J Thorac Cardiovasc Surg.* 1982;84:585-594.
10. Murkin JM, Newman SP, Stump DA, Blumenthal JA. Statement of consensus on assessment of neurobehavioral outcomes after cardiac surgery. *Ann Thorac Surg.* 1995;59:1289-1295.
11. Hammon JW, Stump DA, Kon ND, et al. Risk factors and solutions for the development of neurobehavioral changes after coronary artery bypass grafting. *Ann Thorac Surg.* 1997;63:1613-1618.
12. Newman MF, Kirchner JL, Phillips-Bute B, et al. Longitudinal assessment of neurocognitive function after coronary-artery bypass surgery. *N Engl J Med.* 2001;344: 395-402.
13. Clark RE, Brillman J, Davis DA, Lovell MR, Price TR, Magovern GJ. Microemboli during coronary artery bypass grafting. Genesis and effect on outcome. *J Thorac Cardiovasc Surg.* 1995;109:249-257.
14. Borger MA, Peniston CM, Weisel RD, Vasiliou M, Green REA, Feindel CM. Neuropsychological impairment after coronary bypass surgery: effect of gaseous emboli during perfusionist interventions. *J Thorac Cardiovasc Surg.* 2001;121:743-749.
15. Murkin JM. Cardiopulmonary bypass and the inflammatory response: a role for serine protease inhibitors? *J Cardiothorac Vasc Anesth.* 1997;11:19-23.
16. Selnes OA, Grega MA, Borowicz LM, et al. Cognitive outcomes three years after coronary artery bypass surgery: a comparison of on-pump coronary artery bypass graft surgery patients and nonsurgical controls. *Ann Thorac Surg.* 2005;79:1201-1209.
17. Selnes OA, Grega MA, Bailey MM, et al. Neurocognitive outcomes three years after coronary artery bypass graft surgery: a controlled study. *Ann Thorac Surg.* 2007;84: 1885-1896.
18. Sweet JJ, Finnin E, Wolfe PL, et al. Absence of cognitive decline one year after coronary bypass surgery: comparison to nonsurgical and healthy controls. *Ann Thorac Surg.* 2008;85:1571-1578.
19. Borger MA, Peniston CM, Weisel RD, et al. Decreasing incidence of stroke during valvular surgery. *Circulation.* 1998;98:II137-II143.
20. Bucerius J, Gummert JF, Borger MA, et al. Stroke after cardiac surgery – a risk factor analysis in 16, 184 consecutive adult patients. *Ann Thorac Surg.* 2003;75:472-478.
21. John R, Choudhri AF, Weinberg AD, et al. Multicenter review of preoperative risk factors for stroke after coronary artery bypass grafting. *Ann Thorac Surg.* 2000;69:30-36.
22. Bucerius J, Gummert JF, Borger MA, et al. Predictors of delirium after cardiac surgery delirium: effect of beating-heart (off-pump) surgery. *J Thorac Cardiovasc Surg.* 2004;127:57-64.
23. McKhann GM, Grega MA, Borowicz LM, et al. Encephalopathy and stroke after coronary artery bypass grafting: incidence, consequences and prediction. *Arch Neurol.* 2002;59:1422-1428.
24. Baumgartner WA. Neuroprotection in cardiac surgery. *Ann Thorac Surg.* 2005;79:S2254-S2256.
25. Prasongsukarn K, Borger MA. Reducing cerebral emboli during cardiopulmonary bypass. *Sem Cardiothorac Vasc Anesth.* 2005;9:153-158.

26. Barbut D, Yi-Wen L, Gold JP, et al. Impact of embolization during coronary artery bypass grafting on outcome and length of stay. *Ann Thorac Surg*. 1997;63:998-1002.
27. Blauth CI, Arnold JV, Schulenberg WE, McKhann GM, Taylor KM. Cerebral microembolism during cardiopulmonary bypass: retinal microvascular studies in vivo with fluorescein angiography. *J Thorac Cardiovasc Surg*. 1988;95: 668-676.
28. Blauth CI, Smith PL, Arnold JV, Jagoe JR, Wootton R, Taylor KM. Influence of oxygenator type on the prevalence and extent of microembolic retinal ischemia during cardiopulmonary bypass. Assessment by digital image analysis. *J Thorac Cardiovasc Surg*. 1990;99:61-69.
29. Cavarocchi NC, Pluth JR, Schaff HV, et al. Complement activation during cardiopulmonary bypass: comparison of bubble and membrane oxygenators. *J Thorac Cardiovasc Surg*. 1986;91:252-258.
30. Videm V, Fosse E, Mollnes TE, Ellingsen O, Pedersen T, Karlsen H. Different oxygenators for cardiopulmonary bypass lead to varying degrees of human complement activation in vitro. *J Thorac Cardiovasc Surg*. 1989;97: 764-770.
31. Baker RA, Willcox TW. Australian and New Zealand perfusion survey: equipment and monitoring. *J Extra Corpor Technol*. 2006;38:220-229.
32. Loop FD, Szabo J, Rowlinson RD, Urbanek K. Events related to microembolism during extracorporeal perfusion in man: effectiveness of in-line filtration recorded by ultrasound. *Ann Thorac Surg*. 1976;21:412-420.
33. Padayachee TS, Parsons S, Theobold R, Gosling RG, Deverall PB. The effect of arterial filtration on reduction of gaseous microemboli in the middle cerebral artery during cardiopulmonary bypass. *Ann Thorac Surg*. 1988;45: 647-649.
34. Shann KG, Likosky DS, Murkin JM, et al. An evidence-based review of the practice of cardiopulmonary bypass in adults: a focus on neurologic injury, glycemic control, hemodilution, and the inflammatory response. *J Thorac Cardiovasc Surg*. 2006;132:283-290.
35. Whitaker DC, Newman SP, Stygall J, Hope-Wynne C, Harrison MJ, Walesby RK. The effect of leucocyte-depleting arterial line filters on cerebral microemboli and neuropsychological outcome following coronary artery bypass surgery. *Eur J Cardiothorac Surg*. 2004;25:267-274.
36. Whitaker DC, Stygall JA, Newmann SP, Harrison MJ. The use of leucocyte-depleting and conventional arterial line filters in cardiac surgery: a systematic review of clinical studies. *Perfusion*. 2001;16:433-446.
37. Warren O, Alexiou C, Massey R, et al. The effects of various leucocyte filtration strategies in cardiac surgery. *Eur J Cardiothorac Surg*. 2007;31:665-676.
38. Schoenburg M, Kraus B, Muehling A, et al. The dynamic air bubble trap reduces cerebral microembolism during cardiopulmonary bypass. *J Thorac Cardiovasc Surg*. 2003;126:1455-1460.
39. Sauren LDC, la Meir M, Palmen M, et al. New ultrasonic radiation reduces cerebral emboli during extracorporeal circulation. *Eur J Cardiothorac Surg*. 2007;32:274-280.
40. Heyer EJ, Lee KS, Manspeizer HE, et al. Heparin-bonded cardiopulmonary bypass circuits reduce cognitive dysfunction. *J Cardiothorac Vasc Anesth*. 2002;16:37-42.
41. Baufreton C, Allain P, Chevailler A, et al. Brain injury and neuropsychological outcome after coronary artery surgery are affected by complement activation. *Ann Thorac Surg*. 2005;79:1597-1605.
42. Svenmarker S, Sandstrom E, Karlsson T, et al. Neurological and general outcome in low-risk coronary artery bypass patients using heparin coated circuits. *Eur J Cardiothorac Surg*. 2001;19:47-53.
43. Morgan IS, Codispoti M, Sanger K, Mankad PS. Superiority of centrifugal pump over roller pump in paediatric cardiac surgery: prospective randomised trial. *Eur J Cardiothorac Surg*. 1998;13:526-532.
44. Scott DA, Silbert BS, Doyle TJ, et al. Centrifugal versus roller head pumps for cardiopulmonary bypass: effect on early neuropsychologic outcomes after coronary artery surgery. *J Cardiothorac Vasc Anesth*. 2002;16:715-722.
45. Parolari A, Alamanni F, Naliato M, et al. Adult cardiac surgery outcomes: role of the pump type. *Eur J Cardiothorac Surg*. 2000;18:575-582.
46. Mitchell SJ, Willcox T, Gorman DF. Bubble generation and venous air filtration by hard-shell venous reservoirs: a comparative study. *Perfusion*. 1997;12:325-333.
47. Liu JF, Su ZK, Ding WX. Quantitation of particulate microemboli during cardiopulmonary bypass: experimental and clinical studies. *Ann Thorac Surg*. 1992;54:1196-1202.
48. Brooker RF, Brown WR, Moody DM, et al. Cardiotomy suction: a major source of brain lipid emboli during cardiopulmonary bypass. *Ann Thorac Surg*. 1998;65:1651-1655.
49. Brown WR, Moody DM, Challa VR, Stump DA, Hammon JW. Longer duration of cardiopulmonary bypass is associated with greater numbers of cerebral microemboli. *Stroke*. 2000;31:707-713.
50. Kincaid EH, Jones TJ, Stump DA, et al. Processing scavenged blood with a cell saver reduces cerebral lipid microembolization. *Ann Thorac Surg*. 2000;70:1296-1300.
51. Hogue CW, Palin CA, Arrowsmith JE. Cardiopulmonary bypass management and neurologic outcomes: an evidence-based appraisal of current practices. *Anesth Analg*. 2006;103:21-37.
52. Rubens FD, Boodhwani M, Mesana T, et al. The cardiotomy trial: a randomized, double-blind study to assess the effect of processing of shed blood during cardiopulmonary bypass on transfusion and neurocognitive function. *Circulation*. 2007; 116(Suppl):I89-I97.
53. Djaiani G, Fedorko L, Borger MA, et al. Continuous flow cell saver reduces cognitive decline in elderly patients after coronary bypass surgery. *Circulation*. 2007;116:1888-1895.
54. Benaroia M, Baker AJ, Mazer CD, Erret L. Effect of aortic cannula characteristics and blood velocity on transcranial doppler-detected microemboli during cardiopulmonary bypass. *J Cardiothorac Vasc Anesth*. 1998;12:266-269.
55. Banbury MK, Kouchoukos NT, Allen KB, et al. Emboli capture using the Embol-X intraaortic filter in cardiac surgery: a multicentered randomized trial of 1, 289 patients. *Ann Thorac Surg*. 2003;76:508-515.
56. Reichenspurner H, Navia JA, Berry G, et al. Particulate emboli capture by an intra-aortic filter device during cardiac surgery. *J Thorac Cardiovasc Surg*. 2000;119:233-241.
57. Eifert S, Reichenspurner H, Pfefferkorn T, et al. Neurological and neuropsychological examination and outcome after use of an intra-aortic filter device during cardiac surgery. *Perfusion*. 2003;18(Suppl):55-60.

58. Borger MA, Taylor RL, Weisel RD, et al. Decreased cerebral emboli during distal aortic arch cannulation: a randomized clinical trial. *J Thorac Cardiovasc Surg*. 1999;118:740-745.
59. Willcox TW, Mitchell SJ, Gorman DF. Venous air in the bypass circuit: A source of arterial line emboli exacerbated by vacuum-assisted drainage. *Ann Thorac Surg*. 1999;68: 1285-1289.
60. Jones TJ, Deal DD, Vernon JC, Blackburn N, Stump DA. Does vacuum-assisted venous drainage increase gaseous microemboli during cardiopulmonary bypass? *Ann Thorac Surg*. 2002;74:2132-2137.
61. Carrier M, Cyr A, Voisine P, et al. Vacuum-assisted venous drainage does not increase the neurological risk. *Heart Surg Forum*. 2002;5:285-288.
62. Norman MJ, Sistino JJ, Acsell JR. The effectiveness of low-prime cardiopulmonary bypass circuits at removing gaseous emboli. *J Extra Corpor Technol*. 2004;36:336-342.
63. Myung RJ, Kirshbom PM, Petko M, et al. Modified ultrafiltration may not improve neurologic outcome following deep hypothermic circulatory arrest. *Eur J Cardiothorac Surg*. 2003;24:243-248.
64. Stump DA, Rogers AT, Hammon JW, Newman SP. Cerebral emboli and cognitive outcome after cardiac surgery. *J Cardiothorac Vasc Anesth*. 1996;10:113-118.
65. Boivie P, Hansson M, Engstrom KG. Embolic material generated by multiple aortic crossclamping: a perfusion model with human cadaveric aorta. *J Thorac Cardiovasc Surg*. 2003;125:1451-1460.
66. Hammon JW, Stump DA, Butterworth JF, et al. Single cross-clamp improves 6-month cognitive outcome in high-risk coronary bypass patients: The effect of reduced aortic manipulation. *J Thorac Cardiovasc Surg*. 2006;131:114-121.
67. Taylor RL, Borger MA, Weisel RD, Fedorko L, Feindel CM. Cerebral microemboli during cardiopulmonary bypass: increased emboli during perfusionist interventions. *Ann Thorac Surg*. 1999;68:89-93.
68. Rodriguez RA, Rubens F, Belway D, Nathan HJ. Residual air in the venous cannula increases cerebral embolization at the onset of cardiopulmonary bypass. *Eur J Cardiothorac Surg*. 2006;29:175-180.
69. Svenarud P, Persson M, van der Linden J. Effect of CO_2 insufflation on the number and behavior of air microemboli in open-heart surgery: a randomized clinical trial. *Circulation*. 2004;109:1127-1132.
70. Martens S, Neumann K, Sodemann C, Deschka H, Wimmer-Greinecker G, Moritz A. Carbon dioxide field flooding reduces neurologic impairment after open heart surgery. *Ann Thorac Surg*. 2008;85:543-547.

Neurological and Cognitive Sequelae of Cardiac Surgery

3

Guy M. McKhann, Rebecca F. Gottesman,
Maura A. Grega, Willam A. Baumgartner, and Ola A. Selnes

3.1 Introduction

Over the last 50 years, heart surgery, and coronary artery bypass grafting (CABG) in particular, has been a remarkable success story. John Gibbon and his wife, who were instrumental in the development of the cardiopulmonary bypass pump, were close family friends of one of us (GMcK), so as a youngster he heard about its early trials and tribulations. Years later, as a neurologist, he became increasingly aware of the neurological problems associated with CABG and other heart surgery procedures. This review is based primarily on our group's prospective analyses of the neurological problems associated with heart surgery at Johns Hopkins Hospital, initiated in 1992, and carried out continuously since that time. We have confined our remarks primarily to CABG and valve surgery, and we do not comment on pediatric heart surgery, aortic surgery, or heart transplantation. We have divided these potential neurologic outcomes as: stroke; encephalopathy; short-term cognitive problems; and long-term cognitive problems, and the incidence of each in our patient population is shown in Fig. 3.1.

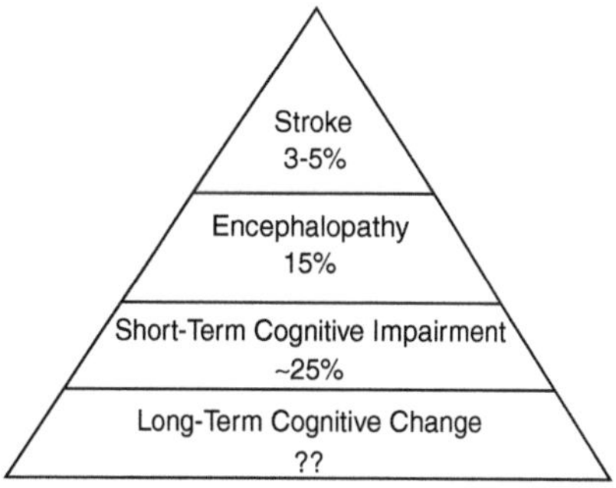

Fig. 3.1 Incidence of adverse neurological and cognitive outcomes in cardiac surgical patients

In comparing this series of patients to those from other institutions and/or different time periods, one must be aware of ongoing changes in both the procedure and patient populations. There are continuing changes in surgical, perfusion, and anesthesia techniques; and current patients are older, and have a higher incidence of risk factors such as hypertension and diabetes, as well as more severe coronary artery disease. Several years ago there was a period in which the advent of angioplasty and percutaneous stenting procedures displaced CABG as a preferred therapeutic approach for many patients. However, recent data have raised questions about the efficacy of these interventional procedures, and the pendulum has started to swing back toward surgery, particularly for those with more severe coronary artery disease. These patients are also often at greatest risk for neurological problems after surgery.

Our analyses, and those of others, have moved beyond merely documenting outcomes. We must also ask questions about mechanisms and possible preventive or interventional approaches. Therefore, we must establish whether the observed outcomes are specific to the procedure under investigation. We have taken a strong stand on the need for control groups for comparison.[1] Without such control groups for comparison, one can be misled in attributing adverse outcomes as being specific to a given procedure. The control group one selects depends on the question being asked. If the emphasis is on the acute effects of a procedure, for example, CABG, then other surgical groups are needed to control for use of the cardiopulmonary bypass pump, anesthesia,

G.M. McKhann (✉)
Department of Neurology, Johns Hopkins University,
Baltimore, Maryland, USA
e-mail: guy.mckhann@jhu.edu

R.S. Bonser et al. (eds.), *Brain Protection in Cardiac Surgery*,
DOI: 10.1007/978-1-84996-293-3_3,

hypothermia, etc. We have chosen "off-pump surgery" as one appropriate control group.

In evaluating longitudinal cognitive outcomes, we are interested in comparing patients with similar degree of vascular disease of the heart and brain who had surgery with those who did not. Thus, as controls for our CABG patients, we selected a nonsurgical group with documented coronary artery disease. For longer-term studies, comparison with a "heart healthy" group, those without known vascular risk factors, is required to determine what changes in cognition are expected with aging in a population with minimal cardiovascular disease.

3.2 Stroke

Stroke can be defined clinically as a new focal neurologic deficit, or by radiographic criteria assessed by modern neuroimaging techniques. At our institution, those individuals suspected clinically of having a postoperative stroke are evaluated by our research team, by a neurology consultation and with neuroimaging. We have found that stroke rate varies depending on the type of surgical procedure, with higher rates noted when standard CABG surgery is combined with other procedures (Table 3.1).

Stroke is one of the most devastating neurologic outcomes after cardiac surgery and has negative consequences during the early postoperative period (see effect of stroke on length of stay [LOS] and mortality in Table 3.1) and during the longer-term recovery period.

Table 3.1 Stroke rates and in-hospital outcomes by cardiac procedure

Procedure	Stroke rate	Mortality for stroke patients	LOS for stroke patients (days)
CABG	3.7%	17.6%	18.6
Valve	2.9%	19.5%	21.4
CABG/valve	6.2%	26.4%	24.1
CABG/other	6.9%	14.3%	20.9
Aortic procedure	7.0%	23.6%	28.1
Other	5.3%	53.6%	20.1
Average	4.7%		

CABG – coronary artery bypass grafting, LOS – postoperative length of hospital stay

Until the mid-to-late 1990s, imaging in patients who had undergone cardiac surgery was primarily performed with computed tomography (CT) scanning. Since that time, magnetic resonance imaging (MRI) with diffusion-weighted imaging (DWI) has been introduced. DWI MRI has the advantage of showing acute infarction within minutes of injury, and in general allows better differentiation between old injury, which is quite prevalent in this population, and new strokes. This discrepancy between CT and MRI is evident when we compare the findings obtained from CT scanning with those from MRI scanning with DWI. Comparing these two techniques in 98 patients with clinically diagnosed strokes, we found that the incidence of "watershed strokes" was twice as high with MRI (37% unilateral watershed stroke detected by CT versus 68% by MRI).[2] The term "watershed stroke" has been applied to ischemic damage to the brain in the distribution between the major vascular territories. It is typically associated with hypoperfusion, such as may occur globally with cardiac arrest, or to focal parts of the brain distal to a high-grade carotid or intracranial stenosis. In noncardiac stroke populations, watershed strokes are fairly rare, occurring only 2–5% of the time.[3–5] In our study of patients with clinical stroke after cardiac surgery, however, they were identified in over half of individuals with clinical stroke, based on DWI MRI imaging.

Identifying these types of strokes may be important for assessing the prognosis of individuals with stroke after cardiac surgery. Compared with patients with other types of postoperative stroke, those with bilateral watershed strokes after heart surgery were 6 times as likely to go to inpatient rehabilitation, 12 times as likely to go to a chronic nursing facility, and 19 times more likely to die in the hospital than they were to be discharged home.[2] Because watershed strokes are typically due to hypoperfusion, one of the factors associated with watershed stroke in the cardiac surgery setting may be drop in blood pressure from preoperative levels during surgery. We are currently exploring this relationship in prospective studies.

3.2.1 *Mechanism of Stroke*

Stroke after cardiac surgery is most likely due to a combination of embolization and hypoperfusion. Although past technologies have emphasized the role of embolization, and have been geared toward the reduction of embolization, we think that it is likely that a combination of embolization and hypoperfusion may lead to stroke and other neurologic injury, and thus both of these mechanisms must be considered in the development of approaches to reduce these adverse outcomes. Caplan has hypothesized that watershed strokes, for instance, are due to embolization in the context of hypoperfusion, suggesting that hypoperfusion causes decreased washout of emboli.[6,7]

3.2.2 Embolization

Micro- and macroemboli during cardiac surgery consist of atherosclerotic debris, particulate matter including fat or other surgical debris, as well as air. These emboli are quite frequent, although whether they are all clinically relevant is still not entirely clear.[8,9] Their presence has been confirmed with transcranial Doppler studies, as well as retinal fluorescein angiography and autopsy studies.[10–12] Autopsy studies have suggested that most, if not all, individuals undergoing CABG surgery, have evidence of cerebral embolization in the form of SCADs (small capillary and arteriolar dilatations). These SCADs are mainly lipid and may occur primarily during cardiotomy suctioning.[9,13]

Macroembolization can also result from disruption of aortic atheroma during surgery or from large vessels in the head or neck or from atrial fibrillation after surgery, among other sources. Aortic atherosclerotic disease has been associated with postoperative stroke,[14] and when it is identified by epiaortic ultrasound and avoided during clamp placement, stroke risk may be reduced.[15,16] Strokes in the later postoperative period are frequently due to atrial fibrillation. One third of individuals undergoing CABG develop atrial fibrillation postoperatively, which increases risk of cardiac thrombus formation and resultant stroke.[17]

3.2.3 Hypoperfusion

Significant hypotension during cardiac surgery increases the odds of postoperative stroke and other neurologic injury. Tufo reported that patients who had a drop in systolic blood pressure to 50 mmHg or below for at least 10 min had four times higher rates of postoperative neurologic complications.[18] Hypoperfusion can also take the form of anemia; Karkouti reported that each additional 1% drop in nadir hematocrit increased the odds of postoperative stroke by 10%.[19] The effect of lesser degrees of hypoperfusion, however, and their relation to an individual's baseline level of blood pressure and anemia still requires further study. In a normal individual, there should not be ischemia unless cerebral perfusion pressures drop below 50 mmHg.[20,21] This does not, however, apply to all individuals who may have chronic hypertension and altered cerebral autoregulation compared with individuals without chronic hypertension. We suspect that change in blood pressure from baseline may be an important factor in predicting risk of postoperative stroke. This may also apply to relationships between baseline and intraoperative hematocrit. Karkouti reported that the degree of anemia an individual tolerates is dependent on his/her baseline level of anemia.[22]

3.2.4 Silent Infarcts

In addition to clinically evident strokes after cardiac surgery, studies have identified new (silent) infarcts on imaging. Acute infarcts by DWI MRI have been found in anywhere from 18–26% of low-risk patients[23,24] and 45–62% of high-risk patients.[25,26] The clinical significance, however, of these infarcts is still unclear; in some studies they have been associated with early encephalopathy or cognitive dysfunction,[27,28] whereas in others this association has not been found.[24,26,29]

3.2.5 Defining the "High Risk" Patient

An important contribution in the field has been the ability to identify those at higher risk for stroke prior to surgery. There have been a number of paradigms for this prediction, which share several predictive factors: age; risk factors for vascular disease such as hypertension, diabetes, or smoking; and evidence of existing vascular disease such as peripheral vascular disease, evidence of aortic or carotid disease, or previous stroke. An example of such a predictive paradigm is shown in Fig. 3.2, and highlights the cumulative effects of vascular risk factors with age.

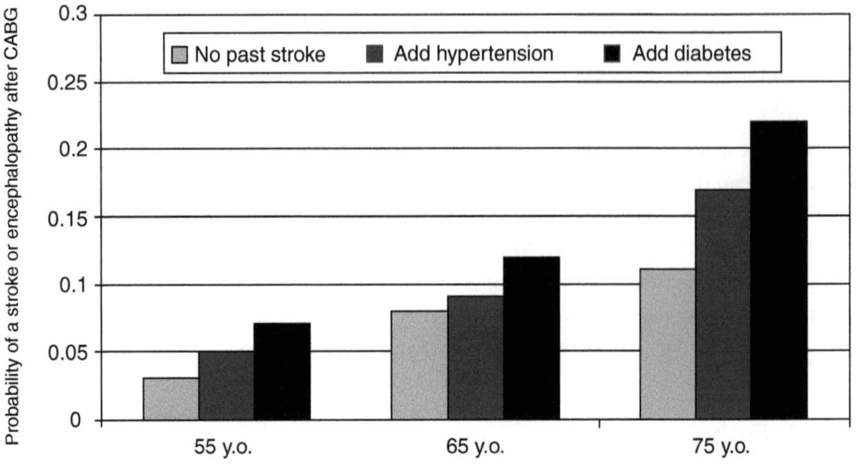

Fig. 3.2 Cumulative effect of risk factors on the probability of having a stroke or encephalopathy after CABG. For example, in a 55-year-old patient with no risk factors, the probability of a postoperative neurological event is quite low at 0.03. For a comparable patient with a history of hypertension, the probability is 0.05. If the patient has both a history of hypertension and diabetes mellitus, the probability increases to 0.07

The advantage of these predictive paradigms is that they are based on data available prior to surgery. Identifying these at-risk patients preoperatively is helpful in both deciding when or if to modify therapeutic approaches as well as for recruiting higher-risk patients for neuroprotective trials.

3.3 Postoperative Encephalopathy

Encephalopathy is a term used to characterize those patients with evidence of more diffuse involvement of the brain, manifesting as confusion, delirium, combativeness, being slow to awaken after surgery, or prolonged stupor or coma. These symptoms can be quite transient, particularly episodes of confusion. The prospective rates of encephalopathy by cardiac surgical procedure are shown in Table 3.2.

Table 3.2 Encephalopathy rates and in-hospital outcomes by cardiac procedure

Procedure	Encephalopathy rate	Mortality for enceph. pts.	LOS for enceph. pts. (days)
CABG	13.7%	10.0%	18.1
Valve	14.4%	20.8%	18.8
CABG/valve	23.8%	10.6%	31.0
CABG/other	14.8%	7.7%	37.3
Aortic procedure	14.7%	5.1%	20.7
Other	13.8%	32.7%	40.0
Average	15.1%		

CABG – coronary artery bypass grafting, LOS – postoperative length of hospital stay

The causes of encephalopathy are multiple, and may vary with age. Clearly certain medications, metabolic derangements, and intercurrent infections can lead to encephalopathy. In the context of cardiac surgery, an important question is whether encephalopathy is part of a continuum of vascular insult to the brain that ranges from stroke to episodic confusion.[30]

Those with encephalopathy are often dismissed by hospital staff as older patients who "normally" have this reaction to surgery. The outcomes after encephalopathy suggest that this group should be taken more seriously, as these patients have longer LOS and higher mortality rates. Unlike stroke, the predictive factors for encephalopathy in the setting of CABG surgery have not been well determined. In other hospitalized patients with delirium, age is the single most predictive factor, followed by a history of preexisting neurological damage.[10,31] However, more work needs to be done in this area.

3.4 Cognitive Outcomes

Complaints about changes in memory and other aspects of cognitive functioning are common after CABG. In early studies, because patients with such subjective cognitive complaints often had coexisting depression, these symptoms were dismissed as being a side effect of postoperative depression. Later studies focused on the role of procedure-related variables, such as the duration of cardio-pulmonary bypass, blood pressure management, and intraoperative emboli as possible causes of postoperative cognitive decline. Despite a large number of investigations carried out to date, no single procedure-related variable has been identified as the principal cause of adverse postoperative cognitive outcomes. More recent studies have attempted to take into account patient-related variables as well, including the patient's preoperative cognitive status. Patients undergoing CABG today are not only older, but they also have a greater prevalence of comorbid diseases, some of which are known to be associated with increased risk of cerebrovascular disease.

3.4.1 Short-Term Cognitive Changes

Estimates of short-term cognitive change after CABG have been highly variable because of differences in choice of time points postoperatively, lack of control groups, as well as differences in the statistical criteria used for defining decline. Not surprisingly, the incidence of short-term cognitive changes varies according to the interval between surgery and follow-up testing. Neurocognitive deficits at the time of hospital discharge after CABG are common, but may be related to adverse effects of anesthetic drugs, narcotics for pain control, or other clinical issues.[32] Therefore, some investigators have chosen to defer follow-up testing until at least 3–4 weeks after surgery.

Another factor of critical importance for estimating the incidence of postoperative cognitive decline after CABG is the choice of statistical criteria for defining postoperative decline. In studies that have not included a comparison group, criteria for decline have been largely arbitrary definitions such as 20% decline on 20% of the tests. Such criteria cannot distinguish between true decline versus normal variability associated with repeated measurements and therefore typically overestimate the degree of postoperative decline. Studies with one or more comparison groups can avoid this limitation by directly comparing the degree of change in pre- to postoperative performance between the treatment group and the controls. Some studies have controlled for the effect of age on cognitive performance,[33] while others have chosen control patients with diagnosed coronary artery disease[34] or hospitalized inpatients having noncardiac procedures.[35]

In a prospective study from our own group, we compared a group of 140 CABG patients with 92 demographically similar patients with diagnosed coronary artery disease but no surgery.[34] Both groups improved from baseline to 12 weeks, and there was no evidence of statistically significant differences between the CABG patients and the comparison group. Our study, and those of others with earlier postoperative follow-up times,[33,36] demonstrate that cognitive decline after CABG is transient and reversible and that most patients return to their baseline cognitive performance between 3 and 12 months after surgery.

There is little information available about which specific aspect of cognition is most vulnerable during the immediate postoperative period. Some studies have reported early decline in memory, psychomotor speed, executive functions and visuo-constructional abilities, suggesting that multiple brain regions may be involved.[37] Based on reports from patients and family members, the most common complaint involves changes in concentration and memory.[38] It is well known, however, that subjective cognitive symptoms do not always correlate with performance on objective neuropsychological tests; thus some investigators have attributed such subjective complaints to depression. There is evidence from noncardiac populations, however, that subjective memory complaints may sometimes reflect changes in memory that may not necessarily be detected by standardized tests of new verbal memory and delayed recall.[39]

3.4.2 Mechanisms

No single procedure-related factor that can account for the early postoperative cognitive changes has been identified. The focus of most investigations has been on neurologic injury secondary to microemboli, hypoperfusion, and the systemic inflammatory response. It has proven surprisingly difficult, however, to find strong evidence that any of these variables, either individually or in combination with other risk factors, can account for the short-term cognitive changes.

Patients with atherosclerosis are known to be at increased risk for cerebral microemboli during the surgery.[14] The clinical consequences of these emboli, however, remain poorly understood. Some earlier studies reported an association between embolic counts and short-term cognitive outcomes,[8,40] but more contemporary studies have not replicated these findings.[41–43] It has been hypothesized that the cognitive manifestations of microemboli may depend as much on patient-related risk factors, such as the degree of preexisting cerebrovascular disease, as on the number and size of the embolic load.[44] Patients without significant preexisting cerebrovascular disease may have a higher threshold for embolic injury than those with such disease. Consistent with this possibility, predictors of cognitive decline in a large multicenter Veterans Administration study included cerebrovascular disease, peripheral vascular disease, and a history of chronic disabling neurological illness.[45]

Long-standing hypertension and aging can be associated with alterations of the brain vascular supply that may make elderly patients more vulnerable to effects of hypoperfusion. Certain regions of the brain, including the hippocampus, periventricular white matter areas, and watershed areas, may be particularly susceptible to the effects of hypoperfusion. Abildstrom and colleagues found that candidates for CABG had lower global cerebral blood flow preoperatively than did controls, but found no association between neuropsychological test performance and postoperative global or regional blood flow.[46] As discussed above, these emboli and hypoperfusion may act synergistically, in that decreased flow during the surgery may result in reduced washout of embolic materials from the brain, particularly in the watershed areas of the brain.[6]

Some elderly patients undergoing major noncardiac surgery with general anesthesia also experience short- or long-term cognitive dysfunction. In a study of patients in the 40–60 year age range, 19% were found to have cognitive decline 1 week after surgery with general anesthesia.[47] Studies comparing regional versus general anesthesia have not found any difference in cognitive outcomes 3 months after surgery, thus questioning a causal relationship between general anesthesia and postoperative cognitive dysfunction.[48] Regardless of the specific etiology of postoperative cognitive impairment after general anesthesia, there is evidence of some degree of short-term cognitive decline even after major *noncardiac surgery* with general anesthesia.[49]

3.4.3 Long-Term Cognitive Changes

While most studies have focused on short-term cognitive outcomes after CABG, a study from Duke University found that at 5 years, an unexpected 42% of patients available for follow-up performed below their baseline levels on a global measure of cognition.[50] Predictors of late cognitive decline included older age, fewer years of education, higher baseline score, and cognitive decline at the time of discharge. Some other studies have replicated these findings[51,52] but in a small study from Germany, none of their patients had what was considered to be clinically significant cognitive decline 5 years after surgery.[35] The authors suggested that the lack of late decline in their study might be related to stricter control of hypertension, hypercholesterolemia, and other risk factors for cerebrovascular disease during the 5-year follow-up period *after* surgery. If these findings can be replicated in larger cohorts, they suggest that late cognitive decline after CABG might be reduced by improved postoperative control of risk factors for progression of underlying cerebrovascular disease.[53]

In contrast with the findings from the above uncontrolled studies, investigations that have included a comparison group have not found evidence of disproportionate late decline associated with the use of cardiopulmonary bypass.[54,55] This finding is highlighted in our recent work shown in Fig. 3.3.

This suggests that the late cognitive changes are related to factors other than cardiopulmonary bypass. Other possible causes of late cognitive decline in a population of elderly patients with cerebrovascular disease might include progression of subcortical small vessel disease, or development of silent infarctions or Alzheimer's disease during the follow-up period.

There is evidence from several epidemiological studies that a history of one or more risk factors for cerebrovascular disease may be associated with accelerated cognitive decline even without cardiac surgery.[56–59] Some studies have found that nearly one third of otherwise asymptomatic individuals have silent brain infarcts on MRI, and older age and hypertension are significant risk factors for having such MRI abnormalities.[60] In the Rotterdam Scan Study, of 1,015 individuals without history of clinical stroke, 21% had at least one silent infarct by screening MRI. These individuals had at least a threefold increased risk of clinical stroke when followed over the next 4 years.[61] Additionally, the presence of silent infarcts may be associated with progressive cognitive decline or late dementia.[60,62] Given the high prevalence of silent infarcts in community based cohorts, one would expect such MRI findings to be even more common among candidates for CABG. In a study from Japan,

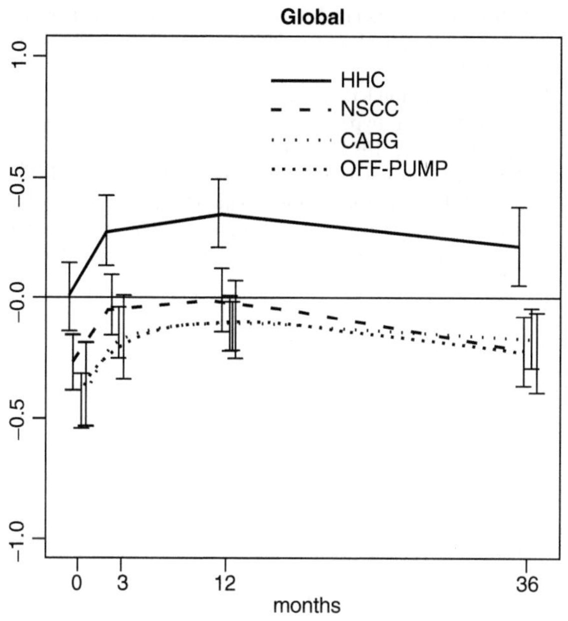

Fig. 3.3 Comparison of coronary artery disease groups versus a healthy comparison group. This graph plots the z-score changes in cognitive test performance over 36 months. The global domain is a combination of eight separate cognitive areas. HHC is the heart healthy comparison group; NSCC is the nonsurgical cardiac comparison group; CABG is the conventional coronary artery bypass surgical group; and off pump is the coronary artery bypass surgical group who had surgery without the use of the cardiopulmonary bypass pump

preoperative MRI was performed in a group of 421 candidates for CABG[63]; and an unexpected half of this group had evidence of silent brain abnormalities *before* surgery. Additionally, patients with single or multiple infarctions had lower baseline cognitive performance, and were more likely to have decline in cognitive test performance postoperatively.

3.4.4 Off-Pump CABG (OPCAB)

The development of techniques for performing coronary artery bypass surgery without the use of cardiopulmonary bypass was motivated largely by expectations that such techniques might reduce the incidence of postoperative adverse neurological and cognitive outcomes. Several studies have demonstrated that the use of off-pump surgery is associated with a reduction in the number of emboli to the brain,[64,65] but clear-cut benefits in terms of neurocognitive outcomes have not been demonstrated. In a recent meta-analysis of eight prospective randomized studies, better cognitive outcomes at 1 and 3 months were found for the off-pump patients. There was no benefit of off-pump surgery for later follow-up times.[66] More recent studies have not demonstrated an early cognitive benefit of having off-pump surgery, however.[67] Prospective long-term follow-up studies of cognition in off-pump patients have now been reported, and there appears to be no evidence of greater cognitive decline associated with conventional on-pump than off-pump surgery 5 years after the procedure.[68] This is perhaps the most direct evidence that although some degree of late cognitive decline does occur after CABG, it is not specifically related to the use of cardiopulmonary bypass.

From a cognitive standpoint, therefore, CABG, as currently practiced, appears to be safe for the great majority of patients. Transient changes involving memory, executive functions, and motor speed may still occur in a subset of patients during the first few days to weeks after CABG. The etiology of these early cognitive changes is most likely multifactorial, and includes a synergistic effect of microemboli, hypoperfusion, anesthesia, and other variables associated with major surgery. Older age and degree of preexisting cerebrovascular disease have been identified as important risk factors. The short term cognitive changes appear to be reversible by 3 months after surgery for the great majority of patients. Late cognitive decline after CABG, occurring between 1 and 5 years after the surgery, has been well documented, but controlled studies have demonstrated that this decline is not specifically attributable to the use of cardiopulmonary bypass itself, but may be secondary to progression of underlying cerebrovascular disease or other age-related changes.

Other possible causes of late cognitive decline in a population of elderly patients with cerebrovascular disease might include progression of subcortical small vessel disease, development of silent infarctions, or Alzheimer's disease during the follow-up period.

3.5 Future Directions

One of the implications of our findings as well as those of others is that the status of the brain before surgery is an important determinant of both acute and subsequent long-term outcomes. In our studies, and most in the literature, we know little about the degree of cerebrovascular disease of the brain prior to surgery.

As mentioned previously, there have been a few studies suggesting that the degree of vascular disease detected by preoperative imaging is predictive of postoperative stroke or cognitive change. There is no good measure of the overall burden of cerebrovascular disease of the brain. Such a measure would be a valuable indicator of the effects of hypertension and diabetes on the brain. Some have suggested that preoperative cognitive assessment may be a reasonable surrogate for the degree of preexisting vascular disease of the brain.

Acknowledgements We wish to thank Dr. Pamela Talalay and Ms. Maryanne M. Bailey for their assistance in preparation of this document. In addition, our work over the years has been supported by the following grants: National Institute of Neurological Disorders and Stroke (#35610), National Institutes of Health, Bethesda, MD; the Charles A. Dana Foundation (#90030633), New York, N.Y.; and the Johns Hopkins Medical Institution GCRC grant RR 00052.

References

1. Selnes OA, Pham L, Zeger S, McKhann GM. Defining cognitive change after CABG: decline versus normal variability. *Ann Thorac Surg*. 2006;82(2):388-390.
2. Gottesman RF, Sherman PM, Grega MA, et al. Watershed strokes after cardiac surgery: diagnosis, etiology, and outcome. *Stroke*. 2006;37(9):2306-2311.
3. Del Brutto OH, Mosquera A, Sanchez X, Santos J, Noboa CA. Stroke subtypes among Hispanics living in Guayaquil Ecuador. Results from the Luis Vernaza Hospital Stroke Registry. *Stroke*. 1993;24(12):1833-1836.
4. Paciaroni M, Silvestrelli G, Caso V, et al. Neurovascular territory involved in different etiological subtypes of ischemic stroke in the Perugia Stroke Registry. *Eur J Neurol*. 2003;10(4):361-365.
5. Yamamoto Y, Georgiadis AL, Chang HM, Caplan LR. Posterior cerebral artery territory infarcts in the New England Medical Center Posterior Circulation Registry. *Arch Neurol*. 1999;56(7):824-832.
6. Caplan LR, Hennerici M. Impaired clearance of emboli (washout) is an important link between hypoperfusion, embolism, and ischemic stroke. *Arch Neurol*. 1998;55(11): 1475-1482.
7. Caplan LR, Wong KS, Gao S, Hennerici MG. Is hypoperfusion an important cause of strokes? If so, how? *Cerebrovasc Dis*. 2006;21(3):145-153.
8. Clark RE, Brillman J, Davis DA, Lovell MR, Price TR, Magovern GJ. Microemboli during coronary artery bypass grafting. Genesis and effect on outcome. *J Thorac Cardiovasc Surg*. 1995;109:249-257. discussion 257-8.
9. Moody DM, Brown WR, Challa VR, Stump DA, Reboussin DM, Legault C. Brain microemboli associated with cardiopulmonary bypass: a histologic and magnetic resonance imaging study. *Ann Thorac Surg*. 1995;59:1304-1307.
10. Babikian VL, Caplan LR. Brain embolism is a dynamic process with variable characteristics. *Neurology*. 2000;54(4): 797-801.
11. Barbut D, Hinton RB, Szatrowski TP, et al. Cerebral emboli detected during bypass surgery are associated with clamp removal. *Stroke*. 1994;25:2398-2402.
12. Barbut D, Yao FS, Hager DN, Kavanaugh P, Trifiletti RR, Gold JP. Comparison of transcranial Doppler ultrasonography and transesophageal echocardiography to monitor emboli during coronary artery bypass surgery. *Stroke*. 1996;27(1):87-90.
13. Brooker RF, Brown WR, Moody DM, et al. Cardiotomy suction: a major source of brain lipid emboli during cardiopulmonary bypass. *Ann Thorac Surg*. 1998;65(6):1651-1655.
14. Goto T, Baba T, Matsuyama K, Honma K, Ura M, Koshiji T. Aortic atherosclerosis and postoperative neurological dysfunction in elderly coronary surgical patients. *Ann Thorac Surg*. 2003;75(6):1912-1918.
15. Suojaranta-Ylinen RT, Roine RO, Vento AE, Niskanen MM, Salmenpera MT. Improved neurologic outcome after implementing evidence-based guidelines for cardiac surgery. *J Cardiothorac Vasc Anesth*. 2007;21(4):529-534.
16. Di EM, Schepens MA, Morshuis WJ, et al. Brain protection using antegrade selective cerebral perfusion: a multicenter study. *Ann Thorac Surg*. 2003;76(4):1181-1188.
17. Mathew JP, Fontes ML, Tudor IC, et al. A multicenter risk index for atrial fibrillation after cardiac surgery. *JAMA*. 2004;291(14):1720-1729.
18. Tufo HM, Ostfeld AM, Shekelle R. Central nervous system dysfunction following open-heart surgery. *JAMA*. 1970; 212(8):1333-1340.
19. Karkouti K, Djaiani G, Borger MA, et al. Low hematocrit during cardiopulmonary bypass is associated with increased risk of perioperative stroke in cardiac surgery. *Ann Thorac Surg*. 2005;80(4):1381-1387.
20. Johnsson P, Algotsson L, Ryding E, Stahl E, Messeter K. Cardiopulmonary perfusion and cerebral blood flow in bilateral carotid artery disease. *Ann Thorac Surg*. 1991;51(4):579-584.
21. Lazar HL, Menzoian JO. Coronary artery bypass grafting in patients with cerebrovascular disease. *Ann Thorac Surg*. 1998;66(3):968-974.
22. Karkouti K, Wijeysundera DN, Yau TM, McCluskey SA, Van RA, Beattie WS. The influence of baseline hemoglobin concentration on tolerance of anemia in cardiac surgery. *Transfusion*. 2008;48(4):666-672.
23. Floyd TF, Shah PN, Price CC, et al. Clinically silent cerebral ischemic events after cardiac surgery: their incidence, regional vascular occurrence, and procedural dependence. *Ann Thorac Surg*. 2006;81(6):2160-2166.
24. Bendszus M, Reents W, Franke D, et al. Brain damage after coronary artery bypass grafting. *Arch Neurol*. 2002;59(7): 1090-1095.
25. Djaiani G, Fedorko L, Borger M, et al. Mild to moderate atheromatous disease of the thoracic aorta and new ischemic brain lesions after conventional coronary artery bypass graft surgery. *Stroke*. 2004;35(9):e356-e358.
26. Knipp SC, Matatko N, Wilhelm H, et al. Evaluation of brain injury after coronary artery bypass grafting. A prospective study using neuropsychological assessment and diffusion-weighted magnetic resonance imaging. *Eur J Cardiothorac Surg*. 2004;25(5):791-800.

27. Barber PA, Hach S, Tippett LJ, Ross L, Merry AF, Milsom P. Cerebral ischemic lesions on diffusion-weighted imaging are associated with neurocognitive decline after cardiac surgery. *Stroke* 2008 March 6.
28. Wityk RJ, Goldsborough MA, Hillis A, et al. Diffusion- and perfusion-weighted brain magnetic resonance imaging in patients with neurologic complications after cardiac surgery. *Arch Neurol.* 2001;58(4):571-576.
29. Cook DJ, Huston J III, Trenerry MR, Brown RD Jr, Zehr KJ, Sundt TM III. Postcardiac surgical cognitive impairment in the aged using diffusion-weighted magnetic resonance imaging. *Ann Thorac Surg.* 2007;83(4):1389-1395.
30. Taggart DP, Westaby S. Neurological and cognitive disorders after coronary artery bypass grafting. *Curr Opin Cardiol.* 2001;16(5):271-276.
31. Rudolph JL, Jones RN, Rasmussen LS, Silverstein JH, Inouye SK, Marcantonio ER. Independent vascular and cognitive risk factors for postoperative delirium. *Am J Med.* 2007;120(9):807-813.
32. Johnson RG. Abnormal neuropsychometrics early after coronary artery bypass grafting. *Crit Care Med.* 2000;28(6): 2142-2143.
33. Keith JR, Puente AE, Malcolmson KL, Tartt S, Coleman AE, Marks HF Jr. Assessing postoperative cognitive change after cardiopulmonary bypass surgery. *Neuropsychology.* 2002;16(3):411-421.
34. Selnes OA, Grega MA, Borowicz LM Jr, Royall RM, McKhann GM, Baumgartner WA. Cognitive changes with coronary artery disease: a prospective study of coronary artery bypass graft patients and nonsurgical controls. *Ann Thorac Surg.* 2003;75(5):1377 1384.
35. Mullges W, Babin-Ebell J, Reents W, Toyka KV. Cognitive performance after coronary artery bypass grafting: a follow-up study. *Neurology.* 2002;59:741-743.
36. Mullges W, Berg D, Schmidtke A, Weinacker B, Toyka KV. Early natural course of transient encephalopathy after coronary artery bypass grafting. *Crit Care Med.* 2000;28(6): 1808-1811.
37. Selnes OA, Goldsborough MA, Borowicz LM, Enger C, Quaskey SA, McKhann GM. Determinants of cognitive change after coronary artery bypass surgery: a multifactorial problem. *Ann Thorac Surg.* 1999;67:1669-1676.
38. Bergh C, Backstrom M, Jonsson H, Havinder L, Johnsson P. In the eye of both patient and spouse: memory is poor 1 to 2 years after coronary bypass and angioplasty. *Ann Thorac Surg.* 2002;74(3):689-693.
39. Bassel C, Rourke SB, Halman MH, Smith ML. Working memory performance predicts subjective cognitive complaints in HIV infection. *Neuropsychology.* 2002;16(3):400-410.
40. Fearn SJ, Pole R, Wesnes K, Faragher EB, Hooper TL, McCollum CN. Cerebral injury during cardiopulmonary bypass: emboli impair memory. *J Thorac Cardiovasc Surg.* 2001;121(6):1150-1160.
41. Braekken SK, Reinvang I, Russell D, Brucher R, Svennevig JL. Association between intraoperative cerebral microembolic signals and postoperative neuropsychological deficit: comparison between patients with cardiac valve replacement and patients with coronary artery bypass grafting. *J Neurol Neurosurg Psychiatry.* 1998;65(4):573-576.
42. Neville MJ, Butterworth J, James RL, Hammon JW, Stump DA. Similar neurobehavioral outcome after valve or coronary artery operations despite differing carotid embolic counts. *J Thorac Cardiovasc Surg.* 2001;121(1):125-136.
43. Browndyke JN, Moser DJ, Cohen RA, et al. Acute neuropsychological functioning following cardiosurgical interventions associated with the production of intraoperative cerebral microemboli. *Clin Neuropsychol.* 2002;16(4):463-471.
44. Andrell P, Jensen C, Norrsell H, et al. White matter disease in magnetic resonance imaging predicts cerebral complications after coronary artery bypass grafting. *Ann Thorac Surg.* 2005;79(1):74-79.
45. Ho PM, Arciniegas DB, Grigsby J, et al. Predictors of cognitive decline following coronary artery bypass graft surgery. *Ann Thorac Surg.* 2004;77(2):597-603.
46. Abildstrom H, Hogh P, Sperling B, Moller JT, Yndgaard S, Rasmussen LS. Cerebral blood flow and cognitive dysfunction after coronary surgery. *Ann Thorac Surg.* 2002;73(4):1174-1178.
47. Johnson T, Monk T, Rasmussen LS, et al. Postoperative cognitive dysfunction in middle-aged patients. *Anesthesiology.* 2002;96(6):1351-1357.
48. Rasmussen LS, Johnson T, Kuipers HM, et al. Does anaesthesia cause postoperative cognitive dysfunction? A randomised study of regional versus general anaesthesia in 438 elderly patients. *Acta Anaesthesiol Scand.* 2003;47(3): 260-266.
49. Monk TG, Weldon BC, Garvan CW, et al. Predictors of cognitive dysfunction after major noncardiac surgery. *Anesthesiology.* 2008;108(1):18-30.
50. Newman MF, Kirchner JL, Phillips-Bute B, et al. Longitudinal Assessment of Neurocognitive function after coronary artery bypass surgery. *N Engl J Med.* 2001;344: 395-402.
51. Selnes OA, Royall RM, Grega MA, Borowicz LM Jr, Quaskey S, McKhann GM. Cognitive changes 5 years after coronary artery bypass grafting: is there evidence of late decline? *Arch Neurol.* 2001;58(4):598-604.
52. Stygall J, Newman SP, Fitzgerald G, et al. Cognitive change 5 years after coronary artery bypass surgery. *Health Psychol.* 2003;22(6):579-586.
53. Denton TA, Fonarow GC, LaBresh KA, Trento A. Secondary prevention after coronary bypass: The American Heart Association "get with the guidelines" program. *Ann Thorac Surg.* 2003;75(3):758-760.
54. Hlatky MA, Bacon C, Boothroyd D, et al. Cognitive function 5 years after randomization to coronary angioplasty or coronary artery bypass graft surgery. *Circulation.* 1999;96 (suppl II):11-15.
55. Potter GG, Plassman BL, Helms MJ, Steffens DC, Welsh-Bohmer KA. Age effects of coronary artery bypass graft on cognitive status change among elderly male twins. *Neurology.* 2004;63(12):2245-2249.
56. Bennett HP, Piguet O, Grayson DA, et al. A 6-year study of cognition and spatial function in the demented and non-demented elderly: the Sydney Older Persons Study. *Dement Geriatr Cogn Disord.* 2003;16(4):181-186.
57. Piguet O, Grayson DA, Creasey H, et al. Vascular risk factors, cognition and dementia incidence over 6 years in the Sydney Older Persons Study. *Neuroepidemiology.* 2003; 22(3):165-171.
58. Saxton J, Ratcliff G, Newman A, et al. Cognitive test performance and presence of subclinical cardiovascular disease in

the cardiovascular health study. *Neuroepidemiology*. 2000; 19(6):312-319.
59. Elwood PC, Pickering J, Bayer A, Gallacher JE. Vascular disease and cognitive function in older men in the Caerphilly cohort. *Age Ageing*. 2002;31(1):43-48.
60. Vermeer SE, Prins ND, Den Heijer T, Hofman A, Koudstaal PJ, Breteler MM. Silent brain infarcts and the risk of dementia and cognitive decline. *N Engl J Med*. 2003;348(13): 1215-1222.
61. Vermeer SE, Hollander M, van Dijk EJ, Hofman A, Koudstaal PJ, Breteler MM. Silent brain infarcts and white matter lesions increase stroke risk in the general population: the Rotterdam Scan Study. *Stroke*. 2003;34(5):1126-1129.
62. Schneider JA, Wilson RS, Cochran EJ, et al. Relation of cerebral infarctions to dementia and cognitive function in older persons. *Neurology*. 2003;60(7):1082-1088.
63. Goto T, Baba T, Honma K, et al. Magnetic resonance imaging findings and postoperative neurologic dysfunction in elderly patients undergoing coronary artery bypass grafting. *Ann Thorac Surg*. 2001;72(1):137-142.
64. Lund C, Hol PK, Lundblad R, et al. Comparison of cerebral embolization during off-pump and on-pump coronary artery bypass surgery. *Ann Thorac Surg*. 2003;76(3): 765-770.
65. Bowles BJ, Lee JD, Dang CR, et al. Coronary artery bypass performed without the use of cardiopulmonary bypass is associated with reduced cerebral microemboli and improved clinical results. *Chest*. 2001;119(1):25-30.
66. Takagi H, Tanabashi T, Kawai N, Umemoto T. A meta-analysis of minimally invasive coronary artery bypass versus percutaneous coronary intervention with stenting for isolated left anterior descending artery disease is indispensable. *J Thorac Cardiovasc Surg*. 2007;134(2):548-549.
67. Hernandez F Jr, Brown JR, Likosky DS, et al. Neurocognitive outcomes of off-pump versus on-pump coronary artery bypass: a prospective randomized controlled trial. *Ann Thorac Surg*. 2007;84(6):1897-1903.
68. van Dijk D, Spoor M, Hijman R, et al. Cognitive and cardiac outcomes 5 years after off-pump vs on-pump coronary artery bypass graft surgery. *JAMA*. 2007;297(7):701-708.

4 Neurocognitive Decline Following Cardiac Surgery: Incidence, Risk Factors, Prevention, and Outcomes

John W. Hammon and David A. Stump

As outcomes from cardiac surgery have been more carefully studied, it is clear that even subtle neurological damage can produce unacceptable declines in physical and social function. Because the brain is such a complex organ, even small injuries may produce symptomatic, functional losses that would not be detectable or important in other organs. Regional hypoperfusion, edema, microemboli, circulating cytotoxins, or subtle changes in blood glucose, insulin, or calcium may result in changes in cognitive function, ranging from subtle to profound. A small 2-mm infarct may cause a disruption of behavioral patterns, physiologic and physical function changes can pass unnoticed, be accepted and dismissed, or profoundly compromise the patient's quality of life. Move the lesion half a centimeter and the same volume lesion may result in a catastrophic stroke. Thus, the brain is the most sensitive organ exposed to damage by cardiac surgery and also the organ that, with the heart, is most important to protect.

4.1 Preoperative Workup

Routine assessment of neurologic injury, which occurs in the setting of cardiac surgery, is not done for most patients because of the priority of the cardiac lesion and because of costs in time and money. General neurologic examinations by members of the surgical team or individuals lacking specialized training are not adequate to rule out subtle neurologic injuries, and this is the principal reason that the incidence of stroke, neurologic, or neuropsychological injury varies widely in the surgical literature.[1–3]

For studies designed to assess or reduce neurologic injury in the setting of cardiac surgery, nonroutine preoperative and postoperative tests are required. These special tests include a complete neurologic examination by a neurologist or a well-trained surrogate. To improve accuracy, a single neurologist should ideally conduct all serial examinations. A standardized protocol of examination should be followed, with uniform reporting of results. The basic, structured examination includes a mental state examination; cranial nerve, motor, sensory, and cerebellar examinations; and examination of gait, station, deep tendon, and primitive reflexes.

The most obvious neurologic abnormalities are paresis, loss of vital brain functions such as speech, vision, comprehension or coma. These are commonly lumped under the general heading of stroke. Disorders of awareness or consciousness can include coma, delirium, and confusion, but transitory episodes of delirium and confusion are often dismissed as due to anesthesia or medications. More subtle losses are determined by comparison of preoperative and postoperative performances using a standard battery of neuropsychological tests prepared by a group of neuropsychologists.[4] A neuropsychological examination is basically an extension of the neurologic examination with a much greater emphasis on higher cortical function. Dysfunction is objectively defined as a deviation from the expected, relative to a large population. For example, although performing at a 95 IQ level is in the normal range, it is low for a physician and a search for a neurologic impairment would be triggered by such a poor performance. A 20% decline in two or more of these tests, compared to the patient's own baseline, suggests a neuropsychological deficit that should be

J.W. Hammon (✉)
Department of Cardiothoracic Surgery, Wake Forest University School of Medicine, Winston-Salem, North Carolina, USA
e-mail: jhammon@wfubmc.edu

R.S. Bonser et al. (eds.), *Brain Protection in Cardiac Surgery*,
DOI: 10.1007/978-1-84996-293-3_4,

followed until resolved or not resolved. This principle was established at a consensus conference of neuropsychologists and clinicians and published in 1997.[5] In studies involving long-term follow-up, the inclusion of a control group of unoperated patients with the same disease and of similar demographics helps define the causes of neuropsychological decline, which occurs later than 3–6 months after surgery.[6]

Many studies have reported neuropsychological outcomes using more than one methodology, often different from the techniques recommended by the consensus conference. In most studies analytic methods for determination of postoperative cognitive decline are: percentage decline, standard deviation decline, factor analysis, and individual test reporting. Using the "percentage decline" definition a patient must decline a percentage (usually 20%) from baseline in a pre-specified number of tests. The "standard deviation decline" definition requires a population (baseline or control) to define the standard deviation (SD) and then create the dichotomous outcome. From the neuropsychology literature, a one standard deviation decline is felt to be clinically significant.[7] However, if the SD is large (i.e., 35%) due to the inclusion of outliers then many patients with a significant impairment may not be classified as having a deficit due to a floor effect: short of death, a patient cannot perform badly enough to lower their score 35%.

The "factor analysis" methodology uses raw neuropsychological data to create several latent cognitive domains which are continuous variables. The latent cognitive domains are frequently dichotomized to produce clinically understandable outcomes, but not readily calculable on an individual patient. "Individual test analysis" assesses performance on individual neuropsychological measures and several continuous outcome variables.[8] Common challenges associated with the use of cognitive testing and clinical challenges to applying the concept to postoperative cognitive decline are: dealing with baseline variabilities in performance, understanding and dealing with the learning effect which complicates multiple testing, accounting for day-to-day variations of the cognitive state in understanding results, and understanding and defining the difference between normal and abnormal cognitive performance.[9] Because of the variation in analysis and reporting, the use of neuropsychological tests is often confusing to those not experienced with these techniques.

Another compounding variable is most small infarctions, both pre- and peri-operatively, occur in the basal ganglia and other subcortical structures. Since most tests of higher cortical function and "cognition" assess the cortical mantle, a patient may have significant problems with postural background movement, balance, and motor memory but still perform adequately on cognitive tests and basic assessment of cranial nerves.[10]

Computed axial tomograms (CAT) or magnetic resonance imaging (MRI) scans are essential for the definitive diagnosis of stroke, delirium, or coma. Preoperative imaging is usually not necessary when new techniques such as diffusion-weighted MRI imaging, MRI spectroscopy, or MRI angiography are used to assess possible new lesions after operation.[11,12] However, recent studies demonstrate patients with cognitive decline have a loss in cell volume due to micro-infarctions that are not detectable with current radiological techniques.[13] Histolologic studies performed on patients who did not survive cardiac surgery have demonstrated millions of small lipid microemboli that may result in cell damage or death, which is evident only in late MRI images and manifested by brain shrinkage and ventricular enlargement.[14]

4.2 Populations at Risk

Advancing age increases the risk of stroke or cognitive impairment in the general population, and surgery, regardless of type, increases the risk still more.[15] In 1986, Gardner and colleagues reported the risk of stroke during coronary artery bypass graft (CABG) surgery to be directly related to age.[16] A European study compared 321 elderly patients without surgery to 1,218 patients who had noncardiac surgery and found a 26% incidence of cognitive dysfunction 1 week after operation and a 10% incidence at 3 months.[17] Between 1974 and 1990 the number of patients undergoing cardiac surgery over age 60 and over age 70 increased twofold and sevenfold, respectively.[18] Genetic factors also influence the incidence of cognitive dysfunction following cardiac surgery.[19]

As the age of cardiac surgical patients increases, the number with multiple risk factors for neurologic injury also increases. Risk factors for adverse cerebral outcomes are listed in Table 4.1.[20] These factors are divided into stroke with a permanent fixed neurologic

Table 4.1 Adjusted odds ratios for Type I and Type II cerebral outcomes associated with selected risk factors

Factor	Model for Type I cerebral outcome	Model for Type II cerebral outcome
Significant factors, $p < 0.05$		
Proximal aortic atherosclerosis	4.52	
History of neurologic disease	3.19	
Use of intra-aortic balloon pump	2.60	
Diabetes mellitus	2.59	
History of hypertension	2.31	
History of pulmonary disease	2.09	2.37
History of unstable angina	1.83	
Age (per additional decade)	1.75	2.20
Systolic blood pressure > 180 mmHg at admission		3.47
History of excessive alcohol consumption		2.64
History of CABG		2.18
Dysrhythmia on day of surgery		1.97
Antihypertensive therapy		1.78
Other factors, p not significant		
Perioperative hypotension	1.92	1.88
Ventricular venting	1.83	
Congestive heart failure on day of surgery		2.46
History of peripheral vascular disease		1.64

Source: With permission from Roach GW et al.[20]

deficit (type 1) and coma or delirium (type 2). Hypertension and diabetes occur in approximately 55% and 25% of cardiac surgical patients, respectively.[21] Fifteen percent have carotid stenosis of 50% or greater, and up to 13% have had a transient ischemic attack or prior stroke. The total number of MRI atherosclerotic lesions in the brachiocephalic vessels adds to the risk of stroke or cognitive dysfunction,[22] as does the severity of atherosclerosis in the ascending aorta as detected by epiaortic ultrasound scanning.[23] Palpable ascending aortic atherosclerotic plaques markedly increase the risk of right carotid arterial emboli as detected by Doppler ultrasound.[24] The incidence of severe aortic atherosclerosis is 1% in cardiac surgical patients less than 50 years old and is 10% in those aged 75–80.[25]

4.3 Mechanisms of Injury

The three major causes of neurologic dysfunction and injury during cardiac surgery are microemboli, hypoperfusion, and a generalized inflammatory reaction, all which can occur in the same patient at the same time for different reasons. The vast majority of intraoperative strokes are due to the embolization of atherosclerotic material from the aorta and brachiocephalic vessels. This occurs as a result of manipulation of the heart and major thoracic vasculature as well as dislodgement of athromata from shearing forces directed at the walls of vessels from inflow cardiopulmonary bypass cannulae.[26] Microemboli are distributed in proportion to blood flow;[27] thus reduced cerebral blood flow reduces microembolic injury but increases the risk of hypoperfusion.[28] During cardiopulmonary bypass (CPB) both alpha-stat acid–base management and phenylepherine reduce cerebral injury in adults, probably by causing cerebral vessel vasoconstriction and reducing the number of microemboli.[28,29] Air,[30] atherosclerotic debris,[31] and fat are the major types of microemboli causing brain injury in clinical practice, and all cause neuronal necrosis by blocking cerebral vessels.[32] Massive air embolism causes a large ischemic injury, but gaseous cerebral microemboli may directly damage endothelium in addition to blocking blood flow.[33] The recent identification of unique small capillary arteriolar dilatations (SCADs) in the brain associated with fat emboli (Fig. 4.1)[34] raises the possibility that these emboli not only block small vessels but also release cytotoxic free radicals, which may significantly increase the damage to lipid-rich neurons.

Anemia and elevated cerebral temperature increase cerebral blood flow but may cause inadequate oxygen delivery to the brain[35]; however, these conditions are easily avoided during clinical cardiac surgery. Although some investigators speculate that normothermic and/or hyperthermic CPB cause cerebral hypoperfusion,[36] experimental studies indicate that cerebral blood flow increases with temperature.[37] Brain injuries associated with this practice are more likely due to increased cerebral microemboli, which produce larger lesions at

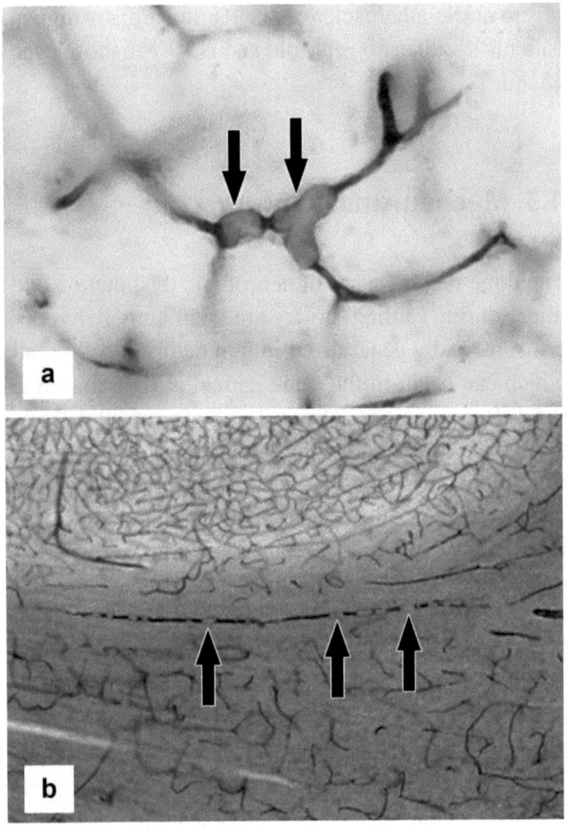

Fig. 4.1 (**a**) High magnification photomicrograph showing small capillary arteriolar dilatations (SCADS) from the brain of a patient dying soon after cardiac surgery. Alkaline phosphatase stained, celloidin imbedded, 50X. (**b**) Experimental fat emboli in the dog. We know now that SCADS seen in patients are fat emboli from wound blood aspirated with cardiotomy suction and redirected to the brain via cardiopulmonary bypass

higher cerebral temperatures.[38] Reduced brain temperature is protective against neural cell injury and remains an important neuroprotective strategy.

All surgery, like accidental trauma, triggers an acute inflammatory response that can result in neurologic injury, but the continuous exposure of heparinized blood to non-endothelial cell surfaces followed by reinfusion of wound blood and recirculation within the body greatly magnifies this response in operations in which CPB is used. Although far from fully described and understood, this primary "blood injury" produces a unique response, which is different in detail from that caused by other threats to homeostasis.

The principal blood elements involved in this acute defense reaction are contact and complement plasma protein systems, neutrophils, monocytes, endothelial cells, and, to a lesser extent, platelets. When activated during CPB, the principal blood elements release vasoactive and cytotoxic substances; produce cell signaling, inflammatory and inhibitory cytokines; express complementary cellular receptors that interact with specific cell signaling substances and other cells; and generate a host of vasoactive and cytotoxic substances that circulate.[39] Normally these reactive blood elements mediate and regulate the defense reaction,[40–42] but during CPB an orderly, targeted response is overwhelmed by the massive activation and circulation of these reactive blood elements. This massive attack damages the endothelium, increases the size of ischemic lesions, and causes organ dysfunction.

4.4 Strategies for Reducing Injury (Table 4.2)

Table 4.2 lists strategies for emboli protection during cardiac surgery. Important methods for reducing emboli deserve emphasis. Principles include adequate anticoagulation, washing blood aspirated from the surgical wound, filtering arterial inflow and venous outflow, strict control of all air entry sites within the perfusion

Table 4.2 Strategies for emboli protection during cardiac surgery

Proven
• Adequate anticoagulation
• Membrane oxygenator
• Closed system CPB
• Wash blood aspirated from surgical wound
• (No need to wash blood from cardiac chambers)
• Filter arterial onflow and venous outflow
• Control all sites of air entry into CPB
• Removal of residual air from heart and great vessels
• Epiaortic ultrasound mapping of ascending aorta
• Minimal aortic manipulation (single aortic cross clamp)
• Retrograde cardioplegia
Experimental
• Off-pump surgery
• Selective filtration of brachiocephalic vessels
• Ultrasonic venous and arterial embolus detection
• Pharmacologic brain protection

circuit, removal of residual air from the heart and great vessels, and avoidance of atherosclerotic emboli.[43–45]

Many intraoperative strategies are available to reduce cerebral atherosclerotic embolization. These include routine epicardial echocardiography of the ascending aorta to detect both anterior and posterior atherosclerotic plaques and to find sites free of atherosclerosis for placing the aortic cannula.[46] Recently, special catheters with or without baffles or screens have been developed to reduce the number of atherosclerotic emboli that reach the cerebral circulation.[47] In patients with moderate or severe ascending aortic atherosclerosis, a single application of the aortic clamp as opposed to partial or multiple applications is strongly recommended and has been shown to reduce postoperative neurocognitive deficits in a large clinical series.[48] Retrograde cardioplegia is preferred over antegrade cardioplegia in these patients to avoid a sandblasting effect of the cardioplegic solution.[49] No aortic clamp may be safe or even possible in some patients with severe atherosclerosis or porcelain aorta. If intracardiac surgery is required in these patients, deep hypothermia may be used with or without graft replacement of the ascending aorta. If only revascularization is needed, pedicled single or sequential arterial grafts,[50] T or Y grafts from a pedicled mammary artery,[51] or vein grafts anastomosed to arch vessels can be used. Patients with intracardiac thrombus or vegetations require aortic cross clamping before cardiac manipulation to avoid dislodging embolic material.

In-depth or screen filters are essential for cardiotomy reservoirs and are usually used in arterial lines. The efficacy of arterial line filters is controversial since screen filters with a pore size less than 20 μm cannot be used because of flow resistance across the filter. However, air and fat emboli can pass through filters although 20 μm screen filters more effectively trap microemboli than larger sizes.[52]

4.5 Neuroprotective Strategies

Recommended conditions for protecting the brain during CPB include mild hypothermia (32–34°C) and hematocrit above 25%.[37] Temporary increases in cerebral venous pressure caused by superior vena cava obstruction and excessive rewarming above blood temperatures of 37°C should be avoided.[38,53] A randomized study in which patients were mildly rewarmed to 35°C core temperature demonstrated improved neurocognitive outcomes over patients rewarmed to 37°C.[53] Either jugular venous bulb oxygen saturation or near-infrared cerebral oximetry are recommended for monitoring cerebral perfusion in patients who may be at high risk for cerebral injury.[54]

Barbiturates reduce cerebral metabolism by decreasing spontaneous synaptic activity[55] and provide a definite neuroprotective effect during clinical cardiac surgery using CPB.[56] The protective effect may be due to decreasing brain blood flow and thereby reducing the embolic load. Unfortunately, these agents delay emergence from anesthesia and prolong intensive care unit stays. High doses of corticosteroids given at least 4 h prior to cardiopulmonary bypass have been shown to be neuroprotective in cases involving circulatory arrest.[57] However, no good evidence of neuroprotection exists in cases of lesser magnitude. NMDA (N-methyl-D aspartate) antagonists, which are effective in animals, provide mild protection compared to control patients, but have a high incidence of neurologic side effects.[58] A small study demonstrated a neuroprotective effect of lidocaine, but this beneficial effect has not been reproduced.[59] Currently no pharmacologic agent is recommended for protection of the central nervous system during CPB.

Off-pump myocardial revascularization theoretically avoids many of the causes of cerebral injury due to CPB, but, as noted above, many causes of neuronal injury are independent of CPB and related to atherosclerosis and air entry sites into the circulation. Nonrandomized measurements of carotid emboli by Doppler ultrasound indicate fewer emboli and slightly improved neurocognitive outcomes in high risk patients who have off-pump surgery.[60] A meta-analysis of off-pump vs. on-pump patients failed to show a significant difference in neurologic outcome between methods.[61]

4.6 Prognosis

Patients with intraoperative stroke or who develop stroke symptoms in the first week after surgery often improve in direct relation to the lesion size and location on imaging studies. Neuropsychological deficits that are present after 3 months are almost always permanent.[62] Assessments after that time are confounded by development of new deficits, particularly in aged patients.[63]

The difficulty of separating intraoperative brain injury from that which occurs in the early or late

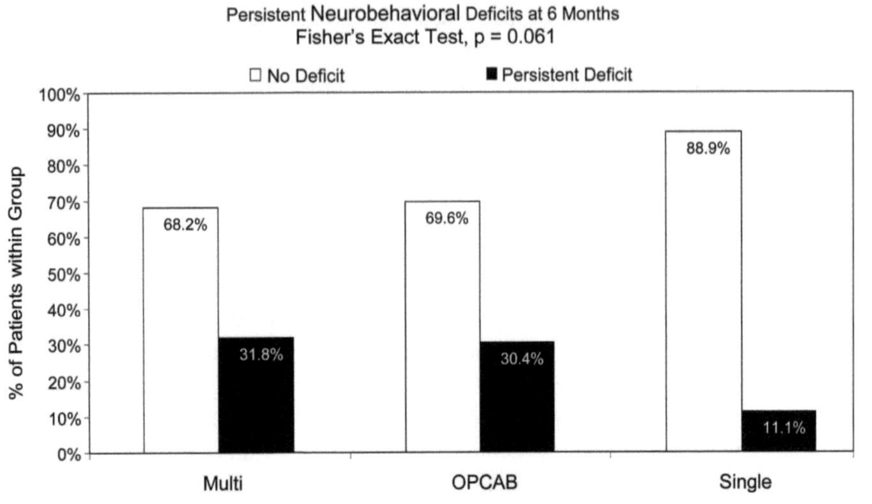

Fig. 4.2 Bar graph with results of neuropsychological testing at 6 months after CABG using three different techniques. Note patients with single aortic clamping have many fewer persistent neuropsychological deficits than patients operated with multiple aortic clamping or OPCAB (From Hammon et al.[64])

postoperative period has been recently addressed by a reanalysis of data published earlier. The authors tracked specific neuropsychological deficits which persisted unchanged for 6 months (persistent deficits) and separated them from new deficits which appeared after surgery (Fig. 4.2).[64] Using this technique it is possible to accurately measure surgical brain injury and design techniques to eliminate this important cause of morbidity. Late follow up studies should include a control group with similar risk factors but not having cardiac operations.[65] This technique demonstrated similar outcomes in surgical and nonsurgical controls at 3 years, putting to rest the previous fear that surgical patients had recurrent neurocognitive deficits, and were thus at greater risk for poor long-term outcomes.[62] In a recent study, a group of surgical patients who were evaluated with pre- and postoperative neuropsychological studies had rigid control of cardiovascular risk factors.[66] They demonstrated no delayed or late cognitive decline, offering hope that aggressive medical therapy following skillful surgery can prevent late neurological injury.

References

1. Shaw PJ et al. Long-term intellectual dysfunction following coronary artery bypass surgery: a six month follow-up study. *J Med*. 1987;62:259-268.
2. Newman S. The incidence and nature of neuropsychological morbidity following cardiac surgery. *Perfusion*. 1989; 4:93-100.
3. Svensson LG, Nadolny EM, Kimmel WA. Multimodal protocol influence on stroke and neurocognitive deficit prevention after ascending/arch aortic operations. *Ann Thorac Surg*. 2002;74:240-246.
4. Newman S, Smith P, Treasure T, et al. Acute neuropsychological consequences of coronary artery bypass surgery. *Curr Psychol Res Rev*. 1987;6:115-124.
5. Murkin JM, Stump DA, Blumenthal JA, et al. Defining dysfunction: group means versus incidence analysis-a statement of consensus. *Ann Thorac Surg*. 1997;64:904-905.
6. Selnes OA, Grega MA, Bailey MM, et al. Neurocognitive outcomes 3 years after coronary artery bypass graft surgery: a controlled study. *Ann Thorac Surg*. 2007;84:1885-1896.
7. Blumenthal JA, Mahanna EP, Madden DJ, et al. Methodological issues in the assessment of neuropsychological function after cardiac surgery. *Ann Thorac Surg*. 1995;59: 1345-1350.
8. Stump DA. Selection and clinical significance of neuropsychologic tests. *Ann Thorac Surg*. 1995;59:1340-1344.
9. Stump DA, Rogers AT, Hammon JW. Neurobehavioral tests are monitoring tools used to improve cardiac surgery outcome. *Ann Thorac Surg*. 1996;61:1295-1296.
10. Das RR, Seshadri S, Beiser AS, et al. Prevalence and correlates of silent cerebral infarcts in the Framingham offspring study. *Stroke*. 2008;39:2929-2935.
11. Baird A, Benfield A, Schlaug G, et al. Enlargement of human cerebral ischemic lesion volumes measured by diffusion-weighted magnetic resonance imaging. *Ann Neurol*. 1997;41:581-589.
12. Bendszus M, Reents W, Franke D, et al. Brain damage after coronary artery bypass grafting. *Arch Neurol*. 2002;59:1090-1095.
13. Vermeer SE, Longstreth WT Jr, Koudstaal PJ. Silent brain infarcts: a systematic review. *Lancet Neurol*. 2007; 6:611-619.
14. Kohn A. Magnetic resonance imaging registration and quantitification of the brain before and after coronary artery bypass graft surgery. *Ann Thorac Surg*. 2002;73:5363-5365.

15. Shaw PJ, Bates D, Cartlidge NE, et al. Neurologic and neuropsychological morbidity following: major surgery: comparison of coronary artery bypass and peripheral vascular surgery. *Stroke*. 1987;18:700-707.
16. Gardner TJ, Horneffer PJ, Manolio TA, et al. Stroke following coronary artery bypass surgery: a ten year study. *Ann Thorac Surg*. 1985;40:574-581.
17. Moller JT, Cluitmans P, Rasmussen LS, et al. Long-term postoperative cognitive dysfunction in the elderly ISPOCD study. ISPOCD investigators, International Study of Post-Operative Cognitive Dysfunction. *Lancet*. 1998;351:857-861.
18. Jones EL, Weintraub WS, Craver JM, et al. Coronary bypass surgery: is the operation different today? *J Thorac Cardiovasc Surg*. 1991;101:108-115.
19. Tardiff BE, Newman MF, Saunders AM, et al. Preliminary report of a genetic basis for cognitive decline after cardiac operations. *Ann Thorac Surg*. 1997;64:715-720.
20. Roach GW, Kanchugar M, Mangano CM, et al. Adverse cerebral outcomes after coronary bypass surgery: multicenter study of perioperative ischemia research groups and the ischemia research and education foundation investigators. *N Engl J Med*. 1996;335:1857-1863.
21. Weintraub WS, Wenger NK, Jones EL, et al. Changing clinical characteristics of coronary surgery patients: differences between men and women. *Circulation*. 1993;88:79-86.
22. Goto T, Baba T, Yoshitake A, et al. Craniocervical and aortic atherosclerosis as neurologic risk factors in coronary surgery. *Ann Thorac Surg*. 2000;69:834-840.
23. Wareing TH, Davila-Roman VG, Daily BB, et al. Strategy for the reduction of stroke incidence in cardiac surgical patients. *Ann Thorac Surg*. 1993;55:1400 1408.
24. Stump DA, Kon NA, Rogers AT, et al. Emboli neuropsychologic outcome following cardiopulmary bypass. *Echocardiography*. 1996;13:555-558.
25. Tuman KJ, McCarthy RJ, Najafi H, et al. Differential effects of advanced age on neurologic and cardiac risks of coronary operations. *J Thorac Cardiovasc Surg*. 1992;104:1510-1517.
26. Lata A, Stump D, Deal D, et al.: Cannula design reduces particulate and gaseous emboli during cardiopulmonary bypass for coronary revascularization. *J Cardiac Surg*. (in press).
27. Jones TJ, Stump DA, Deal D, et al. Hypothermia protects the brain from embolization by reducing and redirecting the embolic load. *Ann Thorac Surg*. 1999;68:1465.
28. Gold JP, Charlson ME, Williams-Russo P. Improvement of outcomes after coronary artery bypass; a randomized trial comparing high verus low mean arterial pressure. *J Thorac Cardiovasc Surg*. 1995;110:1302-1314.
29. Murkin JM, Farrar JK, Tweed WA, et al. Cerebral autoregulation and flow/metabolism coupling during cardiopulmonary bypass: the role of $PaCO_2$. *Anesth Analg*. 1987; 66:665-672.
30. Hill AG, Groom RC, Tewksbury L, et al. Sources of gaseous microemboli during cardiopulmonary bypass. *Proc Am Acad Cardiovasc Perfus*. 1998;9:122-130.
31. Blauth CI. Macroemboli and microemboli during cardiopulmonary bypass. *Ann Thorac Surg*. 1995;59:1300-1303.
32. Stump DA, Brown WR, Moody DM, et al. Microemboli and neurologic dysfunction after cardiovascular surgery. *Semin Cardiothorac Vascular Anesth*. 1999;3:47-54.
33. Helps SC, Parsons DW, Reilly PL, et al. The effect of gas emboli on rabbit cerebral blood flow. *Stroke*. 1990; 21:94-99.
34. Moody DM, Brown WR, Challa VR, et al. Efforts to characterize the nature and chronicle the occurrence of brain emboli during cardiopulmonary bypass. *Perfusion*. 1995; 9:316-417.
35. Cook DJ, Oliver WC, Orsulak TA, et al. Cardiopulmonary bypass temperature, hematocrit, and cerebral oxygen delivery in humans. *Ann Thorac Surg*. 1995;60:1671-1677.
36. Martin TC, Craver JM, Gott MP, et al. Prospective, randomized trial of retrograde warm-blood cardioplegia: myocardial benefit and neurological threat. *Ann Thorac Surg*. 1994;59:298-304.
37. Engelman RM, Pleet AB, Rouson JA, et al. What is the best perfusion temperature for coronary revascularization? *J Thorac Cardiovasc Surg*. 1996;112:1622-1633.
38. Avraamides EJ, Murkin JM. The effect of surgical dislocation of the heart on cerebral blood flow in the presence of a single, two-stage venous cannula during cardiopulmonary bypass. *Can J Anaesth*. 1996;43:A36.
39. Downing SW, Edmunds LH Jr. Release of vasoactive substances during cardiopulmonary bypass. *Ann Thorac Surg*. 1992;54:1236-1243.
40. Warren JS, Ward PA. The inflammatory response. In: Beutler E, Coller BS, Lichtman MA, et al., eds. *Williams Hematology*. 6th ed. New York: McGraw-Hill; 2001:67.
41. Wewers MD. Cytokines and macrophages. In: Remick DG, Friedland JS, eds. *Cytokines in Health and Disease*. 2nd ed. New York: Marcel Dekker; 339.
42. Fantone JC. Cytokines and neutrophils: neutrophil-derived cytokines and the inflammatory response. In: Remick DG, Friedland JS, eds. *Cytokines in Health and Disease*. 2nd ed. New York: Marcel Dekker; 1997:373.
43. Kincaid EH, Jones TJ, Stump DA, et al. Processing scavenged blood with a cell saver reduces cerebral lipid microembolization. *Ann Thorac Surg*. 2000;70:1296-1300.
44. Reichenspurner H, Navia JA, Benny G, et al. Particulate embolic capture by an intra-aortic filter device during cardiac surgery. *J Thorac Cardiovasc Surg*. 2000;119:233-244.
45. Cook DJ, Zehr KJ, Orszulak TA, Slater JM. Profound reduction in brain embolization using an endoaortic baffle during bypass in swine. *Ann Thorac Surg*. 2002;73:198-202.
46. Barzilai B, Marshall WG Jr, Saffitz Je, et al. Avoidance of embolic complications by ultrasonic characterization of the ascending aorta. *Circulation*. 1980;80:1275-1279.
47. Macoviak JA, Hwang J, Boerjan KL, Deal DD. Comparing dual-stream and standard cardiopulmonary bypass in pigs. *Ann Thorac Surg*. 2002;73:203-208.
48. Hammon JW, Stump DA, Butterworth JE, et al. Single cross clamp improves six month cognitive outcome in high risk coronary bypass patients. *J Thorac Cardiovasc Surg*. 2006;131:114-121.
49. Loop FD, Higgins TL, Panda R, et al. Myocardial protection during cardiac operations: decreased morbidity and lower cost with blood cardioplegia and coronary sinus perfusion. *J Cardiovasc Surg*. 1992;104:608-618.
50. Sundt TM, Barner HB, Camillo CJ, et al. Total arterial revascularization with an internal thoracic artery and radial artery T graft. *Ann Thorac Surg*. 1999;68:399-405.

51. Tector AJ, Amundsen S, Schmahl TM, et al. Total revascularization with T grafts. *Ann Thorac Surg*. 1994;57:33-39.
52. Jones TJ, Deal DD, Vernon JC, et al. The propagation of entrained air during cardiopulmonary bypass is affected by circuit design but not by vacuum assisted venous drainage. *Ann Thorac Surg*. 2002;74:2132-2137.
53. Nathan HJ, Wells GA, Munson JL, Wozny D. Neuroprotective effect of mild hypothermia in patients undergoing coronary artery surgery with cardiopulmonary bypass. *Circulation*. 2001;104(I):I-85-I-95.
54. Brown R, Wright G, Royston D. A comparison of two systems for assessing cerebral venous oxyhaemoglobin saturation during cardiopulmonary bypass in humans. *Anaethesia*. 1993;48:697-700.
55. Michenfelder JD. The interdependency of cerebral functional and metabolic effects following massive doses of thiopental in the dog. *Anesthesiology*. 1974;41:231-236.
56. Nussmeier N, Arlund C, Slogoff S. Neuropsychiatric complications after cardiopulmonary bypass: cerebral protection by a barbiturate. *Anesthesiology*. 1986;64:165-170.
57. Shum-Tim D, Tchervenkov CI, Jamal AM, et al. Systemic steroid pretreatment improves cerebral protection after circulatory arrest. *Ann Thorac Surg*. 2001;72:1615-1620.
58. Arrowsmith JE, Harrison MJG, Newman SP, et al. Neuroprotection of the brain during cardiopulmonary bypass: a randomized trial of remacemide during coronary artery bypass in 171 patients. *Stroke*. 1998;29:2357-2362.
59. Mitchell SJ, Pellet O, Gorman DF, et al. Cerebral protection by lidocaine during cardiac operations. *Ann Thorac Surg*. 1999;67:1117-1124.
60. Diegeler A, Hirsch R, Schneider F, et al. Neuromonitoring and neurocognitive outcome in off-pump versus conventional coronary bypass operation. *Ann Thorac Surg*. 2000;69:1162-1166.
61. Puskas J, Cheng D, Knight J, et al. Off-pump versus conventional coronary artery bypass grafting: a meta-analysis and consensus statement from the 2004 ISMICS consensus conference. *Innovations Cardiothorac Surg*. 2005;1:3-27.
62. Newman MF, Kirchner JL, Phillips-Bute B, et al. Longitudinal assessment of neurocognitive function after coronary artery bypass grafting. *N Engl J Med*. 2001;344:395-402.
63. Sotaniemi KA. Cerebral outcome after extracorporeal circulation: comparison between prospective and retrospective evaluations. *Arch Neurol*. 1983;40:75-77.
64. Hammon JW, Stump DA, Butterworth JE, et al. CABG with single cross clamp results in fewer persistent neuropsychological deficits than multiple clamp or OPCAB. *Ann Thorac Surg*. 2007;84:1174-1179.
65. Selnes OA, Grega MA, Bailey MM, et al. Do management strategies for coronary artery disease influence 6-year cognitive outcomes? *Ann Thorac Surg*. 2009;88:445-454.
66. Mullges W, Babin-Ebell J, Reents W, Toyka KV. Cognitive performance after coronary bypass grafting: a follow-up study. *Neurology*. 2002;59:741-743.

Neuropathology of Brain Injury in Cardiac Surgery

5

Colin Smith

5.1 Introduction

Of all the organs of the body, the brain is the most sensitive to perturbations in blood flow; cessation of, or reduction in, cerebral blood flow will, through the accumulation of neurotoxic metabolites, result in potentially irreversible brain injury. The principal mechanisms that underlie these changes to cerebral blood flow related to cardiac surgery are blockage of a vessel through embolic disease, hypotensive brain injury, or brain injury associated with the complete cessation of blood flow, usually as a result of cardiac arrest.

As the techniques of cardiac surgery and intraoperative management and monitoring have improved, fatal outcomes have become less common. Despite the value of autopsy studies in providing additional data in cardiac surgery related deaths,[1] the number of autopsy series addressing the pathology associated with cardiac surgery is limited.[1–9] However, many of the improvements in management reflect the greater understanding of brain injury related to cardiac surgery brought to us by autopsy studies from the previous decades.

This chapter will provide a general introduction to the pathological features associated with occlusion of a vessel through thrombo-embolic disease, brain injury secondary to hypotension, and global ischemic injury after cardiorespiratory arrest; differences between the infant and the adult brain in their responses to perturbations of blood flow; and a review of the literature describing the pathological features associated with cardiac surgery.

C. Smith
Department of Pathology, University of Edinburgh, Edinburgh, Scotland, UK
e-mail: col.smith@ed.ac.uk

5.2 Basic Principles

The underlying problem in brain injury related to cardiac surgery is ischemia; that is reduced cerebral blood flow below a rate at which the metabolic needs of the neuron cannot be sustained. From a purely physiological basis, ischemia needs to be separated from hypoxia, which describes reduced oxygen delivery. While the realities of human disease makes such a distinction mostly irrelevant, with ischemia and hypoxia going hand in hand in many conditions, animal models have shown that hypoxia in the absence of ischemia is insufficient to produce morphological brain injury[10]; however, hypoxia will exacerbate ischemic brain injury.

The neuropathological hallmark of ischemic brain injury is neuronal ischemic cell change, also called "red cell" change (Fig. 5.1). Affected pyramidal neurons lose their normal nuclear structure of an open

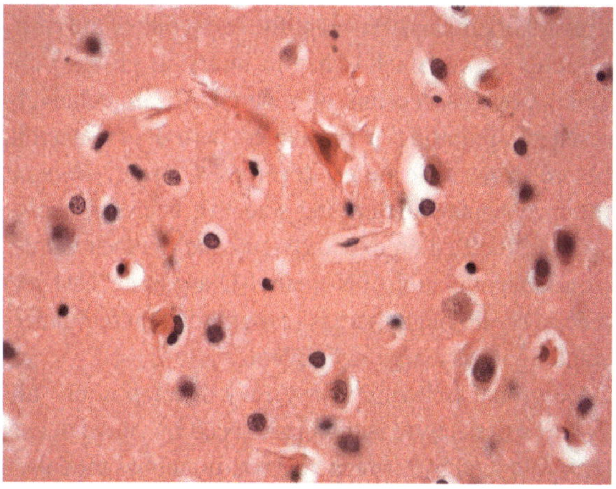

Fig. 5.1 An ischemic neuron showing the typical red cell change, from an area of focal infarction. The neuron has a shrunken nucleus and cytoplasmic eosinophilia (H&E x40)

R.S. Bonser et al. (eds.), *Brain Protection in Cardiac Surgery*,
DOI: 10.1007/978-1-84996-293-3_5,

nucleus with a prominent nucleolus, this being replaced with a shrunken nucleus with little discernable internal structure on light microscopy. Using routine hematoxylin and eosin (H&E) staining of tissue sections, the damaged neurons develop intense eosinophilia of their cytoplasm, resulting in red staining (so-called "red neuron"). It should be noted that the red cell change is not pathognomic of ischemic injury, as other cellular insults, such as hypoglycemia or viral loading of a neuron, may produce a similar appearance.[11] Other stains will also stain the cytoplasm, a common stain being Luxol fast blue (LFB), which results in blue staining of the cytoplasm (luxophilia). Using high-power lenses, incrustations of the ischemic neuronal cytoplasm may be seen, especially using the LFB stain, and this represents irreversible injury to the neuron.

On H&E staining, the ischemic injury is obvious and any experienced neuropathologist will have little difficulty in accurately identifying the process. However, other cellular changes, and in particular dark cell change, catch out the unwary or inexperienced. Dark cell change is a nonspecific microscopic change that may be seen in neurons where ischemia has not been a clinical issue and where the tissue appears otherwise normal. Dark cell change appears to be related to delayed fixation of tissue or excessive handling prior to fixation.[12]

It has been known for many years that all neuronal populations do not respond to a given ischemic insult the same way; selective neuronal necrosis is the term given to this process. For example, two adjacent neuronal populations within the hippocampus, sectors CA1 and CA2, show very differing responses to a given ischemic insult. Neurons within sector CA1 are irreversibly injured very rapidly, being one of the earliest sites of neuronal ischemic injury in global ischemia, whereas neurons of sector CA2 are relatively resistant, requiring a prolonged period of ischemia before irreversible injury develops. Current views on the mechanisms underlying selective neuronal necrosis have focused on excitotoxicity and the overexpression and modulation of N-methyl-D-aspartate (NMDA) receptors, although there is recognition that our understanding is currently incomplete.[13]

Neuronal ischemic injury may develop after only 2–4 min of cerebral ischemia induced by vessel occlusion followed by 1-week survival in animal models.[14] For obvious reasons, the precise timing of neuronal injury in humans has not been studied, but the rodent model gives us some indication of rough timescales involved. The timescale of neuronal ischemic cell change is variable. Prolonged ischemia will produce injury within areas of selective vulnerability rapidly; however, brief periods of ischemia, such as may be seen in cardiac arrest, may result in protracted neuronal ischemic injury, the process developing over several days; this process has been termed delayed neuronal death. There are descriptions of delayed neuronal death in humans.[15,16]

5.3 Focal Ischemic Injury

Neurons are the most vulnerable cell type in the brain and the first cell type to be damaged in ischemia. However, if the ischemic injury is prolonged and significant tissue acidosis develops, the other cell types (astrocytes, oligodendrocytes, vascular smooth muscle cells, endothelial cells) will also be injured and infarction will develop (pan-tissue necrosis). As infarction develops, there is a loss of normal cellular structure with some nuclei undergoing apoptosis. Blood vessels and cell bodies may remain initially as "ghost" outlines, but these structures are removed by infiltrating macrophages, a process known as liquefactive necrosis. The infarcted tissue is removed and in time a gliotic scar develops; this process may take weeks to months to complete.

Focal brain injury is seen after cardiac surgery secondary to emboli, and clinically presents as stroke. Perioperative strokes seen after cardiac surgery have been found to involve the posterior part of the brain and often the posterior circulation more frequently, with cerebellar and posterior cerebral artery territory infarcts being seen.[17] Many sources of emboli have been suggested including cardiac thrombus, atheromatous debris from the aorta, and air emboli.[18,19] Where cardiopulmonary bypass is used, small capillary and arteriolar dilatations (SCADs) have been described.[6] These dilatations were found by examination of thick sections of autopsy human brain tissue from individuals who underwent cardiopulmonary bypass, and from dogs that had experimental cardiopulmonary bypass procedures; they were not seen in humans or dogs that did not undergo cardiopulmonary bypass. The SCADs were described in cortical and deep gray matter, and were postulated as being caused by air or fat microemboli associated with the bypass procedure. They have not been described in cardiac surgery in the absence of bypass support.

Macroscopically, focal infarcts can be difficult to identify less than 24 h after the infarct. As time progresses, the infarcted tissue is soft to touch and will become discolored, having a dusky appearance. Over several weeks, the process of liquefactive necrosis takes place and there is cystic degeneration of the affected area. There may be brown discoloration of the tissues at the edge of the lesion due to blood products.

Microscopically, there is a phase of neutrophil infiltration, which can usually be detected within 12–16 h, and this is followed by macrophage infiltration (Fig. 5.2). The macrophages absorb the necrotic brain tissue and have a foamy appearance. Gliosis is seen around the edge of the cystic cavity that develops. Occasionally, thrombo-embolic material may be seen in vessels related to the site of the infarct.

5.3.1 Air Emboli

Large air emboli are rare and are typically associated with medical procedures; in relation to cardiac surgery, they are described with bypass procedures and with a number of procedures associated with intensive care management involving the insertion of vascular catheters. Microemboli are much more common and are seen in a high proportion of operations using bypass procedures.[20] It has been suggested that gas microemboli may underlie the cognitive impairment seen in a significant number of patients undergoing cardiac surgery.[21] Air emboli may enter both the arterial and venous systems and cause pathology. The pathological appearances of strokes related to air emboli do not significantly differ from those associated with thrombo-emboli; it may be very difficult to definitively identify air emboli at autopsy and pre-autopsy imaging has been recommended.[22]

5.4 Global Ischemic Injury

Global ischemic injury most commonly develops as a consequence of complete cessation of cerebral blood flow after cardiorespiratory arrest. The pattern of brain injury follows a pattern of selective vulnerability, and the pathological changes are directly related to the period of survival following cessation of blood flow. The histological characteristics of neuronal ischemic cell change are typically considered to require a survival of at least 6–8 h post injury to develop, but they have been reported with a survival of only 1 h after the onset of cardiorespiratory arrest.[15]

The earliest cellular changes in global ischemia are seen in sector CA1 of the hippocampi, Purkinje cells of the cerebellum, the striatum, and thalami.[23,24]

Within the neocortical ribbon, neurons of the deeper layers are damaged; the normal cortex has a six-layered architecture and ischemic damage is most pronounced in layers 3, 5, and 6. The injury is also most pronounced within the depths of sulci (Fig. 5.3).

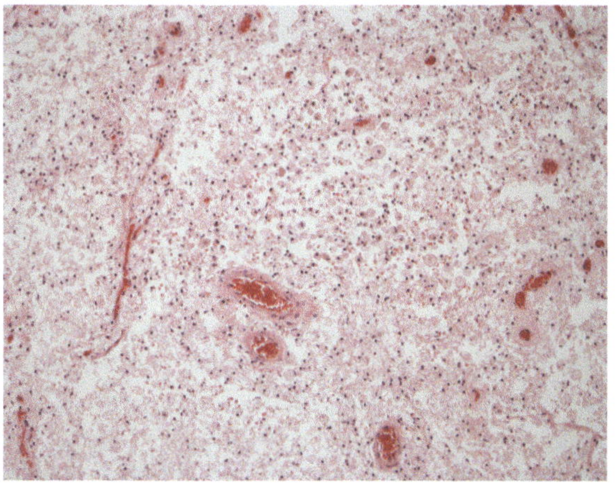

Fig. 5.2 Macrophage infiltration in an established infarct. The macrophages are actively phagocytosing the infracted tissue, the process being termed liquefactive necrosis (H&E x20)

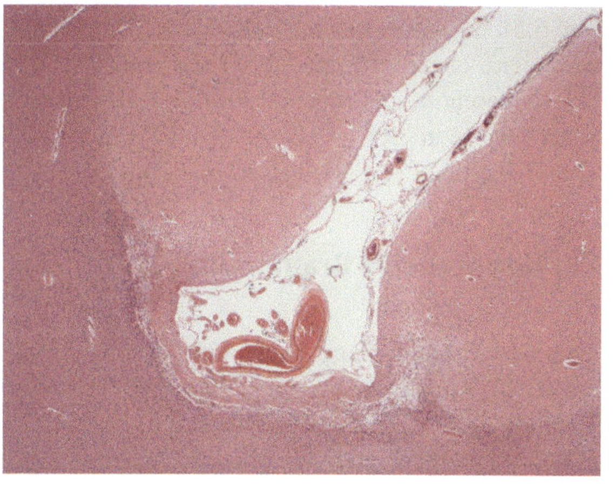

Fig. 5.3 Ischemic damage accentuated at the depths of the sulcus. The adjacent cortex is relatively well preserved, but the tissue at the depths of the sulcus shows established infarction with cystic degeneration (H&E x2)

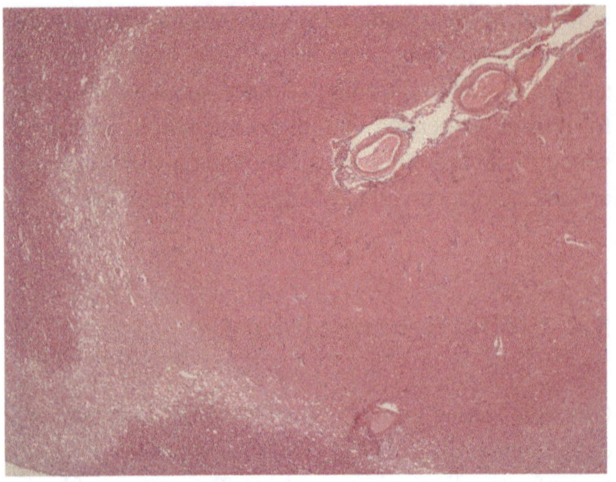

Fig. 5.4 Laminar necrosis. The neurons in the deeper layers of the cortex have undergone ischemic damage and there is a change in the staining intensity within this region when compared to undamaged cortex. The pial surface can be seen towards the top right of the image (H&E x2)

The brainstem is relatively resistant in adults, although when prolonged ischemic injury of the brainstem may be seen.[25]

A survival of at least several days is required before macroscopic changes can be seen. The most consistent macroscopic pathology seen in global ischemia is laminar necrosis of the neocortex (Fig. 5.4). Initially, this is identified as a vague granularity and dusky discoloration of the deeper cortex (in keeping with the microscopic pattern of injury) and by 7–10 days there is obvious linear damage to the neocortex. In prolonged survival (weeks to months) hippocampal sclerosis (Fig. 5.5), neocortical laminar necrosis and cerebellar atrophy are obvious. Secondary to neocortical injury, there is cerebral white matter atrophy with enlargement of the ventricles.

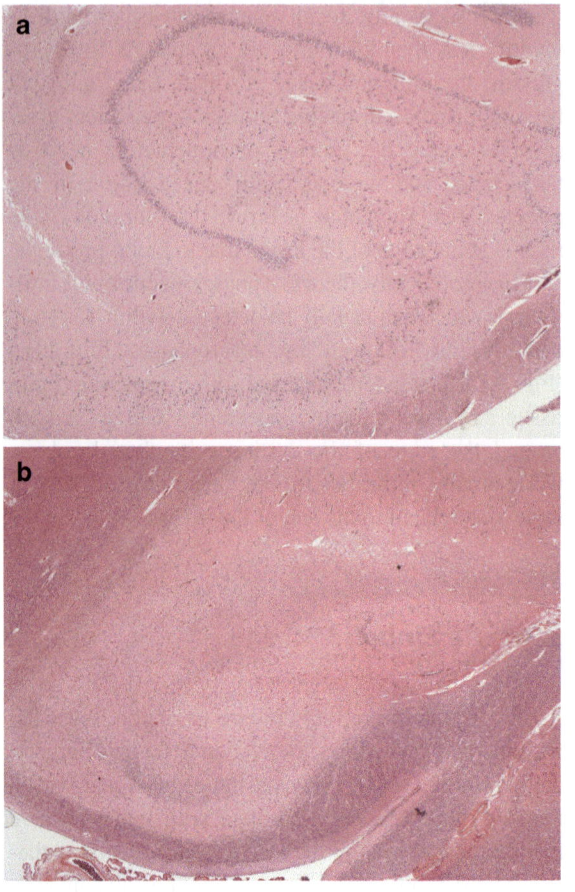

Fig. 5.5 (**a**) A normal section of hippocampus showing the dentate gyrus and sectors CA4, CA3, CA2 and part of CA1 (H&E x2). (**b**) Hippocampal sclerosis. There is extensive neuronal loss throughout the hippocampus, with widespread reactive gliosis (H&E x2)

5.5 Hypotensive Brain Injury

Hypotensive brain injury can follow a similar pattern as global ischemic injury, although the initial brain injury is exacerbated at watershed regions in both the cerebrum and cerebellum. The watershed regions represent the most distal regions supplied by the cerebral end arteries. The most consistent watershed injuries are seen at the parieto-occipital convexity (triple watershed region) and at the dorsal angle of the cerebellum. Microscopically, watershed lesions show a pattern of injury similar to infarction at other sites in the brain.

5.6 Pediatric Brain Injury

While the same general principles apply in pediatric ischemic brain injury (focal lesions, global lesions, hypotensive injury), the pattern of injury may be different. White matter injury is more common in infants, and the pattern of gray matter injury differs from that seen in adults. In the hippocampus, a microglial (rod cell) reaction is seen in relation to the dentate gyrus (Fig. 5.6); damage to sector CA1 is difficult to

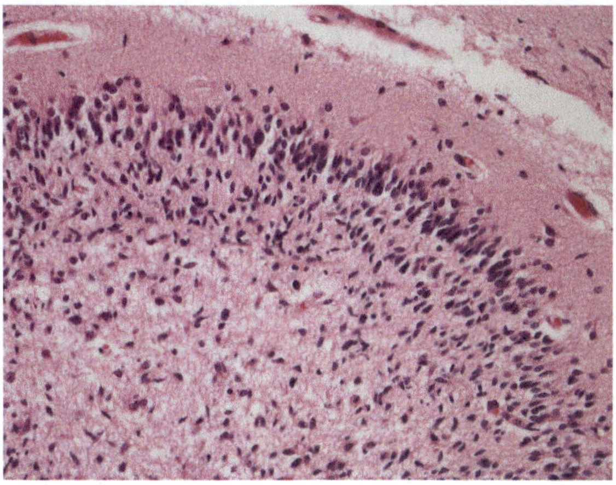

Fig. 5.6 Microglial rod cell reaction seen in relation to the dentate nucleus in a neonate after global ischemic injury (H&E x40)

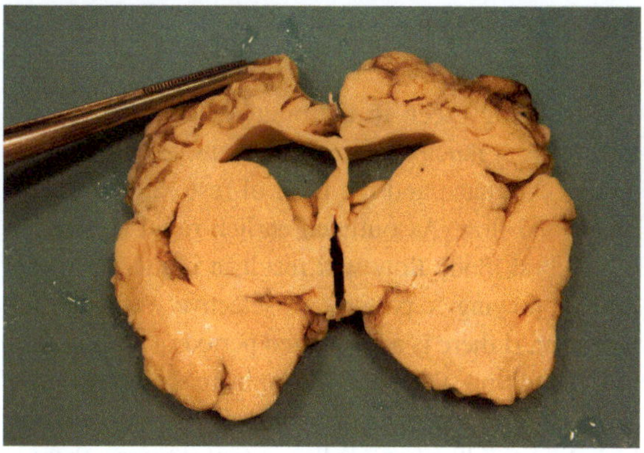

Fig. 5.7 Cystic degeneration of the cerebral cortex in an infant with a survival of several months after global ischemic injury. There is cystic degeneration of the deeper cortex and subcortical tissues, resulting in a mushroom-like appearance of the cortex (ulegyria)

interpret due to the immaturity of these neurons in infants.[26] Basal ganglia damage is common; in some cases, status marmoratus may develop following florid gliosis and mineralization of neurons. The brainstem shows a pattern of injury different from that seen in adults. Nuclei commonly affected include the inferior colliculus and nuclei throughout the basis pontis. The cerebral cortex may also be damaged, showing focal lesions in cases of hypotension, or showing a more diffuse pattern of injury in global ischemia. Damaged neurons have a different appearance determined by the age of the infant; in neonates, much of the loss is by apoptosis, while the typical neuronal ischemic cell change is seen in older infants. Mineralization of neurons and blood vessels may be seen at the edge of infarcts. The damage in the cortex is most pronounced in the deeper layers of cortex and with long-term survival, cystic degeneration of deeper cortex and subcortical white matter results in a mushroom-like appearance termed ulegyria (Fig. 5.7).

White matter injury is seen in the form of focal white matter infarcts, and these are most obvious in the periventricular location, resulting in periventricular leukomalacia (PVL). PVL is an area of white matter necrosis adjacent to the lateral ventricles, with surrounding gliosis, axonal damage, and microglial activation (Fig. 5.8). The anatomical reasons for this typical pattern of white matter injury are not well defined, but many believe that this white matter region represents a border/watershed region in the perinatal period.[27]

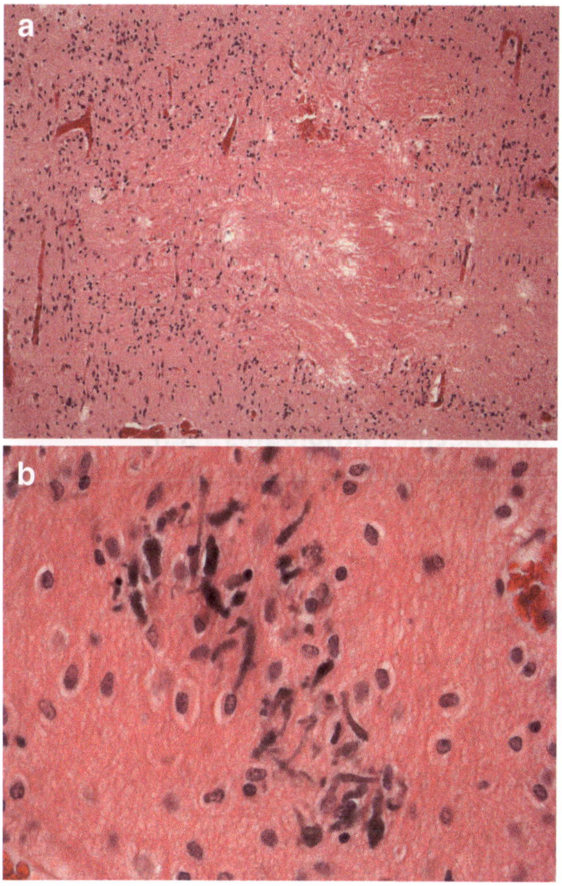

Fig. 5.8 (**a**) An area of white matter injury in a periventricular distribution (periventricular leukomalacia [PVL]) (H&E x20) (**b**) Mineralization of axonal profiles around an area of white matter injury (H&E x40)

5.7 The Respirator Brain

The pathology seen in the brain following a cardiac arrest is very much determined by how rapidly resuscitation is initiated and the level of restoration of cerebral blood flow. As outlined earlier, rapid restoration of cerebral blood flow will result in limited neuronal injury showing a pattern of selective vulnerability. However, if there is a prolonged period of absent cerebral blood flow, there may be an increase in the intrinsic resistance of vessels within the cerebrovascular bed. As a result, when cardiac output resumes, there is no meaningful cerebral blood flow. This will result in a respirator (or nonperfused) brain. The pathology of the respirator brain was first described in detail by Lindenberg[28] and has since been added to over the years. The pathological features are well described by Moseley et al.[29] In summary, the respirator brain undergoes a process of autolysis rather than infarction. Inflammatory cells do not enter the cerebral microenvironment as there is no cerebral blood flow to allow these cells to gain access. At autopsy, the brain is very soft, the degree of decomposition being related to the length of survival post injury.

A recent neuropathological review of brain death confirmed the finding that the respirator brain change was not seen when patients have a relative short period of nonperfusion.[30]

5.8 Specific Pathologies Seen After Cardiac Surgery

Autopsy-based observations have been made in relation to cardiac surgery in both the infants and child population with congenital heart disease,[5,9] and the adult population.[1–4,6–8]

5.8.1 *Surgery for Congenital Heart Disease*

The 1984 study by Bozoky et al.[5] studied 45 cases with congenital heart disease ranging in age from 1 day to 4 years, of which 29 had some form of cardiac intervention. They identified white matter damage particularly in children less than 3 months of age, with gray matter injury being more prevalent in the older age group. The white matter pathology was ischemic and, in approximately 62% of the cases aged less than 3 months with white matter pathology, was in a PVL. Other cases showed gliosis, sometimes associated with macrophage activation. These observations were confirmed by Kinney et al.[9]; their study looked at the brains of 38 infants who died after cardiac surgery and found white matter injury, in the form of PVL and diffuse gliosis, to be a common finding. While the numbers on which to base definitive statements were small, this study concluded that neonates (less than 30 days of age) were at risk for white matter injury, and PVL in particular. They also concluded that the ischemic injury was not directly related to either cardiopulmonary bypass or deep hypothermic circulatory arrest.

5.8.2 *Adult Cardiac Surgery*

Saimanen et al.[8] reviewed 144 cases of adult cardiac surgery with a fatal outcome. These cases had autopsy data and cerebral cast angiography to determine cerebral lesions. 83% of cases died from cardiac causes and 14% from cerebral causes, a higher number of cardiac deaths than reported in other series.[1] Twenty-two cases had recent infarcts, with 12 of these infarcts being thrombo-embolic in nature. The study by Malone et al.[3] which reported 20 cases, found no thrombo-embolic infarcts; the infarcts from this study were all watersheds in nature and associated with reduced cerebral perfusion.

In the study by Orenstein et al.[4] 17 patients who died after cardiopulmonary bypass surgery had refractile particle in capillaries of many organs, including the brain. In some of these cases, there was a survival of up to 8 months after surgery. The microemboli were considered to be from either the polyvinyl chloride tubing used during cardiopulmonary bypass, or from an antifoam agent.

Moody et al.[6] as described earlier, documented SCADs secondary to cardiopulmonary bypass. They studied the cerebral microvasculature using an alkaline phosphatase method; this revealed many thousands of dilatations of the microcirculation, presumed to be microemboli. The lipid within microemboli has been postulated to combine with aluminum or silicon within the oxygenator, forming a complex embolus.[31] The microemboli are cleared with time, with most having disappeared within 1 week after surgery.[32] The secondary pathology related to SCADs is often subtle, although perivascular neutrophil vacuolation has been described.[32]

Clinically significant subdural hemorrhages have been described as a consequence of cardiac surgery.[33–35] Nakajima et al.[33] and later Oka et al.[34] described acute subdural hemorrhage in association with cardiopulmonary bypass. Oka et al.[34] suggested that rapid changes in cerebral blood volume associated with cardiopulmonary bypass procedures may result in tearing of bridging veins. Aoyagi et al.[35] described 4 cases in which subdural hemorrhage complicated valve replacement surgery with associated anticoagulation.

5.9 Summary

Autopsy-based studies have increased our knowledge of the mechanisms underlying acute neurological complications associated with cardiac surgery. Morbidity and mortality have reduced considerably with refinements in cardiac surgery, but longer-term survival may bring new complications, such as long-term cognitive problems. Autopsy studies from long-term survivors may add to our understanding of some of these developing problems in the future.

References

1. Zehr KJ, Liddicoat JR, Salazar JD, et al. The autopsy: still important in cardiac surgery. *Ann Thorac Surg*. 1997;64:380-383.
2. Hill JD, Aguilar MJ, Baranco A, et al. Neuropathological manifestations of cardiac surgery. *Ann Thorac Surg*. 1969;7:409-419.
3. Malone M, Prior P, Scholtz CL. Brain damage after cardiopulmonary by-pass: correlations between neurophysiological and neuropathological findings. *J Neurol Neurosurg Psychiatry*. 1981;44:924-931.
4. Orenstein JM, Sato N, Aaron B, et al. Microemboli observed in deaths following cardiopulmonary bypass surgery. *Hum Pathol*. 1982;13:1082.
5. Bozoky B, Bara D, Kertesz E. Autopsy study of cerebral complications of congenital heart disease and cardiac surgery. *J Neurol*. 1984;231:153-161.
6. Moody DM, Bell MA, Challa VR, et al. Brain microemboli during cardiac surgery or aortography. *Ann Neurol*. 1990;28:477-486.
7. Blauth CI, Cosgrove DM, Webb BW, et al. Atheroembolism from the ascending aorta. An emerging problem in cardiac surgery. *J Thorac Cardiovasc Surg*. 1992;103:1104-1111.
8. Saimanen E, Jarvinen A, Penttila A. Cerebral cast angiography as an aid to medicolegal autopsies in cases of death after adult cardiac surgery. *Int J Legal Med*. 2001;114:163-168.
9. Kinney HC, Panigrahy A, Newburger JW, et al. Hypoxic-ischemic brain injury in infants with congenital heart disease dying after cardiac surgery. *Acta Neuropathol*. 2005;110:563-578.
10. Miyamoto O, Auer RN. Hypoxia, hyperoxia, ischemia, and brain necrosis. *Neurology*. 2000;54:362-371.
11. Auer RN, Dunn JF, Sutherland GR. Hypoxia and related conditions. In: Love S, Louis DN, Ellison DW, eds. *Greenfield's Neuropathology*. 8th ed. London: Hodder Arnold; 2008:63-119.
12. Garman RH. Artifacts in routinely immersion fixed nervous tissue. *Toxicol Pathol*. 1990;18:149-153.
13. Benquet P, Gee CE, Gerber U. Transient brain ischemia: NMDA receptor modulation and delayed neuronal death. *Med Sci (Paris)*. 2008;24:185-190.
14. Smith ML, Auer RN, Siesjö BK. The density and distribution of ischemic brain injury in the rat following 2–10 min of forebrain ischemia. *Acta Neuropathol*. 1984;64:319-332.
15. Petito CK, Feldmann E, Pulsinelli WA, et al. Delayed hippocampal damage in humans following cardiorespiratory arrest. *Neurology*. 1987;37:1281-1286.
16. Horn M, Schlote W. Delayed neuronal death and delayed neuronal recovery in the human brain following global ischemia. *Acta Neuropathol*. 1992;85:79-87.
17. Barbut D, Grassineau D, Lis E, et al. Posterior distribution of infarcts in strokes related to cardiac operations. *Ann Thorac Surg*. 1998;65:1656-1659.
18. Gilman S. Cerebral disorders after open-heart operations. *N Engl J Med*. 1965;272:489-498.
19. Shaw PJ, Bates D, Cartlidge NE, et al. Early neurological complications of coronary artery bypass surgery. *Br Med J*. 1985;291:1384-1387.
20. Padayachee TS, Parsons S, Theobold R, et al. The detection of microemboli in the middle cerebral artery during cardiopulmonary bypass: a transcranial Doppler ultrasound investigation using membrane and bubble oxygenators. *Ann Thorac Surg*. 1987;44:298-302.
21. Borger MA, Feindel CM. Cerebral emboli during cardiopulmonary bypass: effect of perfusionist interventions and aortic cannulas. *J Extra Corpor Technol*. 2002;34:29-33.
22. Plattner T, Thali MJ, Yen K, et al. Virtopsy-postmortem multislice computed tomography (MSCT) and magnetic resonance imaging (MRI) in a fatal scuba diving incident. *J Forensic Sci*. 2003;48:1347-1355.
23. Ng T, Graham DI, Adams JH, et al. Changes in the hippocampus and the cerebellum resulting from hypoxic insults: frequency and distribution. *Acta Neuropathol*. 1989;78:438-443.
24. Cole G, Cowie VA. Long survival after cardiac arrest: case report and neuropathological findings. *Clin Neuropathol*. 1987;6:104-109.
25. Révész T, Geddes JF. Symmetrical columnar necrosis of the basal ganglia and brain stem in an adult following cardiac arrest. *Clin Neuropathol*. 1988;7:294-298.

26. Freide RL. Hemorrhages in asphyxiated premature infants. In: Freide RL, ed. *Developmental Neuropathology*. 2nd ed. Berlin: Springer; 1989:44-58.
27. Rorke LB. Anatomical features of the developing brain implicated in pathogenesis of hypoxic-ischemic injury. *Brain Pathol*. 1992;2:211-221.
28. Lindenberg R. Systemic oxygen deficiencies. In: Minckler J, ed. *Pathology of the Nervous System*, vol. 2. New York: McGraw-Hill; 1971:1583-1617.
29. Moseley JI, Molinari GF, Walker AE. Respirator brain. Report of a survey and review of current concepts. *Arch Pathol Lab Med*. 1976;100:61-64.
30. Wijdicks EF, Pfeifer EA. Neuropathology of brain death in the modern transplant era. *Neurology*. 2008;70:1234-1237.
31. Challa VR, Lovell MA, Moody DM, et al. Laser microprobe mass spectrometric study of aluminum and silicon in brain emboli related to cardiac surgery. *J Neuropathol Exp Neurol*. 1998;57:140-147.
32. Brown WR, Moody DM, Challa VR. Cerebral fat embolism from cardiopulmonary bypass. *J Neuropathol Exp Neurol*. 1999;58:109-119.
33. Nakajima M, Tsuchiya K, Kanemaru K, et al. Subdural haemorrhagic injury after open heart surgery. *Ann Thorac Surg*. 2003;76:614-615.
34. Oka K, Kamota T, Satou M, et al. Subdural hematoma following cardiac surgery. *Kyobu Geka*. 2008;61:868-872.
35. Aoyagi S, Kosuga T, Fukunaga S, et al. Subdural haematoma after open heart surgery. *J Heart Valve Dis*. 2007;16:450-453.

Biochemical Markers of Brain Injury

6

Basel Ramlawi and Frank W. Sellke

6.1 Introduction

Detection of brain injury perioperatively can be a difficult task as it ranges from the very subtle to grossly apparent. Brain injury following cardiopulmonary bypass (CBP) remains a common and serious complication that is often misdiagnosed.[1,2] The American College of Cardiology/American Heart Association guidelines for coronary artery bypass graft (CABG) surgery divide postoperative neurologic deficits into two categories.[3] Type 1 deficits include major focal neurologic events, stupor and coma. Type 2 deficits describe more global cognitive deficits such as deterioration in intellectual function, memory, and confusion without evidence of focal injury. Type 1 deficits are usually caused by identifiable sources of cerebral hypoxia due to intraoperative hypoperfusion or embolic phenomena. In contrast, the etiology of type 2 deficits is unclear and likely multifactorial; where factors such as hypoxia, time on CPB, age, type of procedure, preoperative creatinine levels, and perioperative inflammatory response have been implicated in its pathophysiology.[4] While physical examination and neuroimaging modalities have proven valuable for the detection and treatment of acute focal brain damage postoperatively, mild and diffuse injuries such as neurocognitive decline (NCD) seen in type 2 deficits would benefit from improvements in the early diagnosis and identification of these patients. Neuropsychological tests, the current gold standard for detecting NCD, are complex and difficult to use routinely in the postoperative setting. Identifying biochemical surrogate markers for brain dysfunction would greatly assist in the diagnosis and timely treatments of patients with this complication.

While physical examination and neuroimaging modalities have proven valuable for the detection and treatment of acute focal brain damage postoperatively, mild and diffuse injuries such as neurocognitive decline (NCD) seen in type 2 deficits would benefit from improvements in the early diagnosis and identification of these patients. Neuropsychological tests, the current gold standard for detecting NCD, are complex and difficult to use routinely in the postoperative setting. Identifying biochemical surrogate markers for brain dysfunction would greatly assist in the diagnosis and timely treatments of patients with this complication. Recent studies have focused on proteins that are expressed predominantly in cerebral cells and released into the cerebrospinal fluid and blood following an acute insult to the brain such as CPB.[5–12]

Unlike other areas of medicine where serum markers of end-organ injury is more established in clinical practice (Table 6.1), biochemical markers of brain injury (MBI) have been subject to extensive research with no conclusive marker identified. Unclear pathophysiology of neuronal injury, limited understanding of protein interactions, effect of the blood–brain barrier, heterogeneity of clinical studies, and lack of reliable laboratory assays all contribute to the difficulty in identifying a molecule that would justify widespread clinical applicability. Three patterns of biomarkers emerge in relation to various disease states.[13] First, a biomarker may serve as a risk marker for disease that is present before disease onset and identifies individuals at risk for disease. Second, a biomarker may be a disease marker; that is, it rises with disease onset, and falls with

B. Ramlawi (✉)
Department of Cardiovascular Surgery,
The Methodist DeBakey Heart & vascular Center,
The Methodist Hospital, Houston, TX

R.S. Bonser et al. (eds.), *Brain Protection in Cardiac Surgery*,
DOI: 10.1007/978-1-84996-293-3_6, © Springer-Verlag London Limited 2011

recovery. These may also provide clues about the underlying pathophysiology of disease. Third, a biomarker may be an end product of disease. Such a biomarker rises after onset of disease in proportion to the severity or consequences of disease indicating injury caused by the disease. A list of potential molecules that have been studied is outlined in Table 6.2.

Identifying accurate biomarkers for brain injury following cardiac surgery may shed light on its pathophysiology. Biomarkers may also be helpful in diagnosis, following its time course and severity, and determining potential long-term sequelae. Finally, reliable MBIs may allow for more reliable and consistent research study design of novel perioperative interventions that may improve neurologic outcomes following cardiac surgery.

This Chapter presents an overview of recent findings using commonly investigated MBIs (s100b and neuron-specific enolase [NSE]), the role of inflammation in brain injury following cardiac surgery, novel candidate MBIs as well as the potential for genetic markers of brain injury following cardiac surgery.

Table 6.1 Common clinical organ injury serum markers

End-organ	Serum marker
Kidney	Creatinine, blood urea nitrogen
Heart	Troponin, creatine phosphokinase (CPK-MB)
Pancreas	Amylase, lipase
Liver	Aspartate aminotransferase, alanine aminotransferase, Gamma-Glutamyl transpeptidase
Muscle	Myoglobin, CPK-MM

Table 6.2 Potential markers of brain injury (MBI)

Molecule
S100
Neuron-specific enolase
Creatine kinase BB
Glial fibrillary acidic protein
Myelin basic protein
Tau protein (cleaved)
Fatty acid-binding proteins
NMDA receptor antibodies
Nitric oxide products (Nitrate/Nitrite)
Activin A
Parvalbumin
Thrombomodulin

6.2 Established Markers of Brain Injury Following Cardiac Surgery

The majority of studies involving MBIs within cardiac surgery were restricted to the early postoperative period and involved only markers specific to either neuronal (NSE) or glial (s100) brain tissue. s100 protein has been the most studied of the MBIs within cardiac surgery.[14] It is an acidic calcium-binding protein (molecular weight 21 kDa) found in high concentrations in glial and Schwann cells. It exists in various forms depending on alpha or beta unit configuration. The beta subunit is highly brain specific. The beta-beta (S100bb) units are present in glial and Schwann cells, the alpha-beta (S100ab) subunits appear in glial but not in Schwann cells, whereas alpha-alpha (S100aa) subunits are present in striated muscles, heart, and kidney.[15,16] s100 protein is metabolized in the kidney and excreted in urine, and has a biological half-life of approximately 2 h.[17] The exact functions of s100 proteins are not well known. As s100 proteins are mostly present intracellularly, the majority of the molecules will function as intracellular calcium receptor proteins and modulate intracellular processes including intercell communication, cell structure, growth, energy metabolism, contraction, and intracellular signal transduction. s100b protein has also been involved in promoting axonal growth, glial proliferation, neuronal differentiation, and calcium homeostasis.[18–21]

Neuron-specific enolase (NSE) is a large (78 kDa) dimeric cytoplasmic enzyme that acts in the glycolytic pathway of neurons. It is also present in neuroendocrine tissue and certain tumors such as small-cell lung cancer and melanoma.[22]

Earlier studies focusing on s100 included that of Herrmann et al.; who found that postoperative concentrations and kinetics of s100 and NSE had a high predictive value with respect to the early neuropsychiatric outcome and subtle brain injury after cardiac surgery.[23] S100, and to a lesser extent NSE, have been studied in the cardiac surgical setting with inconclusive results.[1,3,7,8,12,24–28]

Following early enthusiasm about the ability of S100 to predict severity of neuronal damage in cardiac surgical patients, it has been recently discredited due to its lack of specificity. In the setting of CPB, high levels of S100 are found in blood drained from the cardiotomy suction due to its presence in mediastinal fat cells. Jonsson et al. found that S100 levels are decreased significantly by replacing cardiotomy suction with Cell Saver.[5] This implies that blood retransfused from the mediastinum artificially increases serum S100 levels early following CPB without true brain injury. Previous studies that allowed for this confounder have yielded conflicting results when correlating S100 levels with NCD.[12,29,30]

In a recent report, we presented a study comparing s100 and NSE with regard to their association to NCD following cardiac surgical procedures.[31] Forty patients undergoing coronary artery bypass grafting (CABG) and/or valve procedures using CPB were administered a validated neurocognitive battery preoperatively (PRE) and postoperatively at day 4(POD4) and 3 months (3 M). S100, NSE, and tau protein were assayed as MBIs preoperatively and postoperatively at 6 h (6H) and day 4 (P4). Impact of cardiotomy suction and antifibrinolytics on markers of brain injury was assessed. The incidence of early NCD was 40% (16 of 40). NSE and tau protein at the 6H time point were both significantly elevated in the presence of NCD (NCD group) compared to those without NCD (NORM group) (8.69 ± 0.82 vs 5.98 ± 0.61; $p = 0.018$ and 68.8% vs 29.2%; $p = 0.015$, respectively). S100 increase was not different between the NCD and NORM groups (Table 6.3). Cardiotomy suction significantly elevated S100 levels while NSE and tau were not significantly influenced (Table 6.4). Antifibrinolytic therapy did not have an effect on NCD or levels of MBIs. It was concluded that NSE and tau are better associated with NCD and less influenced by cardiotomy suction compared to s100. Other studies have also confirmed this finding.[32]

While cross-reactivity was a significant limitation to s100 use within the CPB setting, efforts have been underway to improve the assay and its specificity.[33] Others have been studying protein stability during long-term storage and establishing reference values for new assays in comparison with the popular Liaison Sangtec 100 test.[34] NSE, however, has also been found to be released from hemolysed erythrocytes,[35] which may lead to false-positive results.

When comparing CABG patients to those undergoing valve replacement, Herrmann et al. found that subjects undergoing VR surgery exhibited higher NSE values during the postoperative course.[36] Furthermore, VR patients showed a higher decline in cognitive performance which was also detectable 6 months after surgery. There was a weak association between the degree of individual postoperative decline of cognitive performance and s100 area under curve values. It was concluded that NSE release and neurobehavioral disorders might be caused by a higher amount of intraoperative cerebral embolic events in VR patients. Also, studies found similar protein s100 levels after cold and warm CPB (32 vs 37°C).[37–41]

Interestingly, Grocott et al. have established a link between elevated s100 levels following CPB and the number of middle cerebral artery microemboli detected by transcranial Doppler following arterial cannulation. Despite their limitations, s100 and NSE remain a valuable tool that may provide clues with regard to subclinical injury that may be due to diffuse microemboli and increased permeability of the blood-brain barrier and not necessarily related to irreversible cerebral damage due to neuronal injury.[42]

Despite their limitations as markers of cerebral damage, s100 and NSE are mostly used to differentiate between the benefits of adverse effects of different intraoperative strategies and surgical techniques. These markers are also being used to evaluate the impact of neuroprotective interventions. Significant improvements, however, are required in the specificity and sensitivity of their assays in order to achieve acceptable results that would make their use applicable to daily clinical practice.

6.3 Inflammatory Markers and Brain Injury

Inflammation has been shown to cause breakdown of the blood-brain barrier and decrease cholinergic transmission. Therefore, inflammatory mediators may become important markers for brain injury.[13,43] The blood–brain barrier is based on the endothelial lining of the vasculature and, under normal circumstances, is not permeable to proteins.[14,44] The systemic inflammatory response syndrome and endothelial cell activation and injury are well known to occur after cardiac

Table 6.3 Correlation between various markers of brain injury and neurocognitive decline (NCD)

Marker of brain injury	Time Point	NCD (16/40)	NORM (24/40)	r	*p* Value	*Adjusted *p* Value
S100b (µg/1)	PRE	0.13±0.02	0.16±0.03	–0.114	0.482	0.661
	6H	0.62±0.10	0.65±0.09	–0.042	0.798	0.445
	P4	0.15±0.03	0.13±0.02	0.113	0.486	0.406
NSE (µg/1)	PRE	5.05±0.92	4.59±0.81	0.060	0.711	0.749
	6H	8.69±0.82	5.98±0.61	0.380	0.016	0.018
	P4	4.65±0.53	3.12±0.57	0.289	0.070	0.078
Tau (% patients positive)	PRE	12.5 (2/16)	8.3 (2/24)	0.068	0.669	0.682
	6H	68.8 (11/16)	29.2 (7/24)	0.390	0.013	0.015
	P4	37.5 (6/16)	25.0 (6/24)	0.134	0.411	0.301

NCD neurocognitive decline group, *NORM* no neurocognitive decline group, *NSE* neuron-specific enolase, *PRE* preoperative, *6H* 6 h postoperatively, *P4* Postoperative day 4

*Logistic regression model with NCD primary outcome. Controlling for age, Aprotinin, cardiotomy suction, CPB time, and preoperative creatinine levels

Source: Adapted from Ramlawi et al.[31]

Table 6.4 Impact of cardiotomy suction compared to cell saver on markers of brain injury

Marker of brain injury	Cardiotomy suction 62.5% (25/40)	Cell saver 37.5% (15/40)	*p* Value
S100b (μg/1)	0.76±0.09	0.43±0.07	0.013
NSE (μg/1)	6.92±0.63	7.31±0.98	0.732
Tau (% patients positive)	44.0 (11/25)	46.7 (7/15)	1.0

Source: Adapted from Ramlawi et al.[31]

operations.[45,46] The endothelium–leukocyte interaction with the release of inflammatory mediators leads to damage to endothelial integrity, sticking of leukocytes in the microcapillary bed, and microcirculatory dysfunction.[47]

Increased endothelial permeability of the blood–brain barrier could explain the augmented release of S100 protein in the blood after CPB. Cardiac surgical patients investigated using MRI within 1 h of surgery all showed signs of brain edema.[48,49] None of the patients experienced any major neurological complications after CPB. Such edema may be regarded as indicative of cytotoxic reactions or vasogenic disorders, both of which are known to compromise the blood–brain barrier.

Brain injury has been associated with increased levels of the serum cytokine inflammatory mediators, interleukin 6 and 8 (IL 6 and IL-8). After congenital cardiac surgery, IL-6 increased at the end of CPB and correlated with S100 at 2 h after CPB ($r=0.55$, $P=0.03$). IL-8 correlated with S100 protein at 24 h after CPB ($r=0.77$, $P=0.002$).[50] It was suggested that increased s100 protein levels after cardiac surgery may be cytokine mediated.

While we still believe that the pathophysiology of type II neurologic injury following CPB is multifactorial, our results among others certainly point to the inflammatory response, a pivotal process in the development of NCD.[31,51] Patients with NCD had significantly higher magnitude early increase compared to those without NCD of CRP(38.01±11.4 vs 16.49±3.5 mg/1, $p=0.042$), IL-1b (2.35±0.3 vs 1.20±0.2 pg/mL, $p=0.002$) and IL-10(29.77±4.7 vs 12.94±2.2 pg/mL, $p<0.001$) as shown in Fig. 6.1. Results from this study are further supported by recent reports that found a correlation between complement activation and brain injury

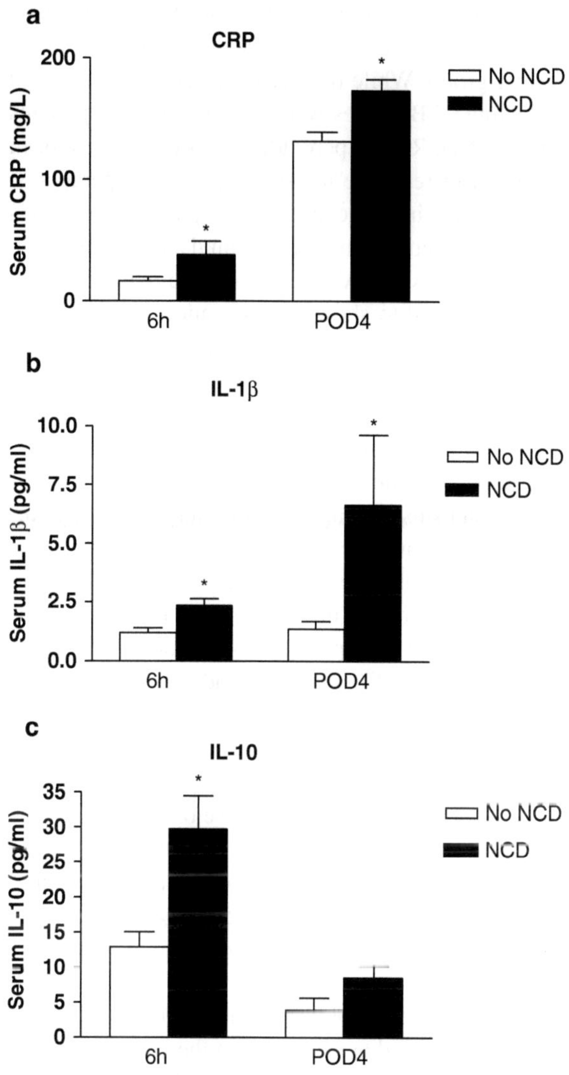

Fig. 6.1 Increased magnitude of the inflammatory response in patients developing NCD post cardiopulmonary bypass as demonstrated by (**a**) CRP, (**b**) IL-1β, and (**c**) IL-10. *Significant (From Ramlawi et al.[51])

as assessed by NCD.[52,53] Moreover, it has also been recently reported that the atheromatous burden from the ascending aorta, an important source of perioperative emboli and possible cause of NCD, was not a primary factor in the pathogenesis of post-CABG cognitive changes.[54]

The association between the acute phase reactant CRP, activated complement mediator C3a, and peroxide levels in relation to early NCD clearly supports the link between inflammation and brain injury.[31] The significant rise in complement activation in patients with

NCD compared to those without NCD certainly points to the increased inflammatory activation present in the former group. While this seems to subside a few days following CPB, values were still higher in the patients with NCD. CRP and peroxide increase may have been triggered in response to brain injury intraoperatively, rather than being the cause of the injury. However, this question cannot be answered from data obtained from that study design. Also, it is unclear why the IL-6 response failed to show an association to early NCD while other mediators were successful. While this study may have been underpowered to detect this difference, this may also be explained by variations of this cytokine within the inflammatory response in relation to blood sampling time.

Mechanisms leading to brain injury following cardiac surgery have been related to humoral and cellular activation of inflammation. First, it is caused by contact activation of the immune system following interaction between the patient's blood and the foreign surfaces of the CPB circuit. Second, ischemia-reperfusion injury of organs such as the heart, lungs, and kidneys after release of the aortic cross-clamp causes immune activation.[24,52,53,55] Attempts to decrease this inflammatory response, via the use of heparin-bonded circuits, corticosteroids, or other pharmacologic agents during CPB, have been shown to decrease brain injury and NCD.[56] With the exception of a few centers, widespread use of such techniques has not yet been established.

Inflammatory cytokines are produced by activated immune cells and are involved in the early amplification of the inflammatory response. Chemokines (such as MIP-1a, MIP-1b, MIG, Eotaxin, RANTES, and CCL2), however, rapidly mediate leukocyte movement to sites of inflammation, including crossing the blood-brain barrier. In a recent study, Rudolph et al. reported that at the 6-h time point, patients who went on to develop delirium had higher increases of chemokines compared to matched controls (class z score 0.3 ± 1.0, $p < .05$).[57] Among five classes of cytokines, there were no other significant differences between patients with or without delirium at either the 6 h or postoperative day 4 assessments. It was concluded that chemokine levels were elevated in patients who developed delirium in the early postoperative period via chemokine-mediated disruption of blood-brain barrier integrity.

In contrast to the above-mentioned inflammatory markers of brain injury, Mielk et al. presented a study that counters the claims that inflammatory cytokines are released by the brain CPB.[58] They measured the plasma concentration of NSE, s100 protein as well as interleukins (IL) IL-6, IL-8, and IL-10 from arterial and cerebral venous blood samples prior to surgery (baseline), during hypothermic CPB at 32 degrees C, after termination of bypass, as well as 2, 4, and 6 h after admission to the intensive care unit. Arterial-cerebral venous concentration gradients of NSE, s100, IL-6, IL-8, and IL-10 were not detectable either during or after CPB. Compared to the baseline period, s100 and NSE significantly increased during hypothermic CPB. After termination of CPB, neuronal-ischemic markers as well as cytokines were increased and remained elevated during the investigated time course without reaching baseline values. They concluded that the increase of investigated parameters associated with the use of CPB are not primarily caused by a cerebral inflammatory response, but rather reflect a release from other sources in the systemic circulation. This, however, does not discount the effect of the systemic inflammatory response on the brain following CPB.

6.4 Investigational Markers of Brain Injury

While our cardiac surgical patients would certainly benefit from a reliable MBI, other branches of medicine have also been investigating potential candidate molecules. Some of the most active groups are researchers in traumatic brain injury, stroke, neurodegenerative diseases, autoimmune deficiency syndrome (AIDS), and oncology. Readily available commercial assays for s100 and NSE have contributed to them being the most investigated MBIs in the literature (Table 6.2). It is likely that as assays for other molecules become more available these will also become equally investigated.

Cleaved tau protein is a microtubule-binding phosphoprotein found in the axons of normal neurons. This molecule, used as a dichotomous variable, was found to be significantly correlated with brain injury as quantified by NCD following cardiac surgery.[51] This molecule was used, with varying results, particularly in the trauma literature.[22,59]

Myelin basic protein (MBP) is an abundant myelin membrane proteolipid produced by oligodendroglia cells and was investigated to assist in the clinical assessment of multiple sclerosis and stroke. Interestingly, higher 24-h peak concentrations of MBP, NSE, and s100 were associated with higher National Institutes of Health Stroke Scale baseline scores ($r=0.186$, $P<0.0001$; $r=0.117$, $P=0.032$; and $r=0.263$, $P<0.0001$, respectively).[60] Higher peak concentrations of MBP and 100 ($r=0.209$, $P<0.0001$; $r=0.239$, $P<0.0001$) were associated with larger computed tomography lesion volumes. Patients with favorable outcomes had smaller changes in MBP and s100 ($P<0.05$) concentrations in the first 24 h. Soluble thrombomodulin (endothelial cell membrane-bound glycoprotein that binds thrombin, potential marker of endothelial injury) was not associated with any severity or outcome measure.

Bokesch et al. studied *N*-methyl-D-aspartate (NMDA) receptor antibodies in the setting of CPB. NMDA receptor peptides and their antibodies have been proposed as MBIs caused by cerebral ischemia and stroke.[61] With neuronal death or ischemia, subunits (NR2) of the NMDA receptor are degraded, and proteolytic fragments appear in the bloodstream. Many subjects generate an antibody response to the NR2A subunit fragments (NR2Ab) that can be assayed in blood samples. Adult patients who experience acute ischemic stroke have elevated blood levels of NR2Ab that correlate with the amount of brain damage on brain scans (MRI) and neurocognitive status. Ninety-six percent (24/25) of patients with NR2Ab concentrations ≥2.0 ng/mL preoperatively had neurological complications within 48 h post-CPB, versus only 5.4% (20/373) of patients with NR2Ab concentrations <2.0 ng/mL, resulting in a 17.9-fold increase (95% CI, 11.6–27.6) in postoperative neurological complications for patients with high levels of NR2A antibodies.

Fatty acid-binding proteins (FABPs) are a family of small cytoplasmic lipid-binding proteins with a molecular weight of 15 kDa.[62] In the brain, H-FABP is predominately found in the neuronal cell body whereas B-FABP is found in glial cells. FABPs are non-enzymatic intracellular proteins involved in the buffering and transport of long chain fatty acids. They modulate fatty acid concentration and thus influence function of enzymes, membranes, ion channels and receptors, gene expression, and cellular growth and differentiation. Brain-type fatty acid-binding protein (BFABP) and heart-type fatty acid-binding protein (HFABP) were found to be elevated in patients with mild traumatic brain injury and after electroconvulsive therapy[63], and increased H-FABP was also found in a small series of patients with ischemic and hemorrhagic stroke.[64] Wunderlich et al. reported that H-FABP and B-FABP concentrations showed peak values already 2–3 h after stroke onset and remained elevated up to last measurements at 120 h.[65] Unlike BFABP, early H-FABP concentrations were significantly associated with the severity of the neurological deficit and the functional outcome. High H-FABP release was associated with large infarction on CT.

Parvalbumin is a neuronal calcium-binding protein (12 kDa) that is found in a subpopulation of gamma aminobutyric acid neurons in most regions of the brain, including the cortex, hippocampus, and cerebellum. Activin A, a glycoprotein produced by the central nervous system, has been implicated in neurologic outcomes. Both were studied as MBIs.[66,67] Harmon et al. also studied the association between nitric oxide products, nitrate and nitrite and brain injury following CABG.[68]

6.5 Genetic Markers of Brain Injury

Despite extensive investigation, the pathophysiology of brain injury following cardiac surgery is not entirely clear. Often, we cannot explain subtle neurologic injury by the usual perioperative risk factors (e.g., embolic phenomena, hypoperfusion, etc.). Age and other associated physiologic factors do not explain the majority of occurrences. Unidentified predisposing factors or events contribute to the development of neurologic dysfunction after cardiac operations. Recently, there has been significant interest in exploring the role of patients' genomic profiles as potential clues.

Apolipoprotein E (ApoE), a serum protein that mediates extracellular cholesterol transport, regulates multiple metabolic pathways and is a major susceptibility gene for Alzheimer's disease.[69] Isoform-specific ApoE effects have been implicated in recovery from several types of brain stress, including head trauma, stroke, and cardiac surgery.[70–72] Among the first to report on ApoE in cardiac surgery, Tardiff et al. studied in a multivariable logistic regression, an analysis including ApoE-e4, preoperative score, age, and years of education. A significant association was found between ApoE-e4 and change in cognitive test score in measures of short-term memory at 6 weeks postoperatively. Patients with lower educational levels were more likely to show a decline in cognitive function associated with the ApoE-e4 allele.[71]. Kofke et al. reported that NSE and s100 levels were significantly higher in patients with the ApoE-e4 allele and concluded that patients with the ApoE-e4 allele may be more susceptible to perioperative neural insults.[73]

Transcriptional profiling using high-density microarrays provides unique data about disease mechanisms, drug responses, regulatory pathways, and gene function by comparing the level of mRNA transcribed in cells in a given pathologic state versus a control. This technology has been used to elucidate complex pathophysiologic mechanisms directly at the gene expression level. Recently, we reported on a significant association between genomic expression pathways and brain injury following CPB. Whole blood messenger RNA (mRNA) was isolated preoperatively and at 6 h following surgery for fold-change calculation. Relative gene expression in patients who develop NCD versus normal patients was assessed by Affymetrix GeneChip U133 Plus 2.0 (Affymetrix Inc, Santa Clara, CA) (>40,000 genes) from mRNA samples collected. NCD patients (17 of 42 patients, 40.5%) were associated with a significantly different gene expression response compared to normal patients (Fig. 6.2). Compared to normal patients, NCD patients had significantly different gene expression pathways involving inflammation (including FAS, IL2RB, CD59), antigen presentation (including HLA-DQ1, TAP1, TAP2), and cellular adhesion (including ICAM2, ICAM3, CAD7) among others (Table 6.5). We concluded that NCD patients have inherently different genetic responses to CPB compared to patients without NCD.[74] Such preliminary studies have laid the ground for more extensive work dealing with gene-based identification of potential mechanisms and markers of brain injury perioperatively.

In conclusion, the ideal biochemical serum marker of brain injury would be highly specific for the brain, highly sensitive for brain injury and be released only after irreversible destruction of brain tissue, and have rapid appearance in serum across the blood-brain barrier[28,75]. Importantly, its levels should not be influenced by the CPB apparatus or commonly used drugs such as heparin, protamine, or propfol. Moreover, unlike markers of other organ dysfunction, a marker of brain injury cannot necessarily be correlated with the magnitude of injury as injury to certain regions of the brain (e.g., motor region) will have greater clinical repercussions compared to other areas (e.g., frontal lobe). All these requirements make identifying a marker more challenging. A major difficulty remains the development of reliable assays that could eventually lead to widespread research and clinical use. Inflammatory markers have shown an association to neurologic injury following CPB; however, the nature of this relationship is not entirely clear. Genetic studies, while still preliminary, should help in elucidating the complex pathophysiology of brain injury following CPB. In the future, such studies may form the basis for a database of genomic markers for the prediction of neurologic injury preoperatively.

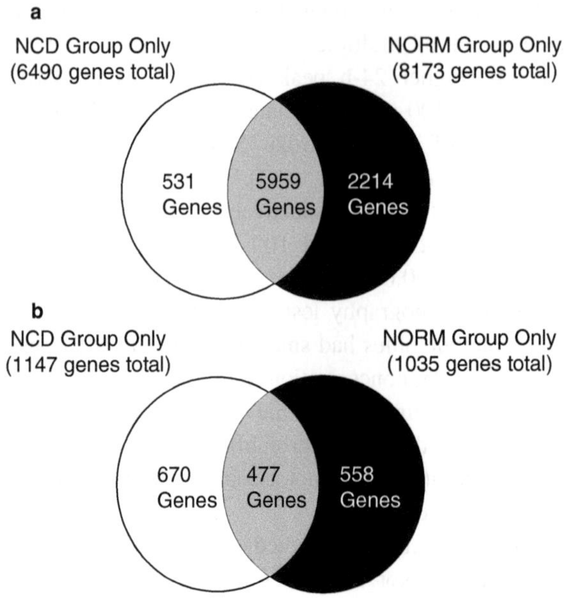

Fig. 6.2 Genes that were differentially expressed after cardiopulmonary bypass (CPB) in patients with (NCD group) and without neurocognitive decline (NORM group). (**a**) Upregulated Genes (6H vs PRE); (**b**) Downregulated Genes (6H vs PRE) (From Ramlawi et al.[74])

Table 6.5 Gene ontology (GO) biologic process (BP) pathways that are differentially expressed at 6 h postoperatively versus preoperatively (PRE) in patients with neurocognitive decline (NCD) compared to patients without NCD

Gene regulation (6H vs PRE)	Patient group	Biologic process #	Gene ontology pathway	Genes observed	p-value
Down	NCD present	6955	Immune response	32	0.000008
		19884	Antigen presentation, exogenous	6	0.000026
		19886	Antigen processing, via MHC II	6	0.00003
		6959	Humoral immune response	5	0.002033
		7166	Cell surface receptor transduction	14	0.003332
		42110	T cell activation	4	0.004954
		16337	Cell-cell adhesion	7	0.006279
	NCD Absent	6952	Defense response	6	0.03404
		7218	Neuropeptide signaling pathway	4	0.046216
Up	NCD Present	7596	Blood coagulation	7	0.001267
		6917	Induction of apoptosis	6	0.048673
	NCD Absent	45454	Cell redox homeostasis	5	0.003162
		6950	Response to stress	19	0.007486
		6916	Antiapoptosis	20	0.010814
		6635	Fatty acid beta-oxidation	4	0.039869

Source: Adapted from Ramlawi et al.[74]

References

1. Ahonen J, Salmenpera M. Brain injury after adult cardiac surgery. *Acta Anaesthesiol Scand*. Jan 2004;48(1):4-19.
2. Arrowsmith JE, Grocott HP, Reves JG, Newman MF. Central nervous system complications of cardiac surgery. *Br J Anaesth*. Mar 2000;84(3):378-393.
3. Eagle KA, Guyton RA, Davidoff R, et al. ACC/AHA guidelines for coronary artery bypass graft surgery: executive summary and recommendations: A report of the American College of Cardiology/American Heart Association Task Force on Practice Guidelines (Committee to revise the 1991 guidelines for coronary artery bypass graft surgery). *Circulation*. Sept 28 1999;100(13):1464-1480.
4. Murkin JM. Etiology and incidence of brain dysfunction after cardiac surgery. *J Cardiothorac Vasc Anesth*. Aug 1999;13(4 Suppl 1):12-17. discussion 36-17.
5. Jonsson H, Johnsson P, Backstrom M, Alling C, Dautovic-Bergh C, Blomquist S. Controversial significance of early S100B levels after cardiac surgery. *BMC Neurol*. Dec 16 2004;4(1):24.
6. Kalman J, Juhasz A, Bogats G, et al. Elevated levels of inflammatory biomarkers in the cerebrospinal fluid after coronary artery bypass surgery are predictors of cognitive decline. *Neurochem Int*. Feb 2006;48(3):177-180.
7. Lloyd CT, Ascione R, Underwood MJ, Gardner F, Black A, Angelini GD. Serum S-100 protein release and neuropsychologic outcome during coronary revascularization on the beating heart: a prospective randomized study. *J Thorac Cardiovasc Surg*. Jan 2000;119(1):148-154.
8. Rasmussen LS, Christiansen M, Hansen PB, Moller JT. Do blood levels of neuron-specific enolase and S-100 protein reflect cognitive dysfunction after coronary artery bypass? *Acta Anaesthesiol Scand*. May 1999;43(5):495-500.
9. Reiber H. Dynamics of brain-derived proteins in cerebrospinal fluid. *Clin Chim Acta*. Aug 20 2001;310(2):173-186.
10. Shaw GJ, Jauch EC, Zemlan FP. Serum cleaved tau protein levels and clinical outcome in adult patients with closed head injury. *Ann Emerg Med*. Mar 2002;39(3):254-257.
11. Vaage J, Anderson R. Biochemical markers of neurologic injury in cardiac surgery: the rise and fall of S100beta. *J Thorac Cardiovasc Surg*. Nov 2001;122(5):853-855.

12. Westaby S, Saatvedt K, White S, et al. Is there a relationship between serum S-100beta protein and neuropsychologic dysfunction after cardiopulmonary bypass? *J Thorac Cardiovasc Surg*. Jan 2000;119(1):132-137.
13. Marcantonio ER, Rudolph JL, Culley D, Crosby G, Alsop D, Inouye SK. Serum biomarkers for delirium. *J Gerontol A Biol Sci Med Sci*. Dec 2006;61(12):1281-1286.
14. Ali MS, Harmer M, Vaughan R. Serum S100 protein as a marker of cerebral damage during cardiac surgery. *Br J Anaesth*. Aug 2000;85(2):287-298.
15. Aurell A, Rosengren LE, Karlsson B, Olsson JE, Zbornikova V, Haglid KG. Determination of S-100 and glial fibrillary acidic protein concentrations in cerebrospinal fluid after brain infarction. *Stroke*. Oct 1991;22(10):1254-1258.
16. Isobe T, Takahashi K, Okuyama T. S100a0 (alpha alpha) protein is present in neurons of the central and peripheral nervous system. *J Neurochem*. Nov 1984;43(5):1494-1496.
17. Usui A, Kato K, Abe T, Murase M, Tanaka M, Takeuchi E. S-100ao protein in blood and urine during open-heart surgery. *Clin Chem*. Sept 1989;35(9):1942-1944.
18. Zimmer DB, Cornwall EH, Landar A, Song W. The S100 protein family: history, function, and expression. *Brain Res Bull*. 1995;37(4):417-429.
19. Fano G, Mariggio MA, Angelella P, et al. The S-100 protein causes an increase of intracellular calcium and death of PC12 cells. *Neuroscience*. Apr 1993;53(4):919-925.
20. Haglid KG, Yang Q, Hamberger A, Bergman S, Widerberg A, Danielsen N. S-100beta stimulates neurite outgrowth in the rat sciatic nerve grafted with acellular muscle transplants. *Brain Res*. Apr 11 1997;753(2):196-201.
21. Selinfreund RH, Barger SW, Pledger WJ, Van Eldik LJ. Neurotrophic protein S100 beta stimulates glial cell proliferation. *Proc Natl Acad Sci USA*. May 1 1991;88(9):3554-3558.
22. Begaz T, Kyriacou DN, Segal J, Bazarian JJ. Serum biochemical markers for post-concussion syndrome in patients with mild traumatic brain injury. *J Neurotrauma*. Aug 2006;23(8):1201-1210.
23. Herrmann M, Ebert AD, Galazky I, Wunderlich MT, Kunz WS, Huth C. Neurobehavioral outcome prediction after cardiac surgery: role of neurobiochemical markers of damage to neuronal and glial brain tissue. *Stroke*. Mar 2000;31(3):645-650.
24. Gao L, Taha R, Gauvin D, Othmen LB, Wang Y, Blaise G. Postoperative cognitive dysfunction after cardiac surgery. *Chest*. Nov 2005;128(5):3664-3670.
25. van Engelen BG, Lamers KJ, Gabreels FJ, Wevers RA, van Geel WJ, Borm GF. Age-related changes of neuron-specific enolase, S-100 protein, and myelin basic protein concentrations in cerebrospinal fluid. *Clin Chem*. June 1992;38(6):813-816.
26. Nygaard O, Langbakk B, Romner B. Neuron-specific enolase concentrations in serum and cerebrospinal fluid in patients with no previous history of neurological disorder. *Scand J Clin Lab Invest*. May 1998;58(3):183-186.
27. Jonsson H, Johnsson P, Alling C, Backstrom M, Bergh C, Blomquist S. S100beta after coronary artery surgery: release pattern, source of contamination, and relation to neuropsychological outcome. *Ann Thorac Surg*. Dec 1999;68(6): 2202-2208.
28. Ingebrigtsen T, Romner B. Serial S-100 protein serum measurements related to early magnetic resonance imaging after minor head injury. Case report. *J Neurosurg*. Nov 1996; 85(5):945-948.
29. Ueno T, Iguro Y, Yamamoto H, Sakata R, Kakihana Y, Nakamura K. Serial measurement of serum S-100B protein as a marker of cerebral damage after cardiac surgery. *Ann Thorac Surg*. June 2003;75(6):1892-1897. discussion 1897-1898.
30. Wang KJ, Wu HH, Fang SY, Yang YR, Tseng AC. Serum S-100 beta protein during coronary artery bypass graft surgery with or without cardiopulmonary bypass. *Ann Thorac Surg*. Oct 2005;80(4):1371-1374.
31. Ramlawi B, Rudolph JL, Mieno S, et al. Serologic markers of brain injury and cognitive function after cardiopulmonary bypass. *Ann Surg*. Oct 2006;244(4):593-601.
32. Rasmussen LS, Christiansen M, Eliasen K, Sander-Jensen K, Moller JT. Biochemical markers for brain damage after cardiac surgery - time profile and correlation with cognitive dysfunction. *Acta Anaesthesiol Scand*. May 2002;46(5): 547-551.
33. Whitaker DC, Green AJ, Stygall J, Harrison MJ, Newman SP. Evaluation of an alternative S100b assay for use in cardiac surgery: relationship with microemboli and neuropsychological outcome. *Perfusion*. July 2007;22(4):267-272.
34. Muller K, Elverland A, Romner B, et al. Analysis of protein S-100B in serum: a methodological study. *Clin Chem Lab Med*. 2006;44(9):1111-1114.
35. Johnsson P, Blomquist S, Luhrs C, et al. Neuron-specific enolase increases in plasma during and immediately after extracorporeal circulation. *Ann Thorac Surg*. Mar 2000;69(3): 750-754.
36. Herrmann M, Ebert AD, Tober D, Hann J, Huth C. A contrastive analysis of release patterns of biochemical markers of brain damage after coronary artery bypass grafting and valve replacement and their association with the neurobehavioral outcome after cardiac surgery. *Eur J Cardiothorac Surg*. Nov 1999;16(5):513-518.
37. Gao F, Harris DN, Sapsed-Byrne S, Sharp S. Neurone-specific enolase and Sangtec 100 assays during cardiac surgery: Part III – dose haemolysis affect their accuracy? *Perfusion*. May 1997;12(3):171-177.
38. Sapsed-Byrne S, Gao F, Harris DN. Neurone-specific enolase and Sangtec 100 assays during cardiac surgery: Part II – must samples be spun within 30 min? *Perfusion*. May 1997;12(3):167-169.
39. Gao F, Harris DN, Sapsed-Byrne S, Sharp S. Neurone-specific enolase and Sangtec 100 assays during cardiac surgery: Part I—The effects of heparin, protamine and propofol. *Perfusion*. May 1997;12(3):163-165.
40. Zeiner A, Holzer M, Sterz F, et al. Mild resuscitative hypothermia to improve neurological outcome after cardiac arrest. A clinical feasibility trial. Hypothermia After Cardiac Arrest (HACA) Study Group. *Stroke*. Jan 2000;31(1):86-94.
41. Shaaban-Ali M, Harmer M, Vaughan RS, et al. Changes in serum S100beta protein and Mini-Mental State Examination after cold (28 degrees C) and warm (34 degrees C) cardiopulmonary bypass using different blood gas strategies (alpha-stat and pH-stat). *Acta Anaesthesiol Scand*. Jan 2002;46(1):10-16.
42. Grocott HP, Croughwell ND, Amory DW, White WD, Kirchner JL, Newman MF. Cerebral emboli and serum S100beta during cardiac operations. *Ann Thorac Surg*. June 1998;65(6):1645-1649. discussion 1649-1650.
43. Jeppsson B, Freund HR, Gimmon Z, James JH, von Meyenfeldt MF, Fischer JE. Blood-brain barrier derangement

in sepsis: cause of septic encephalopathy? *Am J Surg*. Jan 1981;141(1):136-142.
44. Gillinov AM, Davis EA, Curtis WE, et al. Cardiopulmonary bypass and the blood-brain barrier. An experimental study. *J Thorac Cardiovasc Surg*. Oct 1992;104(4):1110-1115.
45. Cremer J, Martin M, Redl H, et al. Systemic inflammatory response syndrome after cardiac operations. *Ann Thorac Surg*. June 1996;61(6):1714-1720.
46. Boyle EM Jr, Pohlman TH, Johnson MC, Verrier ED. Endothelial cell injury in cardiovascular surgery: the systemic inflammatory response. *Ann Thorac Surg*. Jan 1997;63(1):277-284.
47. Lindberg L, Olsson AK, Anderson K, Jogi P. Serum S-100 protein levels after pediatric cardiac operations: a possible new marker for postperfusion cerebral injury. *J Thorac Cardiovasc Surg*. Aug 1998;116(2):281-285.
48. Harris DN, Oatridge A, Dob D, Smith PL, Taylor KM, Bydder GM. Cerebral swelling after normothermic cardiopulmonary bypass. *Anesthesiology*. Feb 1998;88(2):340-345.
49. Harris DN, Bailey SM, Smith PL, Taylor KM, Oatridge A, Bydder GM. Brain swelling in first hour after coronary artery bypass surgery. *Lancet*. Sept 4 1993;342(8871):586-587.
50. Ashraf S, Bhattacharya K, Tian Y, Watterson K. Cytokine and S100B levels in paediatric patients undergoing corrective cardiac surgery with or without total circulatory arrest. *Eur J Cardiothorac Surg*. July 1999;16(1):32-37.
51. Ramlawi B, Rudolph JL, Mieno S, et al. C-Reactive protein and inflammatory response associated to neurocognitive decline following cardiac surgery. *Surgery*. Aug 2006;140(2): 221-226.
52. Bautreton C, Allain P, Chevallier A, et al. Brain injury and neuropsychological outcome after coronary artery surgery are affected by complement activation. *Ann Thorac Surg*. May 2005;79(5):1597-1605.
53. Ben-Abraham R, Weinbroum AA, Dekel B, Paret G. Chemokines and the inflammatory response following cardiopulmonary bypass – a new target for therapeutic intervention? – A review. *Paediatr Anaesth*. Oct 2003;13(8): 655-661.
54. Bar-Yosef S, Anders M, Mackensen GB, et al. Aortic atheroma burden and cognitive dysfunction after coronary artery bypass graft surgery. *Ann Thorac Surg*. Nov 2004;78(5): 1556-1562.
55. Ohata T, Sawa Y, Kadoba K, et al. Normothermia has beneficial effects in cardiopulmonary bypass attenuating inflammatory reactions. *Asaio J*. July–Sept 1995;41(3): M288-291.
56. Aldea GS, Soltow LO, Chandler WL, et al. Limitation of thrombin generation, platelet activation, and inflammation by elimination of cardiotomy suction in patients undergoing coronary artery bypass grafting treated with heparin-bonded circuits. *J Thorac Cardiovasc Surg*. Apr 2002;123(4):742-755.
57. Rudolph JL, Ramlawi B, Kuchel GA, et al. Chemokines are associated with delirium after cardiac surgery. *J Gerontol A Biol Sci Med Sci*. Feb 2008;63(2):184-189.
58. Mielck F, Ziarkowski A, Hanekop G, et al. Cerebral inflammatory response during and after cardiac surgery. *Eur J Anaesthesiol*. May 2005;22(5):347-352.
59. Berger RP. The use of serum biomarkers to predict outcome after traumatic brain injury in adults and children. *J Head Trauma Rehabil*. July-Aug 2006;21(4):315-333.
60. Jauch EC, Lindsell C, Broderick J, Fagan SC, Tilley BC, Levine SR. Association of serial biochemical markers with acute ischemic stroke: the National Institute of Neurological Disorders and Stroke recombinant tissue plasminogen activator Stroke Study. *Stroke*. Oct 2006;37(10):2508-2513.
61. Bokesch PM, Izykenova GA, Justice JB, Easley KA, Dambinova SA. NMDA receptor antibodies predict adverse neurological outcome after cardiac surgery in high-risk patients. *Stroke*. June 2006;37(6):1432-1436.
62. Pelsers MM, Glatz JF. Detection of brain injury by fatty acid-binding proteins. *Clin Chem Lab Med*. 2005;43(8): 802-809.
63. Pelsers MM, Hanhoff T, Van der Voort D, et al. Brain- and heart-type fatty acid-binding proteins in the brain: tissue distribution and clinical utility. *Clin Chem*. Sept 2004;50(9): 1568-1575.
64. Zimmermann-Ivol CG, Burkhard PR, Le Floch-Rohr J, Allard L, Hochstrasser DF, Sanchez JC. Fatty acid binding protein as a serum marker for the early diagnosis of stroke: a pilot study. *Mol Cell Proteomics*. Jan 2004;3(1):66-72.
65. Wunderlich MT, Hanhoff T, Goertler M, et al. Release of brain-type and heart-type fatty acid-binding proteins in serum after acute ischaemic stroke. *J Neurol*. June 2005;252(6):718-724.
66. Florio P, Abella RF, de la Torre T, et al. Perioperative activin A concentrations as a predictive marker of neurologic abnormalities in children after open heart surgery. *Clin Chem*. May 2007;53(5):982-985.
67. Abdul-Khaliq H, Schubert S, Stoltenburg-Didinger G, et al. Release patterns of astrocytic and neuronal biochemical markers in serum during and after experimental settings of cardiac surgery. *Restor Neurol Neurosci*. 2003;21(3-4):141-150.
68. Harmon D, Eustace N, Ghori K, et al. Plasma concentrations of nitric oxide products and cognitive dysfunction following coronary artery bypass surgery. *Eur J Anaesthesiol*. Apr 2005;22(4):269-276.
69. Strittmatter WJ, Bova Hill C. Molecular biology of apolipoprotein E. *Curr Opin Lipidol*. Apr 2002;13(2):119-123.
70. O'Donnell HC, Rosand J, Knudsen KA, et al. Apolipoprotein E genotype and the risk of recurrent lobar intracerebral hemorrhage. *N Engl J Med*. Jan 27 2000;342(4):240-245.
71. Tardiff BE, Newman MF, Saunders AM, et al. Preliminary report of a genetic basis for cognitive decline after cardiac operations. The Neurologic Outcome Research Group of the Duke Heart Center. *Ann Thorac Surg*. Sept 1997;64(3): 715-720.
72. Hsiung GY, Sadovnick AD, Feldman H. Apolipoprotein E epsilon4 genotype as a risk factor for cognitive decline and dementia: data from the Canadian Study of Health and Aging. *Cmaj*. Oct 12 2004;171(8):863-867.
73. Kofke WA, Konitzer P, Meng QC, Guo J, Cheung A. The effect of apolipoprotein E genotype on neuron specific enolase and S-100beta levels after cardiac surgery. *Anesth Analg*. Nov 2004;99(5):1323-1325. table of contents.
74. Ramlawi B, Otu H, Rudolph JL, et al. Genomic expression pathways associated with brain injury after cardiopulmonary bypass. *J Thorac Cardiovasc Surg*. Oct 2007;134(4): 996-1005.
75. Bakay RA, Ward AA Jr. Enzymatic changes in serum and cerebrospinal fluid in neurological injury. *J Neurosurg*. Jan 1983;58(1):27-37.

Pitfalls of Neuropsychometric Assessment and Alternative Investigative Approaches

7

Yasir Abu-Omar and David P. Taggart

7.1 Introduction

Advances in surgical and anesthetic techniques over the last two decades have led to a reduction in the overall mortality following cardiac surgery despite the fact that older patients with more comorbidities constitute an increasing proportion of the surgical population. This reduction in mortality has not been paralleled by a reduction in neurocognitive dysfunction as older patients are potentially more susceptible to all forms of cerebral injury.[1]

Numerous techniques have been used in the investigation of this form of cerebral injury. The most commonly used method of assessment is neuropsychological or neuropsychometric testing. This represents a valuable tool in the assessment of this subtle form of injury and provides a method of systematically and quantitatively studying the behavioral impact of this deficit. However, using neuropsychometric assessment to quantify these perioperative cognitive changes has yielded rates with wide variability, ranging from 14% to 48% at hospital discharge[2] and up to 24% at 6-month follow-up,[3] highlighting the limitations associated with this form of assessment. In this chapter, this technique of assessment is reviewed in detail along with its advantages and limitations. In addition, some of the other more commonly used methods are also outlined.

Y. Abu-Omar (✉)
Department of Cardiothoracic Surgery, Papworth Hospital, Papworth Everard, UK
email: yabuomar@doctors.org.uk

7.2 Assessment of Cerebral Injury

Cerebral injury following cardiac surgery occurs in various forms ranging, with decreasing order of severity and increasing incidence, from stroke to delirium to cognitive dysfunction.[1] Stroke is the most serious and devastating postoperative complication. Its incidence is now reported to be around 1–2% in patients undergoing coronary artery bypass grafting and 2–4% in those undergoing open cardiac and combined procedures.[4,5] Consequently, stroke is no longer a sensitive index of neurological dysfunction following cardiac surgery as it does not measure a significant proportion of surgical patients who suffer some degree of neurological injury manifesting as cognitive impairment. While this may not be life-threatening, it has a significant impact on the patients' quality of life following surgery[6] and has now become the form of injury most frequently targeted for investigative and therapeutic strategies. The increasing interest in neurological sequelae following cardiac surgery witnessed the development and utilization of numerous investigative techniques to define the nature of injury and elicit its etiology (Table 7.1).

7.2.1 Neuropsychometric Assessment

Investigative approaches such as neurological examination and the Mini-Mental State Examination are easy to perform and reproducible. However, their low sensitivity and inability to provide quantitative measures renders them of little use in the assessment of subtle

R.S. Bonser et al. (eds.), *Brain Protection in Cardiac Surgery*,
DOI: 10.1007/978-1-84996-293-3_7,

Table 7.1 Some of the investigative techniques used in the assessment of postoperative neurological outcome

Clinical	Neurological examination Neuropsychological testing
Biochemical	S100β Neuron-specific enolase
Ultrasound	Transcranial Doppler (TCD) Epiaortic ultrasound Transoesophageal ultrasound (TOE)
Brain Imaging	Computed tomography Magnetic resonance imaging Structural: T1, T2 and diffusion-weighted imaging (DWI) Functional (FMRI) Magnetic resonance spectroscopy (MRS) Positron emission tomography (PET)
Electrophysiology	Electroencephalography (EEG) and somatosensory evoked potentials (SSEP)
Others	Near-infrared spectroscopy (NIRS) Jugular bulb oxygen saturation

cognitive dysfunction. Consequently, the most frequently used method of assessment of cognitive impairment is neuropsychometric testing. This classically involves the use of a battery of psychological tests that examine various cognitive domains including memory, attention, visuospatial ability, and motor speed.

In 1995, a statement of consensus was published by a multidisciplinary team of leading experts in the field.[7,8] They made a number of recommendations that include:

- Preoperative neurological and neuropsychometric assessment is essential to identify those with pre-existing neurological abnormality and provide a baseline for comparison.
- The inclusion of a control group.
- Selection of an appropriate battery of tests that examine different cognitive domains.
- Acknowledging the potential influence of environmental, physiological, and psychological factors on test performance.
- Objectivity and reliability should be maximized by ensuring that the tests are carried out by an appropriately trained individual (preferably the same individual on longitudinal follow-up) blinded to the form of treatment the patients have received.
- Attempts to minimize the practice effects with repeated testing should be carried out (e.g., providing multiple practice trials on each test).
- The recommended core neuropsychological battery should include:
  - Rey auditory verbal learning test
  - Trail-making A
  - Trail-making B
  - Grooved pegboard

This consensus was followed up 2 years later with the following recommendations[9]:

- Individual change in scores is the most sensitive means of detecting factors associated with postoperative cognitive decline.
- Group mean scores are affected by real change within the group as well as the relative improvement related to practice effects making them a less useful measure.
- Maximizing reproducibility of the results by ensuring that the assessment is carried out in suitable surroundings with minimal distractions and interruptions and preferably by the same examiner during follow-up.
- The importance of correcting for practice effects when analyzing the data collected.

Blumenthal and colleagues recommended the use of a unified, internationally agreed battery of tests.[8] This is intended to be concise but abbreviated from the complete battery (which may take up to 10 h to complete!). This would provide an agreed definition of impairment and permit comparability between the different studies.

7.2.2 Definition of Cognitive Decline

Once the results of the neuropsychological test battery are available, the next challenge is to identify the patients with cognitive deficit. Many definitions of impairment have been used and include:

- Decline of one level in global impairment rating
- Decline of 20% or more in at least 20% of tests
- Decline of one standard deviation in two or more tests (or in 20% of tests)

Of all the above, the latter is the most frequently used definition of impairment. Another approach is the domain-specific approach, which addresses the proportion of patients who, for example, exhibit impairment of memory or language and which may also shed some light on the pathophysiology of cognitive dysfunction. It must be noted, however, that spatial localization using neuropsychometric testing remains relatively insensitive as many of the tests used require multiple cognitive processes for their execution. Despite that, neuropsychometric assessment may serve as a differentiating feature compared to changes expected to occur with other pathological conditions such as aging or dementia. However, to date, there appears to be no good evidence for a specific "cardiac surgery-related neuropsychological syndrome."

7.3 Limitations

Neuropsychometric assessment has presented researchers with various challenges. The extent to which postoperative cognitive impairment is detected is dependent on numerous factors that include:

- The number and sensitivity of the tests used
- Timing of the assessment
- Methods of analysis
- The surgical procedure performed
- Inclusion and exclusion criteria of the individual study
- The criteria used to define neurocognitive decline or dysfunction
- Regression to the mean

International consensus conferences have addressed these various issues in an attempt to standardize methodology and detection of cognitive impairment.[7,9] As outlined previously, this consensus recommended that assessment of all cognitive domains is carried out. This, however, adds a significant time constraint and very few studies have included tests covering all these domains. The time factor is important as it is laborious for the patient and examiner alike and may result in exhaustion and deterioration in performance.

7.3.1 Definition of Impairment

An important limitation of neuropsychological testing is the varying definitions of impairment.[10] The most commonly used definition of impairment is a decline of one standard deviation in two or more tests. An alternative is to use a decline of 20% from baseline as indicative of significant impairment. Mahanna and colleagues examined the effect of different definitions of impairment on the incidence of postoperative neurocognitive decline and noted large differences in the rates reported.[10] For example, by applying five different arbitrary criteria for decline to the same dataset, the rate of decline at 6 weeks following surgery ranged from as low as 1% to as high as 34%, confirming that the variation between the studies are, at least in part, related to the different "arbitrary" criteria used. Likewise, the statistical method used in the analysis may also result in wide variability in the results obtained. Another possible form of analysis is to examine the change in individual performance compared to baseline in a categorical manner (e.g., 1SD drop) using logistic regression or a continuum using linear multivariate regression. The former method is limited by the arbitrariness of the categorical boundary set of normality versus impairment, whereas the latter is associated with difficulty in interpretation regarding its clinical significance.[8]

7.3.2 Baseline Performance and Regression to the Mean

There is substantial variability in neuropsychological performance at baseline even after adjusting for age and background education. Such variability may be related to the high level of emotional stress in the presurgical period. However, there is evidence that patients with coronary artery disease undergoing CABG may have a significant reduction in preoperative cognitive performance with significantly impaired word fluency, manual dexterity, verbal learning, and psychomotor speed.[11] Further decline in these patients who are already impaired preoperatively may be underestimated. These limitations should be taken into account in choosing the method of analysis and interpretation of results.

Single case definitions are limited by the effects of regression toward the mean, where extreme baseline scores become less extreme with repeat testing in the absence of real change.[12] For example, a high baseline performer is more likely to be wrongly classified as having deteriorated on repeat testing. On the other hand, detecting decline in function following cardiac surgery in patients with poor preoperative scores may be underestimated.

The timing of the postoperative tests may also be important. Decline in the early postoperative period may be related to the transient pharmacological effects of narcotics and other anesthetic agents. On the other hand, later decline may be related to factors that are independent of the perioperative insult such as depression or other neuropsychiatric conditions.

7.3.3 Test Selection

Selection of appropriate tests that are adequately sensitive to detect subtle decline in cognitive function is essential. It is preferable that the battery of tests covers all the major cognitive domains as cognitive changes arise as a consequence of more than one etiological mechanism. For example, if a test battery does not include assessment of parietal lobe function such as spatial and constructional ability, deficits in that area will be missed and the subject may be falsely labeled as normal. Such a comprehensive battery will be very time-consuming, and practical considerations dictate implementation of a core abbreviated battery that assesses domains thought to be most likely affected by cardiac surgery.[8]

7.3.4 Control Group

A major limitation of the studies examining the rate of neurocognitive dysfunction following surgery is the fact that a control group has not been used in the vast majority.[1, 12] This is why the definition of impairment is invariably based on an arbitrary criteria set within the study population. This is illustrated in the study by van Dijk and colleagues. In the original Octopus study comparing cognitive change in patients undergoing on-pump versus off-pump surgery, 31% of patients were classified as having decline at 3 months following surgery.[13] The criterion for decline in this study was 20% decline in 20% of tests. In a follow-up study where healthy controls were recruited, using the same criteria for impairment astonishingly resulted in 28% of these normal subjects being classified as having cognitive decline.[14] They thus concluded that the incidence of cognitive dysfunction after CABG has previously been greatly overestimated. In a recently published follow-up of the same study groups after 5 years, the authors were unable to demonstrate that patients who underwent CABG have more cognitive decline after 5 years than control subjects without coronary artery disease (odds ratio 1.37 [95% confidence interval, 0.65–2.92]).[15]

Although using group mean estimates has been advocated to avoid the effects of regression toward the mean,[12] this still does not account for differences due to practice effects. The latter can only be accounted for by the inclusion of age-matched controls that undergo repeat testing in the absence of any intervention.

Many factors may contribute to the rate of cognitive decline. In patients, the most obvious would be the inherent pathophysiological mechanisms that accompany major surgery. What about in controls? Controls may constitute a healthy age-matched group, a surgical control group undergoing noncardiac surgical procedures or, alternatively, a disease-matched group not undergoing surgery. In the latter, decline in cognitive function may be an index of advancing age and underlying cerebrovascular disease. This is further complicated by the fact that this decline may be masked by improvement with time due to the "practice effect" where participants improve their performance with repeated exposure to the same neuropsychological test battery.

So what is the most appropriate group of controls? This will ultimately depend on the research question being asked. Using nonsurgical controls with coronary artery disease, Selnes and colleagues reported no difference between the two groups in cognitive performance at 3 months or 1 year after baseline examination.[16] In a follow-up study, the longitudinal neuropsychological performance of CABG patients did not differ from that of a comparable nonsurgical control group of patients with coronary artery disease at 1- or 3-year follow-up concluding that previously reported late cognitive decline after coronary artery bypass grafting may not be specific to the use of cardiopulmonary bypass, but may also occur in patients with similar risk factors for cardiovascular and cerebrovascular disease.[17] The same group conducted a study using a "heart-healthy" control group with no risk factors for vascular disease and therefore minimizing or eliminating the effect of cerebrovascular disease progression. They reported similar distribution of within subject change in scores in this heart-healthy group as in the CABG and disease-matched controls confirming that the major factor may be test–retest variability rather than disease-related decline.[18]

The within-subjects preoperative and postoperative research design recommended in the initial Statement of Consensus in 1995 has been criticized by Keith and colleagues.[19] They suggested that the use of a control group cannot entirely account for the effects of repeated administration of the neuropsychological tests because of an interaction between the cardiac surgery and practice effects. By addressing the relative merits of between-groups versus within-groups research designs, they recommended use of between-groups designs, dispensing with the preoperative baseline assessment, and instead relying on comparison of postoperative cross-sectional assessment of cardiac surgical patients with well-matched controls to evaluate possible adverse cognitive effects of surgery. In response to this, Selnes suggested that, from a statistical perspective, the proposal to rely on cross-sectional comparisons ignoring baseline values is likely to increase both bias and variance of the estimated surgical effect.[20] By comparing the change from baseline, any differences between the CABG and control groups that persist with time are eliminated. Selnes concluded that longitudinal change in performance should still be considered the method of choice for studying cognitive outcomes after cardiac surgery.

7.3.5 Attrition and Follow-Up

As with any clinical follow-up study, an expected proportion of cases will be lost to follow-up through withdrawal, further illness, disability, or death. This is particularly true in long-term longitudinal studies where data are reported on a subset of patients. Such loss to follow-up may represent selective attrition where those at highest risk of morbidity are the ones that have not been assessed and thus excluded from the study. There is evidence that those who drop out at longer-term follow-up have greater cognitive decline at hospital discharge.[8] This would subsequently underestimate the rate and degree of the reported impairment.

7.4 Summary

Neuropsychometric testing is currently the most frequently used mechanism for assessing perioperative cognitive change. Its numerous limitations, outlined above, coupled with the importance of cognitive outcomes impose a degree of urgency in improving the current methods or, ideally, developing better measures of cognitive assessment. Until such time, quantification of the criteria for impairment, baseline assessment, appropriate data analytical techniques, and use of a control group is essential if results of neuropsychometric tests are to be interpretable and of any clinical significance.

7.5 Alternative Investigative Approaches

While numerous methods of assessments have been used in the investigation of postoperative cognitive impairment in search of a "gold standard," none have thus far demonstrated adequate ease of administration, sensitivity, specificity, and reproducibility to allow routine use. Numerous investigative approaches have been used and are summarized in Table 7.1. Many of those approaches are discussed in detail in the appropriate sections in this book.

The authors have utilized a novel imaging investigation, namely functional magnetic resonance imaging of the brain (FMRI).[21,22] Since the inception of its basic principles over 15 years ago, use of FMRI has rapidly evolved and is now a well-established technique for studying brain function in health and disease. It allows mapping of networks in the brain responsible for sensory, motor, and cognitive processing and allows quantification of brain activation with higher spatial and temporal resolution compared to older techniques.[23]

This technique depends on the fact that the microvascular magnetic resonance signal is strongly influenced by the oxygenation state of the blood. This effect is known as "blood oxygenation level dependent" or "BOLD" effect.[24] Performing a certain task (motor, sensory, or cognitive) during the acquisition of FMRI images results in local increases in the metabolic rate in the regions concerned due to neuronal activation.[25] This demands an increase in substrate delivery and is met by an increase in local blood flow.[26] This increase in blood flow exceeds demand resulting in a *reduction* in oxygen extraction with greater neuronal activity. Thus, the ratio of oxyhemoglobin to deoxyhemoglobin increases in areas of increased neuronal activity. Deoxyhemoglobin is slightly paramagnetic relative to brain tissue, whereas oxyhemoglobin is isomagnetic. The former therefore causes distortion of the magnetic field.[27] The field inhomogeneities associated with deoxyhemoglobin results in shortening of the T2* relaxation time and is detected as an increase in MRI signal intensity relative to baseline. This forms the basis of the BOLD signal (Fig. 7.1). Evidence of the relation between the BOLD response and neural activity comes from electrophysiological data from single-unit microelectrode recordings. Studies with simultaneous FMRI and electrophysiological recordings suggest that the BOLD contrast mechanism directly reflects local increase in neural activity elicited by a stimulus.[28] Comparison of serial brain images before and after initiation of a specific cognitive task allows detection of small signal changes in activation and thus localization of the responsible areas of the brain. This is now a well-established technique for mapping brain functions involved in many cognitive tasks including verbal working memory. Recent work has demonstrated that cognitive activation can be followed serially in patients to identify even subtle changes.[29] This technique has now been used in the assessment of cerebral injury following cardiac surgery.[21,22]

In a recent study, using a verbal working memory task of increasing complexity (*n*-back task) in patients undergoing off-pump and on-pump surgery, a relative reduction in FMRI signal intensity in the latter group was identified in a prefrontal region of interest (Fig. 7.2). In contrast, activation patterns were unaltered in the off-pump group. These changes occurred

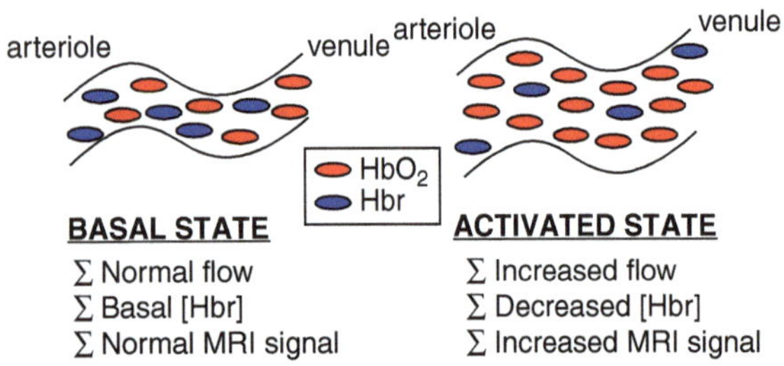

Fig. 7.1 The BOLD response. With neuronal activation, there is an increase in blood flow that exceeds demand. This results in a relative reduction in the proportion of deoxyhemoglobin (Hbr), which consequently causes an increase in the MRI signal intensity. *HbO_2* Oxyhemoglobin, *Hbr* Deoxyhemoglobin

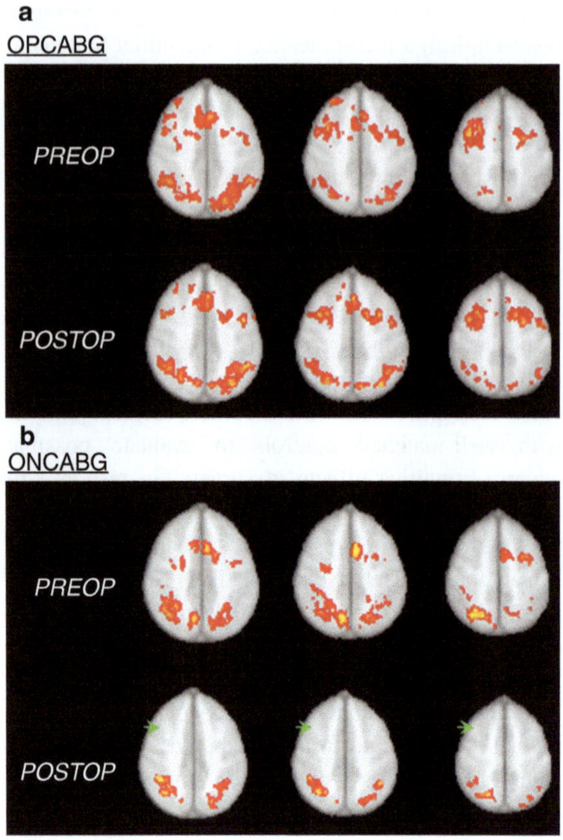

Fig. 7.2 Mean group activation images in the two groups; a) Off-pump CABG and b) On-pump CABG. These show no postoperative difference in the activation pattern in patients undergoing off-pump surgery but a significant reduction in activation in the prefrontal regions postoperatively in the on-pump group (*arrows*)

in the absence of any detectable differences in task performance, highlighting the poor sensitivity associated with use of isolated cognitive tests. This alteration in activity observed in the on-pump group was correlated with the degree of intraoperative microembolization. Moreover, and most alarming, is that the observed changes persisted over the follow-up period of 11 months, which suggests that these may be irreversible in the longer term. Variations in the intensity of activation detected using FMRI may be related to neuroaxonal injury or, alternatively, a reflection of an imbalance between excitatory and inhibitory inputs. Recovery is more likely to occur following the latter mechanism as neuroaxonal injury may be permanent. Whatever the mechanism may be, the results demonstrate significant functional impairment as evident by impaired hemodynamic coupling.

FMRI may prove to be more sensitive than neuropsychological testing in assessing perioperative cerebral injury and may offer additional insights into its pathophysiology and into potential therapeutic approaches.

7.6 Conclusions

Techniques and technologies associated with cardiac surgery continue to evolve. These provide an opportunity for the evaluation of possible neuroprotective agents, and studies comparing the effects of such novel interventions on postoperative neurological outcomes are needed. However, accurate definition and detection of postoperative neurological injury is imperative prior to such an evaluation.

Identification of patients at the highest risk of postoperative neurological morbidity would increase the power of studies aimed at evaluating novel interventions. An exciting prospect is the potential for targeting this high-risk group by identification of genetic predisposition to cerebral injury – alleles of apolipoprotein ε4 [epsilon4], C-reactive protein, and interleukin 6 have been associated with a significant increase in postoperative neurological morbidity.[30, 31]

An enormous amount of work is still needed to further enhance the understanding of this complex multifactorial problem. Large prospective trials with appropriate controls are necessary to further define the impact of various etiological factors, disease progression, and the effect of surgical and anesthetic techniques on postoperative cognitive decline. It is hoped that strategies under development will help reduce the neurological morbidity associated with cardiac surgery.

References

1. Taggart DP, Westaby S. Neurological and cognitive disorders after coronary artery bypass grafting. *Curr Opin Cardiol.* 2001;16(5):271-276.
2. van Dijk D et al. Neurocognitive dysfunction after coronary artery bypass surgery: a systematic review. *J Thorac Cardiovasc Surg.* 2000;120(4):632-639.
3. Taggart DP et al. Is cardiopulmonary bypass still the cause of cognitive dysfunction after cardiac operations? *J Thorac Cardiovasc Surg.* 1999;118(3):414-420, discussion 420-421.
4. Anyanwu AC et al. Epidemiology of stroke after cardiac surgery in the current era. *J Thorac Cardiovasc Surg.* 2007; 134(5):1121-1127.
5. Sedrakyan A et al. Off-pump surgery is associated with reduced occurrence of stroke and other morbidity as compared with traditional coronary artery bypass grafting: a meta-analysis of systematically reviewed trials. *Stroke.* 2006;37(11):2759-2769.
6. Newman MF et al. Report of the substudy assessing the impact of neurocognitive function on quality of life 5 years after cardiac surgery. *Stroke.* 2001;32(12):2874-2881.
7. Murkin JM et al. Statement of consensus on assessment of neurobehavioral outcomes after cardiac surgery. *Ann Thorac Surg.* 1995;59(5):1289-1295.
8. Blumenthal JA et al. Methodological issues in the assessment of neuropsychologic function after cardiac surgery. *Ann Thorac Surg.* 1995;59(5):1345-1350.
9. Murkin JM et al. Defining dysfunction: group means versus incidence analysis – a statement of consensus. *Ann Thorac Surg.* 1997;64(3):904-905.
10. Mahanna EP et al. Defining neuropsychological dysfunction after coronary artery bypass grafting. *Ann Thorac Surg.* 1996;61(5):1342-1347.
11. Vingerhoets G, Van Nooten G, Jannes C. Neuropsychological impairment in candidates for cardiac surgery. *J Int Neuropsychol Soc.* 1997;3(5):480-484.
12. Browne SM et al. Cognitive performance after cardiac operation: implications of regression toward the mean. *J Thorac Cardiovasc Surg.* 1999;117(3):481-485.
13. Van Dijk D et al. Cognitive outcome after off-pump and on-pump coronary artery bypass graft surgery: a randomized trial. *JAMA.* 2002;287(11):1405-1412.
14. Keizer AM et al. The incidence of cognitive decline after (not) undergoing coronary artery bypass grafting: the impact of a controlled definition. *Acta Anaesthesiol Scand.* 2005;49(9):1232-1235.
15. van Dijk D et al. Cognitive outcomes five years after not undergoing coronary artery bypass graft surgery. *Ann Thorac Surg.* 2008;85(1):60-64.
16. Selnes OA et al. Cognitive changes with coronary artery disease: a prospective study of coronary artery bypass graft patients and nonsurgical controls. *Ann Thorac Surg.* 2003;75(5):1377-1384, discussion 1384-1386.
17. Selnes OA et al. Cognitive outcomes three years after coronary artery bypass surgery: a comparison of on-pump coronary artery bypass graft surgery and nonsurgical controls. *Ann Thorac Surg.* 2005;79(4):1201-1209.
18. McKhann GM et al. Is there cognitive decline 1 year after CABG?Comparison with surgical and nonsurgical controls. *Neurology.* 2005;65(7):991-999.
19. Keith JR, Cohen DJ, Lecci LB. Why serial assessments of cardiac surgery patients' neurobehavioral performances are misleading. *Ann Thorac Surg.* 2007;83(2):370-373.
20. Selnes OA, Zeger SL. Coronary artery bypass grafting baseline cognitive assessment: essential not optional. *Ann Thorac Surg.* 2007;83(2):374-376.
21. Abu-Omar Y et al. Short-term changes in cerebral activity in on-pump and off-pump cardiac surgery defined by functional magnetic resonance imaging and their relationship to microembolization. *J Thorac Cardiovasc Surg.* 2006; 132(5):1119-1125.

22. Abu-Omar Y et al. The role of microembolisation in cerebral injury as defined by functional magnetic resonance imaging. *Eur J Cardiothorac Surg*. 2004;26(3):586-591.
23. Jezzard P, Matthews PM, Smith SS. *Functional MRI: an introduction to methods*. Oxford: Oxford University Press; 2001.
24. Ogawa S et al. Functional brain mapping by blood oxygenation level-dependent contrast magnetic resonance imaging. A comparison of signal characteristics with a biophysical model. *Biophys J*. 1993;64(3):803-812.
25. Attwell D, Laughlin SB. An energy budget for signaling in the grey matter of the brain. *J Cereb Blood Flow Metab*. 2001;21(10):1133-1145.
26. Attwell D, Iadecola C. The neural basis of functional brain imaging signals. *Trends Neurosci*. 2002;25(12):621-625.
27. Ogawa S et al. Brain magnetic resonance imaging with contrast dependent on blood oxygenation. *Proc Natl Acad Sci USA*. 1990;87(24):9868-9872.
28. Logothetis NK. The underpinnings of the BOLD functional magnetic resonance imaging signal. *J Neurosci*. 2003;23(10):3963-3971.
29. Matthews PM, Clare S, Adcock J. Functional magnetic resonance imaging: clinical applications and potential. *J Inherit Metab Dis*. 1999;22(4):337-352.
30. Grocott HP et al. Genetic polymorphisms and the risk of stroke after cardiac surgery. *Stroke*. 2005;36(9):1854-1858.
31. Tardiff BE et al. Preliminary report of a genetic basis for cognitive decline after cardiac operations. The Neurologic Outcome Research Group of the Duke Heart Center. *Ann Thorac Surg*. 1997;64(3):715-720.

8 Imaging of the Brain in Cardiac Surgery as a Tool in Brain Protection Studies

Martin Bendszus

8.1 Methods for Assessing Brain Injury After Cardiac Surgery

Computed tomography (CT) is based on the absorption of X-rays in tissue. Tissue density is correlated with the amount of radiation being absorbed. Tissue absorption values are expressed as Hounsfield units (HU). Per definition, water has an HU of 0. In brain tissue, acute hemorrhage results in an increase of absorption caused by the cellular components of the blood. In contrast to normal absorption values of brain tissue (35–45 HU), acute hemorrhage features absorption values of approximately 60–70 HU. Thus, acute hemorrhage appears as a hyperdense lesion (that is, bright lesion compared with brain tissue) with a mass effect. Due to the marked difference in tissue density, CT features a high sensitivity in the detection of blood and is the method of choice to rule out acute hemorrhage. In acute ischemic infarction of the brain, diagnosis on CT is based on increased water content in brain tissue resulting in a decrease of tissue density. Thereby, acute cerebral infarction presents as hypodense (i.e., dark) lesion relative to brain parenchyma. In the hyperacute phase (i.e., <2 h), acute cerebral infarction, in general, escapes diagnosis from CT since water shifts from the extra- to the intracellular space precede a significant increase in absolute water content. Large territorial infarction later on presents as hypodense space-occupying lesions 2 h after onset at the earliest, whereas small ischemic lesions may be identified only at later stages or not at all, especially if preexisting microangiopathy of the brain with diffuse white matter hypodensity is present. Therefore, CT, in general, is not suitable in monitoring the overall ischemic lesion load in studies assessing brain protection in cardiac surgery.

Magnetic resonance imaging (MRI) including conventional T1-weighted (T1-w) and T2-weighted (T2-w) sequences is a sensitive technique for the detection of focal brain lesions. However, the nature of these signal alterations on MRI is non-specific.[18] Signal abnormalities may be caused by different pathophysiological processes encompassing inflammation, ischemia, demyelination, axonal injury, and edema. Moreover, based on standard MRI, it is impossible to distinguish specific stages of CNS lesions such as acute injury, reactive inflammation, and glial responses, and finally healing processes and scar formation. In ischemic stroke, a gross differentiation between acute and chronic infarction is feasible only in large acute infarcts presenting with mass effect, whereas in small lesions, this temporal differentiation is often impossible on the basis of T2-w images.[28] Diffusion-weighted MR sequences specifically visualize acute ischemia and have become clinical routine in the evaluation of acute stroke.[32] Pulse sequences for DWI are available on all modern MR scanners and, for common diagnostic purposes, generally take less than a minute. In ischemic brain tissue, cytotoxic edema develops within minutes after vessel occlusion resulting in a rapid decline in proton diffusion capacity.[25,30] This reduced proton diffusion capacity is detectable in vivo by applying additional strong magnetic field gradient pulses to a regular MR pulse sequence.[25,30] On diffusion-weighted images, acute ischemia with reduced proton diffusion capacity presents as a hyperintense (i.e., bright) area against the dark background of normal tissue, thus facilitating detection of even small lesions with high specificity and sensitivity (Fig. 8.1). The average sensitivity and specificity of

M. Bendszus
Director, Department of Neuroradiology,
University of Heidelberg, Heidelberg, Germany
e-mail: martin.bendszus@med.uni-heidelberg.de

R.S. Bonser et al. (eds.), *Brain Protection in Cardiac Surgery*,
DOI: 10.1007/978-1-84996-293-3_8, © Springer-Verlag London Limited 2011

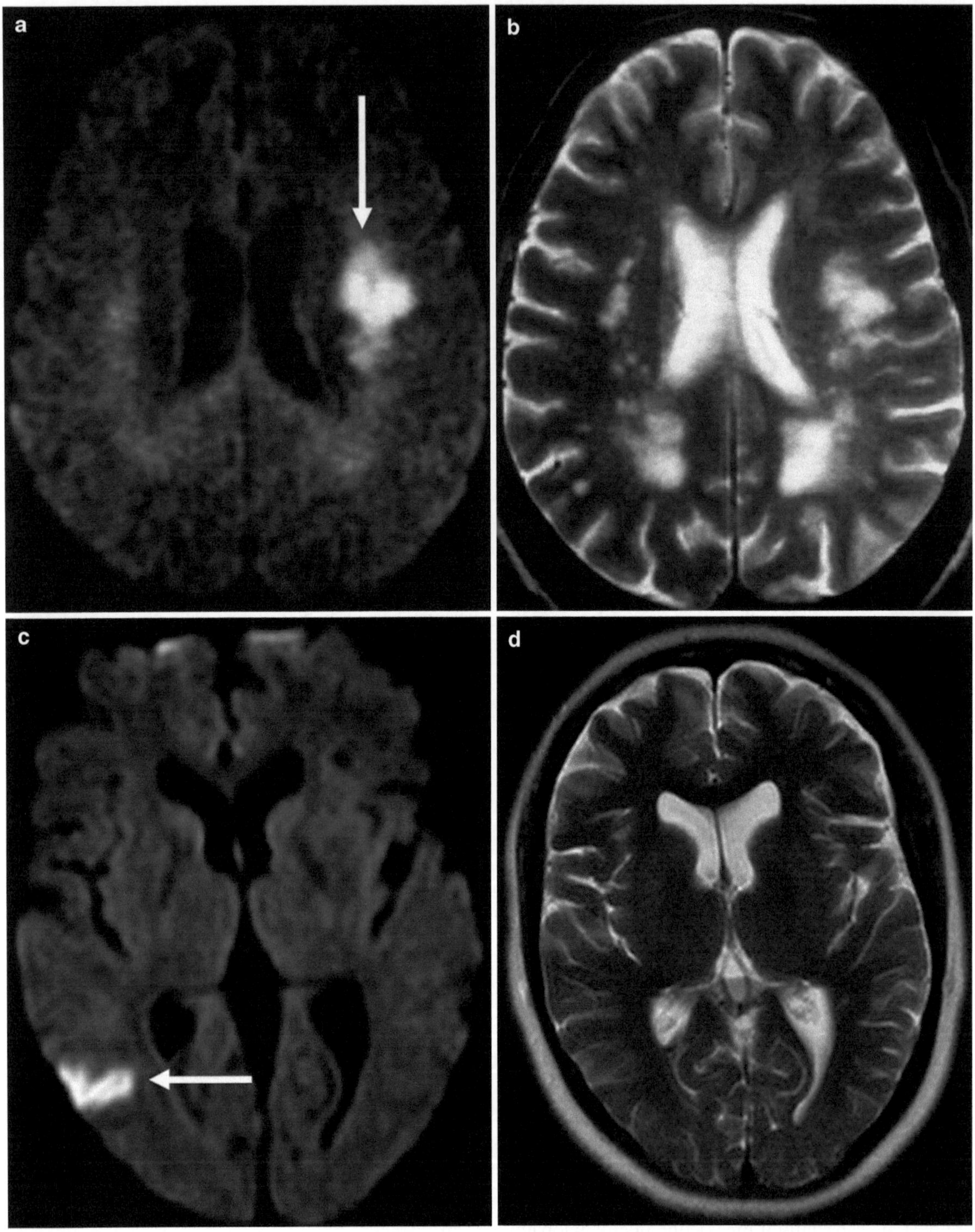

Fig. 8.1 Sensitivity and specificity of diffusion-weighted MRI. Hyperintense lesion on diffusion-weighted MRI (**a**) demonstrates the acute ischemic event in the left frontal lobe (*arrow*). On standard T2-w MRI (**b**), preexisting vascular lesions in both hemispheres cannot be separated from the acute event indicating the lack of specificity of standard MR-techniques. Acute ischemic lesion appearing bright on diffusion-weighted MRI (**c**, *arrow*) shortly after the ischemic event, whereas T2-w MRI fails to depict the ischemic lesion at this stage (**d**)

DWI in detecting acute human stroke are up to 94% and 97%, respectively.[32] Upon acute infarction, a signal increase on DWI becomes visible within 24 h in nearly all patients and, importantly, disappears within 14 days after onset.[7] In contrast, T2-w abnormalities develop later, but persist. Thus, a bright DWI signal indicates an early or subacute, but not a chronic (>14 days old) stage of an ischemic lesion.[7] Detection of ischemic lesions on DWI is limited by spatial resolution. At commonly applied acquisition parameters, a voxel volume measures about 10–15 mm^3 which represents the threshold for detection of an ischemic focus. Technical factors such as the gradient, the magnetic field strength, and the diffusion-weighted sequence used further affect the sensitivity of DWI for acute ischemia[9] and may explain divergent rates of ischemic events reported in different studies.

8.2 MRI of the Brain in Cardiac Surgery

Coronary artery bypass grafting (CABG) is the most frequent major surgical procedure with more than half a million operations per year in the USA.[38] Progress in surgical techniques, anesthesia, and postoperative care has markedly lowered overall morbidity and case fatality.[38] Nevertheless, the incidence of neurological complications still amounts to 0.4–5.7% for stroke, 10–28% for delirium, and 33–83% for neuropsychological deficit.[38] Similar rates have been reported for patients undergoing heart valve replacement.[1] These complications increase case fatality and result in substantially raised treatment costs.[36] Cerebral ischemia owing to thrombo-embolism or hypoperfusion has been considered as a major cause for neurological complications.[38] Previous studies have used T2-w MR-sequences to investigate the incidence and the relevance of ischemic lesions pre- and postoperatively. The extent of ischemic brain lesions on preoperative T2-w MR sequences has been reported to be a predictor for postoperative neuropsychological decline[26,27] and physical health status.[29] Before the advance of diffusion-weighted MRI, T2-w MRI has been applied to assess new ischemic lesions postoperatively. These studies have shown highly variable results ranging from no lesions[37] up to an incidence of 42%.[41] The reason for these divergent findings may be the lack of specificity of T2-w MRI especially in depicting new ischemic lesions if preexisting vascular lesions are present. Interestingly, the majority of lesions did not result in overt neurological symptoms. In a pilot study, DWI was applied in patients revealing focal neurological complications postoperatively.[42] The extent of ischemic brain injury on MRI was much more extensive than the clinical symptoms would suggest, indicating that focal neurological signs represent only the tip of the iceberg of the overall postoperative ischemic damage.

The first DWI-based study in a prospective patient cohort reported new ischemic lesions in 26% of patients undergoing CABG[4] (Fig. 8.2). These new postoperative lesions exhibited an embolic type of lesion pattern and were not associated with focal neurological symptoms or a diffuse cognitive decline. Subsequent studies have confirmed a high frequency of ischemic lesions ranging from 31%[34] to 51%[22,24] after CABG. The incidence of acute ischemic lesions after cardiac valve replacement is similar to CABAG ranging from 32%[39] to 47%.[2,10,13,23] Overall, lesions reveal an embolic pattern.[10] Atheromatous disease of the thoracic aorta may be a crucial factor for the development of postoperative lesions on DWI: a recent study observed new DWI foci in 60% in patients with mild to moderate atherosclerosis in the ascending aorta and the aortic arch, whereas in patients without atherosclerosis DWI lesions were absent.[11] Interestingly, off-pump surgery (that is, without cardiopulmonary bypass) did not reduce the ischemic lesion load in a pilot study (31%).[14] Likewise, in a study directly comparing off-pump and on-pump surgery, no significant difference was found between both groups (8.2% in off-pump versus 17.3% in on pump).[26,27] This indicates that extracorporal circulation does not substantially contribute to ischemic DWI lesions. However, microscopic air embolism cannot be excluded since the resolution of DWI is limited to the voxel size which is within the range of several cubic millimeters. Even though the vast majority of these lesions remained clinically silent, a similar lesion appearance has been observed in symptomatic patients,([42,43]). Similar to overt neurological complications, the presence of DWI lesions is closely correlated with a vascular risk profile, including age,[11,39] preexisting cerebral vascular lesions on T2-w MRI,[4,39] and the presence of mild to moderate atheromatous disease of the thoracic aorta.[11] While especially small embolic ischemic lesions frequently do not cause focal neurological deficit, the occurrence of hemodynamic stroke

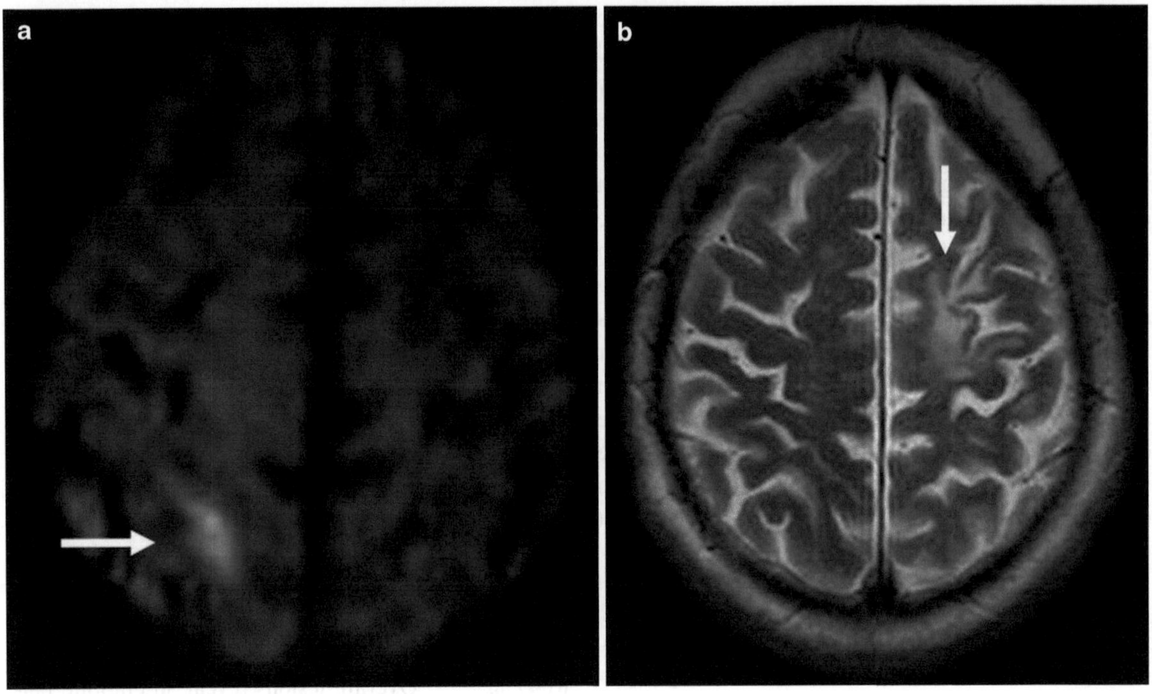

Fig. 8.2 Clinically silent periprocedural cortical ischemia after CABAG. Three days after CABAG, a new ischemic lesion is present in the left parietal cortex on diffusion-weighted MRI (**a**, *arrow*) which did not result in neurological symptoms. The lesion is hardly discernable on T2-w MRI (**b**). Hyperintense ischemic lesion in the left frontal lobe (*arrow* in **b**) which is not bright on diffusion-weighted MRI, indicating that this is not an acute lesion

on diffusion-weighted MRI is generally associated with severe neurological symptoms and adverse clinical outcome (Fig. 8.3).[17]

8.3 Clinical Significance of MRI Lesions

DWI has demonstrated new ischemic lesions in an unexpectedly high number of patients undergoing cardiac surgery. The high proportion of clinically unaffected patients has raised the question on the practical relevance of these DWI lesions.[6] This not only affects cardiac surgery, but a variety of vascular procedures with a risk for cerebral embolization, including cerebral and coronary angiography and carotid endarterectomy. In most studies, new clinically silent DWI lesions after the procedure presented as hyperintense ischemic scars on follow-up T2-w images indicating persistent structural damage to the brain.[3–5,12,31,33] However, there have also been few reports on the regression of post-procedural DWI abnormalities without subsequent ischemic scars on T2-w images.[16,19] These apparent discrepancies can be explained by two confounding factors: first, in these studies, only very small DWI foci did not convert into T2-w lesions, a fact that reflects a lower sensitivity of T2-w images in detecting ischemic lesions. Second, transient cerebral ischemia similarly leads to DWI abnormalities which upon regression do not cause persistent CNS lesions on T2-w images.[21] However, DWI in these patients was performed, on average, within 24 h after onset of symptoms indicating that reversal of DWI abnormalities predominantly affected ultra-early ischemic lesions. Nevertheless, normalization of DWI does not mean absence of neuronal damage. In areas of rapid normalization of DWI abnormalities after transient experimental ischemia structural neuronal damage has been demonstrated.[35] This is probably caused by delayed neuronal cell death by apoptosis developing in the absence of tissue necrosis.[35] Therefore, any DWI lesion which is present 24 h after the event should be considered as an indicator for cerebral infarction.[6]

The vast majority of embolic periprocedural DWI lesions do not cause an obvious neurological deficit. These asymptomatic DWI lesions have the same

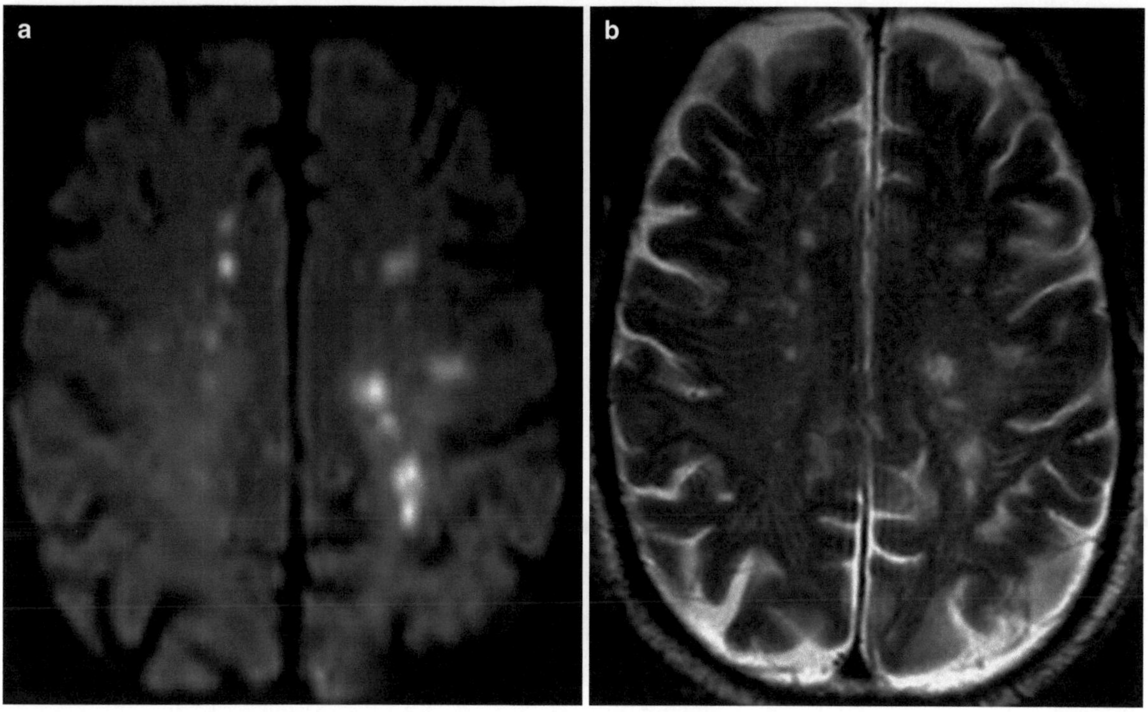

Fig. 8.3 Hemodynamic infarction. Bilateral areas of punctuate hyperintensity in the subcortical fronto-parietal white matter on diffusion-weighted MRI (**a**) and T2-w MRI (**b**) 4 days after aortic valve replacement. This is a typical pattern for hemodynamic infarction. Clinically, this patient revealed bilateral signs of motor deficit and was poorly responsive

characteristics on imaging as symptomatic lesions. Primarily, the lesion location in an "eloquent" brain area determines occurrence and extent of neurological deficits. Even small periprocedural DWI lesions, if located in an "eloquent" brain area, can cause severe neurological deficits (Fig. 8.4). Vice versa, persistent ischemic cerebral deficits have not been described in patients without DWI lesions. These findings also apply to patients who develop strokes independently from a diagnostic or therapeutic procedure. Severe neurological deficit has been described in patients with a small lesion located in an "eloquent" brain area such as the precentral gyrus.[15,40] Moreover, follow-up studies showed that after a symptomatic ischemic lesion, recurrent new DWI lesions developed in 34% of patients, but only 2% of these patients showed new neurological symptoms.[20] Again, subsequent DWI lesions were mostly located in "non-eloquent" brain regions.

Based on the available literature, the key question whether "silent" DWI lesions are really silent on clinical grounds cannot be answered with certainty, yet. Routine clinical examination covers **focal** neurological abnormalities such as paresis, ataxia, hypaesthesia, visual defects, and oculomotor syndromes. It also encompasses focal neuropsychological deficits such as aphasia, apraxia, dyscalculia, etc. Global brain dysfunction such as subtile cognitive decline, memory and mood disturbances, reduction of psychomotor speed, and personality changes may be missed, because they require specific attention by neuropsychological tests. Only five studies have specifically addressed the relation between DWI lesions after vascular procedures with a risk for cerebral embolization and neuropsychological deficits with controversial results. In patients undergoing coronary angiography,[26,27] coronary artery bypass grafting[34], or valve replacement[2], new DWI lesions were associated with a decline in neuropsychological test performance. In a recent study, postoperative neuropsychological impairment was directly related to the overall ischemic lesion load. In contrast, no such correlation was found in three other studies in patients after cardiac surgery.[4,10,14,22] Most recently, long-term cognitive dysfunction after cardiac surgery was not reported to be related to new postoperative lesions on MRI; rather there was a close correlation

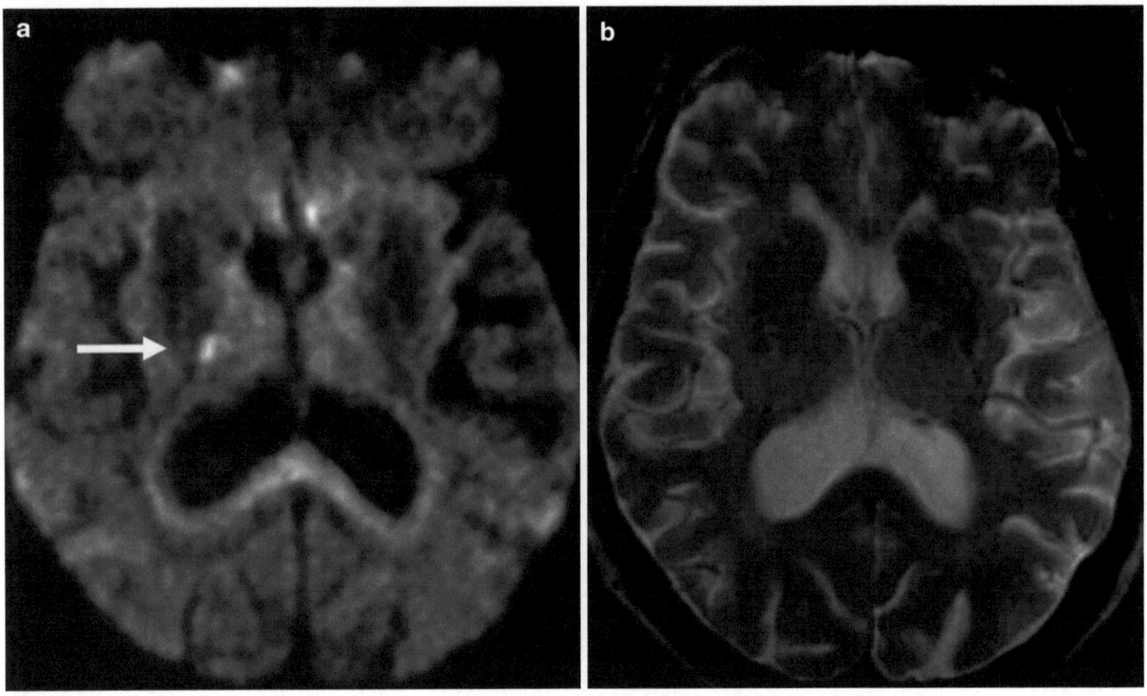

Fig. 8.4 Symptomatic periprocedural ischemia after CABAG. Diffusion-weighted MRI (**a**) of a patient with a mild hemipareses 2 days after CABAG shows a hyperintense lesion in the posterior limb of the right internal capsule in vicinity of the cortico-spinal tract. This lesion is hardly discernable on T2-w MRI (**b**)

between early cognitive deficit and long-term cognitive deficit.[24] These controversial findings may be explained by the relatively small patient samples, but they point to a possible pathophysiological role of DWI lesions in cognitive decline in a subgroup of patients which warrants further investigation in a larger population. The concept that lesion load contributes to cognitive decline is supported by DWI studies of patients with vascular dementia. Patients with a recent deterioration showed a much higher incidence of clinically "silent" diffusion abnormalities compared to those without symptoms.[8]

Cardiac surgery is associated with a relatively low incidence of overt neurological complications. Thus, for assessment of cerebrovascular events on clinical grounds, large and homogeneous patient populations are needed for a reliable comparison of the complication rates of different procedures. As an alternative approach, DWI appears to be a more sensitive read-out parameter to quantify new ischemic events. DWI of the brain has a great potential to serve as a surrogate parameter for future neuroprotective trials. While clinically overt ischemic brain lesions represent only the tip of the iceberg, DWI exhibits the overall lesion load below the waterline. Thereby, the number of patients needed to demonstrate significant treatment effects may dramatically be decreased.

References

1. Ahlgren E, Aren C. Cerebral complications after coronary artery bypass and heart valve surgery: risk factors and onset of symptoms. *J Cardiothorac Vasc Anesth*. 1998;12:270-273.
2. Barber PA, Hach S, Tippett LJ, Ross L, Merry AF, Milsom P. Cerebral ischemic lesions on diffusion-weighted imaging are associated with neurocognitive decline after cardiac surgery. *Stroke*. 2008;39:1427-1433.
3. Bendszus M, Koltzenburg M, Burger R, Warmuth-Metz M, Hofmann E, Solymosi L. Silent embolism in diagnostic cerebral angiography and neurointerventional procedures: a prospective study. *Lancet*. 1999;354:1594-1597.
4. Bendszus M, Reents W, Franke D, et al. Brain damage after coronary artery bypass grafting. *Arch Neurol*. 2002;59:1090-1095.
5. Bendszus M, Koltzenburg M, Bartsch AJ, et al. Heparin and air filters reduce embolic events caused by intra-arterial cerebral angiography: a prospective, randomized trial. *Circulation*. 2004;110:2210-2215.

6. Bendszus M, Stoll G. Silent ischemia: hidden fingerprints of invasive medical procedures. *Lancet Neurol*. 2006;5:364-372.
7. Burdette JH, Ricci PE, Petitti N, Elster AD. Cerebral infarction: time course of signal intensity changes on diffusion-weighted MR images. *AJR Am J Roentgenol*. 1998;171:791-795.
8. Choi SH, Na DL, Chung CS, Lee KH, Na DG, Adair JC. Diffusion-weighted MRI in vascular dementia. *Neurology*. 2000;54:83-89.
9. Conturo TE, McKinstry RC, Aronovitz JA, Neil JJ. Diffusion MRI: precision, accuracy and flow effects. *NMR Biomed*. 1995;8:307-332.
10. Cook DJ, Huston J 3rd, Trenerry MR, Brown RD Jr, Zehr KJ, Sundt TM 3rd. Postcardiac surgical cognitive impairment in the aged using diffusion-weighted magnetic resonance imaging. *Ann Thorac Surg*. 2007;83:1389-1395.
11. Djaiani G, Fedorko L, Borger M, et al. Mild to moderate atheromatous disease of the thoracic aorta and new ischemic brain lesions after conventional coronary artery bypass graft surgery. *Stroke*. 2004;35:356-358.
12. Feiwell RJ, Besmertis L, Sarkar R, Saloner DA, Rapp JH. Detection of clinically silent infarcts after carotid endarterectomy by use of diffusion-weighted imaging. *AJNR Am J Neuroradiol*. 2001;22:646-649.
13. Floyd TF, Shah PN, Price CC, et al. Clinically silent cerebral ischemic events after cardiac surgery: their incidence, regional vascular occurrence, and procedural dependence. *Ann Thorac Surg*. 2006;81:2160-2166.
14. Friday G, Sutter F, Curtin A, et al. Brain magnetic resonance imaging abnormalities following off-pump cardiac surgery. *Heart Surg Forum*. 2005;8:105-109.
15. Gass A, Szabo K, Behrens S, Rossmanith C, Hennerici M. A diffusion-weighted MRI study of acute ischemic distal arm paresis. *Neurology*. 2001;57:1589-1594.
16. Gauvrit JY, Delmaire C, Henon H, et al. Diffusion/perfusion-weighted magnetic resonance imaging after carotid angioplasty and stenting. *J Neurol*. 2004;251:1060-1067.
17. Gottesman RF, Sherman PM, Grega MA, et al. Watershed strokes after cardiac surgery: diagnosis, etiology, and outcome. *Stroke*. 2006;37:2306-2311.
18. Higer HP, Bielke G. *Tissue characterization in MR-imaging*. Berlin/Heidelberg/Paris/London/New York/Tokyo: Springer; 1990.
19. Jaeger HJ, Mathias KD, Hauth E, et al. Cerebral ischemia detected with diffusion-weighted MR imaging after stent implantation in the carotid artery. *AJNR Am J Neuroradiol*. 2002;23:200-207.
20. Kang DW, Latour LL, Chalela JA, Dambrosia J, Warach S. Early ischemic lesion recurrence within a week after acute ischemic stroke. *Ann Neurol*. 2003;54:66-74.
21. Kidwell CS, Alger JR, Di Salle F, et al. Diffusion MRI in patients with transient ischemic attacks. *Stroke*. 1999;30:1174-1180.
22. Knipp SC, Matatko N, Wilhelm H, et al. Evaluation of brain injury after coronary artery bypass grafting. A prospective study using neuropsychological assessment and diffusion-weighted magnetic resonance imaging. *Eur J Cardiothorac Surg*. 2004;25:791-800.
23. Knipp SC, Matatko N, Schlamann M, et al. Small ischemic brain lesions after cardiac valve replacement detected by diffusion-weighted magnetic resonance imaging: relation to neurocognitive function. *Eur J Cardiothorac Surg*. 2005;28:88-96.
24. Knipp SC, Matatko N, Wilhelm H, et al. Cognitive outcomes three years after coronary artery bypass surgery: relation to diffusion-weighted magnetic resonance imaging. *Ann Thorac Surg*. 2008;85:872-879.
25. Kucharczyk J, Mintorovitch J, Asgari HS, Moseley M. Diffusion/perfusion MR imaging of acute cerebral ischemia. *Magn Reson Med*. 1991;19:311-315.
26. Lund C, Nes RB, Ugelstad TP, et al. Cerebral emboli during left heart catheterization may cause acute brain injury. *Eur Heart J*. 2005;26:1269-1275.
27. Lund C, Sundet K, Tennøe B, et al. Cerebral ischemic injury and cognitive impairment after off-pump and on-pump coronary artery bypass grafting surgery. *Ann Thorac Surg*. 2005;80:2126-2131.
28. Marks MP, de Crespigny A, Lentz D, Enzmann DR, Albers GW, Moseley ME. Acute and chronic stroke: navigated spin-echo diffusion-weighted MR imaging. *Radiology*. 1996;199:403-408.
29. Mathisen L, Andersen MH, Hol PK, et al. Preoperative cerebral ischemic lesions predict physical health status after on-pump coronary artery bypass surgery. *J Thorac Cardiovasc Surg*. 2005;130:1691-1697.
30. Moseley ME, Cohen Y, Mintorovitch J, et al. Early detection of regional cerebral ischemia in cats: comparison of diffusion- and T2-weighted MRI and spectroscopy. *Magn Reson Med*. 1990;14:330-346.
31. Muller M, Reiche W, Langenscheidt P, Hassfeld J, Hagen T. Ischemia after carotid endarterectomy: comparison between transcranial Doppler sonography and diffusion-weighted MR imaging. *AJNR Am J Neuroradiol*. 2000;21:47-54.
32. Mullins ME, Schaefer PW, Sorensen AG, et al. CT and conventional and diffusion-weighted MR imaging in acute stroke: study in 691 patients at presentation to the emergency department. *Radiology*. 2002;224:353-360.
33. Omran H, Schmidt H, Hackenbroch M, et al. Silent and apparent cerebral embolism after retrograde catheterisation of the aortic valve in valvular stenosis: a prospective, randomised study. *Lancet*. 2003;361:1241-1246.
34. Restrepo L, Wityk RJ, Grega MA, et al. Diffusion- and perfusion-weighted magnetic resonance imaging of the brain before and after coronary artery bypass grafting surgery. *Stroke*. 2002;33:2909-2915.
35. Ringer TM, Neumann-Haefelin T, Sobel RA, Moseley ME, Yenari MA. Reversal of early diffusion-weighted magnetic resonance imaging abnormalities does not necessarily reflect tissue salvage in experimental cerebral ischemia. *Stroke*. 2001;32:2362-2369.
36. Roach GW, Kanchuger M, Mangano CM, et al. Adverse cerebral outcomes after coronary bypass surgery. Multicenter Study of Perioperative Ischemia Research Group and the Ischemia Research and Education Foundation Investigators. *N Engl J Med*. 1996;335:1857-1863.
37. Schmidt R, Fazekas F, Offenbacher H, et al. Brain magnetic resonance imaging in coronary artery bypass grafts: a pre- and postoperative assessment. *Neurology*. 1993;43:775-778.
38. Selnes OA, Goldsborough MA, Borowicz LM, McKhann GM. Neurobehavioural sequelae of cardiopulmonary bypass. *Lancet*. 1999;353:1601-1606.

39. Stolz E, Gerriets T, Kluge A, Klovekorn WP, Kaps M, Bachmann G. Diffusion-weighted magnetic resonance imaging and neurobiochemical markers after aortic valve replacement: implications for future neuroprotective trials? *Stroke*. 2004;35:888-892.
40. Sudo K, Kishimoto R, Tajima Y, Matsumoto A, Tashiro K. A paralysed thumb. *Lancet*. 2004;363:1364.
41. Toner I, Hamid SK, Peden CJ, Taylor KM, Smith PL. Magnetic resonance imaging and P300 (event-related auditory evoked potentials) in the assessment of postoperative cerebral injury following coronary artery bypass graft surgery. *Perfusion*. 1993;8:321-329.
42. Wityk RJ, Goldsborough MA, Hillis A, et al. Diffusion- and perfusion-weighted brain magnetic resonance imaging in patients with neurologic complications after cardiac surgery. *Arch Neurol*. 2001;58:571-576.
43. Restrepo L, Wityk RJ, Grega MA, et al. Diffusion- and perfusion-weighted magnetic resonance imaging of the brain before and after coronary artery bypass grafting surgery. *Stroke*. 2002; 33: 2909-2915.

Current Techniques of Emboli Detection and Their Utility in Brain Protection Studies

9

Sunil K. Bhudia, David A. Stump, and Timothy J. Jones

9.1 Introduction

The exact etiology of cardiopulmonary bypass (CPB)-associated morbidity and mortality remains unclear and is probably multifactorial resulting from the interactions of a variety of mechanisms: alterations in blood flow, activation of inflammatory processes, temperature manipulations, and emboli. Brain injury, regardless of etiology, can lead to brain edema, further exacerbating the injury.[1]

Operations performed on the circulatory system will always be associated with reported incidents of macroembolization resulting from the introduction of gross air, thrombus, and atherosclerotic debris into the circulation. Usually, such episodes are catastrophic and relate to specific intraoperative problems or events. Over the last 50 years, developments in perfusion apparatus and technique in association with appropriate training and experience have resulted in such episodes occurring infrequently. In contrast, the occurrence of microemboli during cardiac surgery is more common and potentially remains an everyday occurrence.

Emboli generation and extracorporeal circulation has been the focus of much research.[2–7] The number of emboli detected intraoperatively has been demonstrated to be associated with postoperative neurobehavioral deficits. Further work has identified when these emboli occur during surgery, enabling strategies to be developed to reduce the embolic load as well as the effect of the emboli.

S.K. Bhudia (✉)
University Hospital Coventry and Warwickshire, Coventry, United Kingdom
e-mail: sbhudia@doctors.org.uk

Traditionally, emboli are described as macro or micro emboli. This classification is arbitrary mainly due to our inability to size emboli in vivo, but it has been suggested that the ability of an embolus to obstruct a 200-μm vessel should form the basis of this classification. A more useful description is one based upon the composition or source of the emboli[8] with emboli being either biological (blood borne), nonbiological (foreign to host), or gaseous (Table 9.1). Identification of the composition or source of the emboli might help us to develop strategies to reduce their incidence. Biological emboli may consist of debris from disruption of atherosclerotic plaques or calcium, remnants of damaged cells, platelets, neutrophils and cellular aggregates, fibrin, chylomicrons, and lipids from the operative field. Nonbiological emboli may comprise of plastic fragments generated by the pump or flushed from the circuit components, aluminum, silicone antifoam, and glove powder. Gaseous emboli may be inadvertently introduced into the circulation by the surgeon or perfusionist or they may be generated by the components of the circuit by processes of entrainment, cavitation, or temperature and pressure changes.

9.2 Techniques of Emboli Detection and Brain Injury

Methods of embolus detection have been described using visual or optical imaging, ultrasound, histological techniques, cerebral imaging, and at postmortem. No technique has gained widespread acceptance and most remain research tools. This is due to the complex behavior and composition of intravascular emboli. Solid, liquid, and gaseous emboli behave in different

R.S. Bonser et al. (eds.), *Brain Protection in Cardiac Surgery*,
DOI: 10.1007/978-1-84996-293-3_9, © Springer-Verlag London Limited 2011

Table 9.1 Types and classification of emboli reported during cardiopulmonary bypass

Biologic	Nonbiologic	Gaseous
Atherosclerotic plaque	PVC fragments	Air
Calcium fragments	Aluminium debris	Oxygen
Fibrin clumps	Silicone from antifoam linings	Nitrogen
Platelet aggregates	Bone wax	Carbon dioxide
Red blood cell aggregates	Glove powder	Nitrous oxide
Neutrophil aggregates	Cotton fibers	
Chylomicrons		
Lipid		

ways which is further influenced by physiological conditions such as flow rate and pattern, pressure, and temperature. To date, most methods of detection have relied upon a degree of subjectivity in their interpretation with a low specificity. Frequently, a balance exists due to increased sensitivity resulting in an increased false positive rate. Several manufacturers now claim to reliably and reproducibly be able to count emboli mainly using ultrasound-based technology. The ability to discriminate between types of emboli and to reliably size emboli remains a difficult area.

9.2.1 Retinal Fluorescein Angiography

Using the technique of retinal fluorescein angiography (RFA) [9,10] Blauth and colleagues observed microembolic events occurring during CPB.[11]

Embryologically, the retina develops from central nervous tissue and receives its blood supply from the internal carotid artery. It is therefore regarded by many as "a window to the brain." Following enhancement of the microvasculature using injections of fluorescein dye, they took pictures of the fundus in 64 patients[12] undergoing coronary artery surgery who were randomized to either a bubble or membrane oxygenator. RFA performed 5 min prior to the termination of CPB demonstrated microembolic perfusion defects in 100% of the bubble oxygenator group compared to 44% of the membrane oxygenator group. An earlier study of 21 patients,[13] using bubble oxygenators, revealed 100% incidence of microembolic perfusion defects, the majority of which resolved by 8 days. There was a direct association between the number of occlusions and neurobehavioral deficit. A subsequent canine study[13] demonstrated the emboli to be intravascular platelet-fibrin micro aggregates.

9.2.2 Ultrasound

Using transcranial Doppler (TCD) examination, emboli have been demonstrated in vivo and these findings have been verified in the laboratory.[14,15]

The Doppler effect enables the use of ultrasound to study the velocity of red blood cells. The Doppler shift or the change in frequency of reflected sound waves due to the movement of blood is proportional to the blood velocity. Most embolic material possesses a higher acoustic contrast with plasma than red blood cells and so produces a signal of greater amplitude. The frequency, amplitude, intensity, and spectral array of the reflected signal are analyzed to make assumptions about embolic numbers, size, and material. The technique may be prone to error due to noise artifacts, orientation of the transducer, and variations in power and gain settings.[16]

Advanced ultrasound technology and complex counting algorithms including neural networking systems such as EDAC® or the EMBODOP®, which is based on multifrequency analysis, are capable of counting emboli up to 1,000 per second and estimate size in a range from 10 μm to 12.7 mm. Both systems claim to differentiate air from solid emboli in vitro but this is harder to validate in vivo.

Traditionally, the TCD probe is placed over the thin temporal bone and the sound waves are focused on the middle cerebral artery via a process called insonation. An alternative transducer location to detect emboli is over the common carotid artery which reduces the problems of insonation and allows the study of a larger proportion of the circulating cerebral blood volume.[15] Changes in an individual's TCD velocity will mirror relative changes in cerebral blood flow (CBF), but TCD is unable to provide a direct measurement of CBF.[17]

This simple, noninvasive technique provides immediate detection of emboli enabling the study of the intraoperative timing of emboli.[5,18–20] Such studies have identified manipulation of the aorta as one risk factor for the generation of emboli. Similarly using TCD, items of CPB equipment and technique have been identified as sources of emboli.[12,21,22] Most significantly, several research groups have demonstrated a positive association between the number of emboli detected intraoperatively and the incidence of postoperative brain injury.[5–7]

9.2.3 Echocardiography

Transthoracic (TTE) and transesophageal echocardiography (TOE) have also demonstrated the occurrence of emboli during cardiac surgery. TTE is limited in its usefulness intraoperatively due to the presence of an air–tissue interface. TOE utilizing the acoustic window provided by the anatomical relationship of the esophagus to the posterior aspect of the heart has further demonstrated the occurrence of gaseous emboli both during and after CPB.[23–25]

9.2.4 Pathoradiology

Using a histochemical technique, Moody and colleagues[26,27] studied the cerebral microvasculature in dogs and postmortem specimens of humans who had recently undergone CPB. The technique involves staining for endothelial alkaline phosphatase in thick celloidin sections of the brain. Subsequently, prepared slides may be viewed under the light microscope or processed for high-resolution micro radiography. They discovered focal small capillary and arteriolar dilatations or microaneurysms which they termed SCADs. The SCADs stained positive for lipid and they postulated that they represented microemboli.[28] With the development of a dog model, the group determined the timing of the microemboli[29] and an association between the number of SCADs and the return of mediastinal blood to the circulation.

9.3 Brain Imaging

Various imaging modalities are available to evaluate and quantify degree of brain damage. Computed tomography (CT),[30–32] magnetic resonance imaging (MRI),[29,33–36] single photon emission computed tomography (SPECT),[37] and cerebral ultrasound scan[38] have been used in cardiac surgery. CT and MRI are well established for examining cerebral ischemia and evaluating cerebral vascular disease.

9.3.1 Computerized Tomography

Muraoka and colleagues demonstrated with CT early reduction in brain mass following CPB conducted with bubble oxygenators; however, no clinically apparent neurologic deficit was detected.[32] In their patients, all pediatric, CT appearance returned to normal within 6–11 months. Introduction of membrane oxygenators and arterial filters into the CPB circuit reduced the occurrence of this finding, implicating ischemia secondary to emboli as the cause of the brain injury.[32]

Most brain infarcts in cardiac surgery are embolic rather than hemorrhagic.[39] Brain infarcts may not be detected by conventional CT scanning in patients with clinical evidence of stroke.[30,31] In these studies, 60–70% of patients with clinically apparent neurologic deficits have abnormal CT scan results. On the other hand, abnormalities may be detected on the CT scan without apparent clinical deficits.

9.3.2 Magnetic Resonance Imaging

In patients undergoing coronary artery bypass graft (CABG) with CPB, new brain lesions have been reported in 0% to over 40% postoperatively using MRI.[34,35,40,41] In patients undergoing valve surgery, this occurrence is almost 60%.[33] In pediatric patients undergoing repair of congenital heart disease, new infarcts were detected in over 5% of patients using MRI; however, almost all had cerebral ventricular enlargement.[42] As with CT scanning, there is a subset of patients with neurologic deficit clinically, but normal MR images.

Because conventional CT scanning and MRI are not specific enough to identify subtle brain injury, the correlation between embolic load and volume of cerebral ischemia has not yet been demonstrated. Newer radiological techniques appear more promising and may be able to establish this relationship.

9.3.3 Single Photon Emission Computed Tomography

In a group of pediatric patients with postoperative movement disorders, CT scans or MRI were normal. However, perfusion defects were demonstrated using technetium 99m-hexamethyl propylene amine oxime SPECT. These defects were found both in deep and cortical grey matter.

9.3.4 Fluid Attenuated Inversion Recovery

Fluid attenuated inversion recovery (FLAIR) utilizes magnetic resonance, and images are obtained by addition of a 180° inversion pulse prior to a spin-echo sequence allowing longitudinal magnetization of cerebral spinal fluid to reach its null point, where it does not contribute any signal. These images are more sensitive for detecting ischemic changes and edema than conventional MRI.

It is thought that patients develop some degree of brain edema on CPB, which has been shown using FLAIR images.[1] This edema may be secondary to various causes including cytotoxic edema from microemboli or hypoperfusion, hemodilution, and blood-brain barrier opening from inflammation. In most patients, the edema resolves within a week.[1]

New brain lesions may be detected with FLAIR following cardiac surgery, but with no apparent accompanying clinical neurologic deficit.[1]

9.3.5 Diffusion-Weighted Imaging

Diffusion-weighted imaging (DWI) detects disturbances in diffusion of water molecules within the brain parenchyma. Water molecules diffuse at different rates depending on the area of the brain. Diffusion is rapid through the extracellular space and is impeded by the cytoskeleton and cell membranes within cells. Brain injury causes intracellular edema resulting in focal redistribution of extracellular water into intracellular space. This redistribution of water results in restricted water diffusion potential. Restriction in diffusion causes an abnormally bright signal on DWI.

It has been shown in both animal models[43,44] and humans[45–47] that DWI detects abnormalities in the brain before manifestations of infarct on conventional MRI became apparent. Abnormalities can be identified within an hour of ischemia in experimental animals[43,44] and persist for nearly 2 weeks, at which time, conventional MRI would be expected to be abnormal.[48] Also DWI is more sensitive than conventional MRI in the acute setting[46,47] and can aid in separating acute from chronic lesions.[46] To date, there are no studies correlating DWI to embolic load during cardiac surgery.

9.3.6 Perfusion Imaging

MRI can be utilized to investigate regional brain perfusion by several methods. Selective radiofrequency inversion pulse can be used to rephase protons in a volume of blood. Inversion pulse images are then subtracted from noninverted images to obtain images of blood flow.[49]

9.3.7 Nuclear Magnetic Resonance Spectroscopy

Nuclear magnetic resonance (NMR) spectroscopy is widely used in structure analysis of chemicals. In medicine, it provides noninvasive biochemical information in-vivo utilizing conventional MRI. Nuclei of atoms spin and generate a magnetic field. When an external magnetic field is applied to the nucleus, the spin state where the magnetic field is aligned with the external field has a different, lower, energy from that spin state that gives rise to an opposing field. Because the two states have different energy levels, it is possible to convert from lower energy state to a higher state by input of suitable energy. This energy difference is such that radiofrequency waves can perform the switch. The NMR spectrum arises because nuclei in different parts of the molecule experience different local magnetic fields according to molecular structure, and so have different frequencies at which they absorb. These absorptions are plotted on a graph where the frequency differences are plotted relative to some standard compound which defines the zero baseline.

A tissue generates signals from the protons present at the intersection of slices excited by the radiofrequency pulses.[50] The spectrum generated is predominantly from water protons and is therefore suppressed by chemical-shift selective radiofrequency pulses. Various nuclei can be used for spectroscopy, including carbon-13, fluorine-19, and sodium-32. However, hydrogen [^{1}H] (proton), more commonly, and phosphorous-31 are used to evaluate brain injury.[51–53]

In proton spectroscopy, tetramethylsilane is used as the standard compound to define the zero baseline. In normal individuals, resonance peaks from lipids and lactate are not identified.[54] However, in infracted tissue there is an elevation of lactate peaks.[52,54] Other findings include a diminished *N*-acetyl aspartate peak and decrease in choline-containing compounds versus creatine ratio.[54]

9.4 Techniques and Studies to Reduce Embolization

9.4.1 *Perfusion*

The use of CPB will always be associated with the potential for intravascular embolization. Improvements in our understanding and management of the clotting system have reduced the earlier incidence of blood-derived emboli. Subsequent work has identified the type and design of CPB equipment as well as the way in which it is used to be of importance in the amount of emboli delivered to the patient. The CPB circuit may act as a source of emboli or it may potentiate embolic activity by not adequately removing circulating emboli and returning them to the arterial circulation.

Arterial line filters were an early attempt to reduce the incidence of neurobehavioural (NB) complications, arising from the well-documented occurrence of particulate embolism during CPB.[55–57] The incorporation of a micropore filter in the arterial return line of the CPB circuit not only reduces particle counts in the arterial line downstream from the filter,[58,59] but it also reduced the number of emboli detected in the middle cerebral artery[60] with an associated reduction in postoperative cerebral dysfunction.[6] Similarly, the use of membrane oxygenators as opposed to bubble oxygenators has been associated with a decrease in the number of microemboli and an improvement in NB outcome.[2,12] Leucocyte-depleting arterial filters and dynamic bubble traps may also contribute to emboli reduction.[61,62]

The design and shape of the circuit components such as the hard shell reservoir may result in the production of gaseous microemboli.[21,63] There is a difference between manufacturers as to the ability of their circuit components to remove gaseous microemboli during CPB.[64]

The perfusionist plays a key role in minimizing embolization during cardiac surgery. It has been shown that the number of times the perfusionist intervenes with the circuit to give drugs or take blood samples is positively correlated with the incidence of embolization [22,65] and neurocognitive outcome.[66] Circuit interventions should be kept to a minimum using techniques aimed at reducing the potential for air embolization. Other important associations include purging of sampling lines, high flow rates, low reservoir volumes, and bolus injections.[65]

Air entrained in the venous line either at the start of CPB or due to a nonocclusive purse string is a source of microembolization.[67,68] It is therefore key to minimize this, particularly in low prime circuits.[69] Similarly, the use of vacuum-assisted venous drainage at high levels of suction will impede the ability of the circuit components to remove entrained air.[67,68]

9.4.2 *Pharmacological*

The main therapeutic intervention to reduce emboli during CPB is adequate heparinization.[70,71] The use of platelet activation inhibitor substances such as prostacyclin[72,73] and the treatment of carotid occlusive disease is also aimed at reducing the number of intraoperative emboli.

Investigation of a pharmacological approach to reduce NB complications of open-ventricle operations requiring CPB was carried out by Slogoff[74] and Nussmeir.[75] Randomized patients received thiopental to maintain electroencephalogram (EEG) silence from before arterial cannulation to termination of CPB with significantly fewer patients exhibiting NB complications. The overall incidence of NB complications in their second study[75] was one fourth of their first study.[74] This may be due, in part, to fewer emboli being delivered to the brain because of reduced CBF secondary to thiopental decreasing metabolic function. Cerebral protection with thiopental was not, however, entirely benign. Patients receiving the drug required more frequent inotropic support than the control group; in addition, the larger dose of thiopental led to longer sleeping times, delayed endotracheal extubation, and obviously increased sedation during the first three postoperative days.

Isoflurane has been demonstrated to confer neuroprotection during periods of hypoxia and ischemia[76] but the associated increase in CBF may place the patient at increased risk of cerebral embolization.

During CPB, the technique used for acid-base management may influence the cerebral embolic load. Alpha stat management has been shown to be superior to pH stat management with regard to cerebral protection in adults undergoing mild to moderate hypothermic CPB.[77,78] During alpha stat management, the autoregulation of cerebral blood flow is maintained in comparison to pH stat when autoregulation is lost and cerebral blood flow increases. This increase in blood flow may increase the embolic load delivered to the brain.[79]

9.4.3 Surgical

Studies of the timing of intraoperative emboli have identified procedures and interventions such as application and removal of the aortic cross clamp and side clamp at times of high embolic risk.[2,18] The atherosclerotic aorta is increasingly recognized as a source of intraoperative emboli.[80] Intraoperative epiaortic ultrasound scanning or TEE may be used to identify the presence and location of plaque prior to aortic cannulation and application of the aortic cross clamp and help reduce embolization.[81,82] Some have questioned its clinical usefulness; however, this imaging my allow identification of the optimal cross-clamp and cannulation site. Similarly, alternative aortic cannulation and venting techniques have been recommended to reduce the occurrence of intraoperative emboli.[83,84] Modifying surgical technique particularly with regard to reducing the number of aortic manipulations has been associated with an improvement in neurological outcome.[7,85]

Good surgical technique can also help to reduce embolization related to intracardiac thrombus and debris from diseased heart valves. Adequate deairing with active cardiac venting guided by TEE can improve the adequacy of deairing following open heart surgery.

During surgery, blood collecting within the chest is returned to the CPB circuit via cardiotomy suction. This practice allows blood with a high fat and inflammatory mediator content to enter the circulation and an association has been demonstrated between the volume of reinfused blood and the number of cerebral fat emboli or SCADs.[26,27] Experimentally, processing the shed blood using filters and/or washing the blood with a cell saver reduces the number of SCADs.[86,87] This has led to a number of clinical trials. The two largest ones, both from Canada, reported conflicting results, with one study demonstrating no difference and the other demonstrating improved neurological outcome.[88,89] In addition, there are a number of smaller studies reporting a reduction in inflammatory mediators[90] and also a reduction in clotting factors[88,89] with a tendency toward increased postoperative bleeding[89] if shed blood is processed via a cell saver. More recently, cell salvage has been associated with improved postoperative cardiac function in association with decreased pulmonary and systemic vascular resistance.[91]

9.5 Summary

Neurological dysfunction due to embolization continues to be a significant cause of postcardiac surgery morbidity and mortality. Likely sources of emboli are atherosclerotic debris from disruption of plaques, air either entrained, propagated, or generated by the CPB apparatus and biological emboli from the reinfusion of blood lost during surgery. Techniques used to detect emboli to date have mainly been the remit of the researcher, but new techniques make everyday monitoring of patients and CPB circuits for embolic activity a realistic option. The surgical team needs to be aware of the possibility of emboli, and by using appropriate equipment, good techniques, and clear communication, the incidence of embolic damage may be reduced. Further research is needed to reduce and preferably eliminate emboli; however, this goal may be unlikely and therefore research should also focus on techniques to reduce the effects of emboli should they occur.

References

1. Harris DN, Bailey SM, Smith PL, Taylor KM, Oatridge A, Bydder GM. Brain swelling in first hour after coronary artery bypass surgery [see comments]. *Lancet*. 1993; 342(8871):586-587.
2. Padayachee TS, Parsons S, Theobold R, Linley J, Gosling RG, Deverall PB. The detection of microemboli in the middle cerebral artery during cardiopulmonary bypass: a transcranial Doppler ultrasound investigation using membrane and bubble oxygenators. *Ann Thorac Surg*. 1987;44(3):298-302.
3. Blauth C, Smith P, Newman S, et al. Retinal microembolism and neuropsychological deficit following clinical cardiopulmonary bypass: comparison of a membrane and a bubble oxygenator. A preliminary communication. *Eur J Cardio-Thorac Surg*. 1989;3(2):135-138. discussion 139.
4. Kurusz M. Gaseous microemboli: sources, causes, and clinical considerations. *Med Instrument*. 1985;19:73-75.
5. Clark RE, Brillman J, Davis DA, Lovell MR, Price TR, Magovern GJ. Microemboli during coronary artery bypass grafting. Genesis and effect on outcome [see comments]. *J Thorac Cardiovasc Sur*. 1995;109(2):249-257. discussion 257-248.
6. Pugsley W, Klinger L, Paschalis C, Treasure T, Harrison M, Newman S. The impact of microemboli during cardiopulmonary bypass on neuropsychological functioning. *Stroke*. 1994;25(7):1393-1399.
7. Hammon JW Jr, Stump DA, Kon ND, et al. Risk factors and solutions for the development of neurobehavioral changes after coronary artery bypass grafting. *Ann Thorac Surg*. 1997;63(6):1613-1618.
8. Butler BD, Kurusz M. Embolic Events. In: Gravlee GP, Davis RF, Kurusz M, Utley J, eds. *Cardiopulmonary Bypass: Principles and Practice*. 2nd ed. Philadelphia, PA: Lippincott Williams & Wilkins; 2000:320-341.
9. Williams IM. Intravascular changes in the retina during open-heart surgery. *Lancet*. 1971;2(7726):688-691.
10. Williams IM. Retinal vascular occlusions in open heart surgery. *Brit J Ophthalmol*. 1975;59(2):81-91.
11. Blauth C, Arnold J, Kohner EM, Taylor KM. Retinal microembolism during cardiopulmonary bypass demonstrated by fluorescein angiography. *Lancet*. 1986;2(8511):837-839.
12. Blauth CI, Smith PL, Arnold JV, Jagoe JR, Wootton R, Taylor KM. Influence of oxygenator type on the prevalence and extent of microembolic retinal ischemia during cardiopulmonary bypass Assessment by digital image analysis. *J Thorac Cardiovasc Sur*. 1990;99(1):61-69.
13. Blauth CI, Arnold JV, Schulenberg WE, McCartney AC, Taylor KM. Cerebral microembolism during cardiopulmonary bypass Retinal microvascular studies in vivo with fluorescein angiography. *J Thorac Cardiovasc Surg*. 1988;95(4):668-676.
14. Pugsley W. The use of Doppler ultrasound in the assessment of microemboli during cardiac surgery. *Perfusion*. 1989;4:115-122.
15. Stump DA, Stein CS, Tegeler CH, et al. Validity and reliability of a device for detecting carotid emboli. *J Neuroimag*. 1991;1:18-22.
16. Deal DD, Stump DA, Brooker MD. Ultrasonic monitoring for emboli in the operating room: errors of detection. *J Neuroimag*. 1997;7:254 (Abstract).
17. Trivedi UH, Patel RL, Turtle MR, Venn GE, Chambers DJ. Relative changes in cerebral blood flow during cardiac operations using xenon-133 clearance versus transcranial Doppler sonography [see comments] [published erratum appears in Ann Thorac Surg 1997 Oct;64(4):1228]. *Ann Thorac Surg*. 1997;63(1):167-174.
18. van der Linden J, Casimir-Ahn H. When do cerebral emboli appear during open heart operations? A transcranial Doppler study [see comments]. *Ann Thorac Surg*. 1991;51(2): 237-241.
19. Stump DA, Rogers AT, Hammon JW, Newman SP. Cerebral emboli and cognitive outcome after cardiac surgery. *J Cardiothorac Vasc Anesth*. 1996;10(1):113-118. quiz 118-119.
20. Yao FS, Barbut D, Hager DN, Trifiletti RR, Gold JP. Detection of aortic emboli by transesophageal echocardiography during coronary artery bypass surgery. *J Cardiothorac Vasc Anest*. 1996;10(3):314-317.
21. Mitchell SJ, Willcox T, McDougal C, Gorman DF. Emboli generation by the Medtronic Maxima hard-shell adult venous reservoir in cardiopulmonary bypass circuits: a preliminary report. *Perfusion*. 1996;11(2):145-155.
22. Taylor RL, Borger MA, Weisel RD, Fedorko L, Feindel CM. Cerebral microemboli during cardiopulmonary bypass: increased emboli during perfusionist interventions. *Ann Thorac Surg*. 1999;68(1):89-93.
23. Duff HJ, Buda AJ, Kramer R, Strauss HD, David TE, Berman ND. Detection of entrapped intracardiac air with intraoperative echocardiography. *Am J Cardiol*. 1980; 46(2):255-260.
24. Oka Y, Moriwaki KM, Hong Y, et al. Detection of air emboli in the left heart by M-Mode transesophageal echocardiography following cardiopulmonary bypass. *Anesthesiology*. 1985;63:109-113.
25. Oka Y, Inoue T, Hong Y, Sisto DA, Strom JA, Frater RW. Retained intracardiac air. Transesophageal echocardiography for definition of incidence and monitoring removal by improved techniques. *J Thorac Cardiovasc Surg*. 1986;91(3): 329-338.
26. Moody DM, Bell MA, Challa VR, Johnston WE, Prough DS. Brain microemboli during cardiac surgery or aortography [see comments]. *Ann Neurol*. 1990;28(4):477-486.
27. Brown WR, Moody DM, Challa VR, Stump DA. Histologic studies of brain microemboli in humans and dogs after cardiopulmonary bypass. *Echocard J Cardiovasc Ultra Allied Technol*. 1996;13(5):559-565.
28. Challa VR, Moody DM, Troost BT. Brain embolic phenomena associated with cardiopulmonary bypass. *J Neurol Sci*. 1993;117(1-2):224-231.
29. Moody DM, Brown WR, Challa VR, Stump DA, Reboussin DM, Legault C. Brain microemboli associated with cardiopulmonary bypass: a histologic and magnetic resonance imaging study. *Ann Thorac Surg*. 1995;59(5):1304-1307.
30. Libman RB, Wirkowski E, Neystat M, Barr W, Gelb S, Graver M. Stroke associated with cardiac surgery. Determinants, timing, and stroke subtypes. *Arch Neurol*. 1997; 54(1):83-8.
31. Aberg T, Ronquist G, Tyden H, et al. Adverse effects on the brain in cardiac operations as assessed by biochemical, psychometric, and radiologic methods. *J Thorac Cardiovasc Surg*. 1984;87(1):99-105.

32. Muraoka R, Yokota M, Aoshima M, et al. Subclinical changes in brain morphology following cardiac operations as reflected by computed tomographic scans of the brain. *J Thorac Cardiovasc Surg*. 1981;81(3):364-369.
33. Steinberg GK, De La Paz R, Mitchell RS, Bell TE, Albers GW. MR and cerebrospinal fluid enzymes as sensitive indicators of subclinical cerebral injury after open-heart valve replacement surgery. *Am J Neuroradiol*. 1996;17(2):205-212. discussion 213-205.
34. Simonson TM, Yuh WT, Hindman BJ, Embrey RP, Halloran JI, Behrendt DM. Contrast MR of the brain after high-perfusion cardiopulmonary bypass. *Am J Neuroradiol*. 1994; 15(1):3-7.
35. Vik A, Brubakk AO, Rinck PA, Sande E, Levang OW, Sellevold O. MRI: a method to detect minor brain damage following coronary bypass surgery? *Neuroradiology*. 1991; 33(5):396-398.
36. Sellman M, Hindmarsh T, Ivert T, Semb BK. Magnetic resonance imaging of the brain before and after open heart operations [see comments]. *Ann Thorac Surg*. 1992;53(5): 807-812.
37. Marochnik S, Alexandrov AV, Anthone D, Lewin C, Caldwell CB, Pullicino PM. Feasibility of SPECT for studies of brain perfusion during cardiopulmonary bypass. *J Neuroimag*. 1996;6(4):243-245.
38. Krull F, Latta K, Hoyer PF, Ziemer G, Kallfelz HC. Cerebral ultrasonography before and after cardiac surgery in infants. *Pediatr Cardiol*. Jul-Aug 1994;15(4):159-162.
39. Stump DA, Kon NA, Rogers AT, Hammon JW. Emboli and neuropsychological outcome following cardiopulmonary bypass. *Echocardiography*. 1996;13:1.
40. Schmidt R, Fazekas F, Offenbacher H, et al. Brain magnetic resonance imaging in coronary artery bypass grafts: a pre- and postoperative assessment. *Neurology*. Apr 1993; 43(4):775-778.
41. Toner I, Hamid SK, Peden CJ, Taylor KM, Smith PL. Magnetic resonance imaging and P300 (event-related auditory evoked potentials) in the assessment of postoperative cerebral injury following coronary artery bypass graft surgery. *Perfusion*. 1993;8(4):321-329.
42. McConnell JR, Fleming WH, Chu WK, et al. Magnetic resonance imaging of the brain in infants and children before and after cardiac surgery. A prospective study [see comments]. *Am J Dis Child*. 1990;144(3):374-378.
43. Mintorovitch J, Moseley ME, Chileuitt L, Shimizu H, Cohen Y, Weinstein PR. Comparison of diffusion- and T2-weighted MRI for the early detection of cerebral ischemia and reperfusion in rats. *Magn Reson Med*. 1991;18(1):39-50.
44. Moseley ME, Cohen Y, Mintorovitch J, et al. Early detection of regional cerebral ischemia in cats: comparison of diffusion- and T2-weighted MRI and spectroscopy. *Magn Reson Med*. May 1990;14(2):330-346.
45. Marks MP, de Crespigny A, Lentz D, Enzmann DR, Albers GW, Moseley ME. Acute and chronic stroke: navigated spin-echo diffusion-weighted MR imaging [published erratum appears in Radiology 1996 Jul;200(1):289]. *Radiology*. 1996;199(2):403-408.
46. Lutsep HL, Albers GW, DeCrespigny A, Kamat GN, Marks MP, Moseley ME. Clinical utility of diffusion-weighted magnetic resonance imaging in the assessment of ischemic stroke [see comments]. *Ann Neurol*. 1997;41(5):574-580.
47. Warach S, Dashe JF, Edelman RR. Clinical outcome in ischemic stroke predicted by early diffusion-weighted and perfusion magnetic resonance imaging: a preliminary analysis. *J Cereb Blood Flow Metab*. Jan 1996;16(1):53-59.
48. Baird DL, Murkin JM, Lee DL. Neurologic findings in coronary artery bypass patients: perioperative or preexisting? *J Cardiothorac Vasc Anesth*. 1997;11(6):694-698.
49. Siewert B, Schlaug G, Edelman RR, Warach S. Comparison of EPISTAR and T2*-weighted gadolinium-enhanced perfusion imaging in patients with acute cerebral ischemia. *Neurology*. Mar 1997;48(3):673-679.
50. Brant-Zawadzki M, Weinstein P, Bartkowski H, Moseley M. MR imaging and spectroscopy in clinical and experimental cerebral ischemia: a review. *Am J Roentgenol*. Mar 1987; 148(3):579-588.
51. Frahm J, Bruhn H, Gyngell ML, Merboldt KD, Hanicke W, Sauter R. Localized high-resolution proton NMR spectroscopy using stimulated echoes: initial applications to human brain in vivo. *Magn Reson Med*. Jan 1989;9(1):79-93.
52. Graham GD, Blamire AM, Howseman AM, et al. Proton magnetic resonance spectroscopy of cerebral lactate and other metabolites in stroke patients. *Stroke*. Mar 1992;23(3): 333-340.
53. Gillard JH, Barker PB, van Zijl PC, Bryan RN, Oppenheimer SM. Proton MR spectroscopy in acute middle cerebral artery stroke. *Am J Neuroradiol*. May 1996;17(5):873-886.
54. Bruhn H, Frahm J, Gyngell ML, Merboldt KD, Hanicke W, Sauter R. Cerebral metabolism in man after acute stroke: new observations using localized proton NMR spectroscopy. *Magn Reson Med*. Jan 1989;9(1):126-131.
55. Ehrenhaft JL, Claman MA, Layton JM, Zimmerman GR. Cerebral complications of open-heart surgery. *J Thorac Cardiovasc Surg*. 1961;41:503-508.
56. Lindberg DA, Lucas FV, Sheagren J, Malm JR. Silicone embolization during clinical and experimental heart surgery employing a bubble oxygenator. *Am J Pathol*. 1961;39: 129-144.
57. Miller JA, Fonkalsrud EW, Harrison LL, Maloney JV. Fat embolism associated with extracorporeal circulation and blood transfusion. *Surgery*. 1962;51:448-451.
58. Osborn JJ, Swank RL, Hill JD, Aguilar MJ, Gerbode F. Clinical use of a Dacron wool filter during perfusion for open-heart surgery. *J Thorac Cardiovasc Surg*. 1970;60: 575-581.
59. Loop FD, Szabo J, Rowlinson RD, Urbanek K. Events related to microembolism during extracorporeal perfusion in man: effectiveness of in-line filtration recorded by ultrasound. *Ann Thorac Surg*. 1976;21:412-420.
60. Padayachee TS, Parsons S, Theobold R, Gosling RG, Deverall PB. The effect of arterial filtration on reduction of gaseous microemboli in the middle cerebral artery during cardiopulmonary bypass. *Ann Thorac Surg*. 1988;45(6): 647-649.
61. Whitaker DC, Newman SP, Stygall J, Hope-Wynne C, Harrison MJG, Walesby RK. The effect of leucocyte-depleting arterial line filters on cerebral microemboli and neuropsychological outcome following coronary artery bypass surgery. *Eur J Cardio-Thorac Surg*. Feb 2004;25(2): 267-274.
62. Perthel M, Kseibi S, Bendisch A, Laas J. Use of a dynamic bubble trap in the arterial line reduces microbubbles during

cardiopulmonary bypass and microembolic signals in the middle cerebral artery. *Perfusion.* May 2005;20(3): 151-156.
63. Mitchell SJ, Willcox T, Gorman DF. Bubble generation and venous air filtration by hard-shell venous reservoirs: a comparative study. *Perfusion.* 1997;12(5):325-333.
64. Jones TJ, Deal DD, Vernon JC, Blackburn N, Stump DA. How effective are cardiopulmonary bypass circuits at removing gaseous microemboli?[see comment]. *J Extra-Corporeal Technol.* 2002;34(1):34-39.
65. Rodriguez RA, Williams KA, Babaev A, Rubens F, Nathan HJ. Effect of perfusionist technique on cerebral embolization during cardiopulmonary bypass. *Perfusion.* Jan 2005; 20(1):3-10.
66. Borger MA, Peniston CM, Weisel RD, Vasiliou M, Green RE, Feindel CM. Neuropsychologic impairment after coronary bypass surgery: effect of gaseous microemboli during perfusionist interventions. *J Thorac Cardiovasc Surg.* Apr 2001;121(4):743-749.
67. Willcox TW, Mitchell SJ, Gorman DF. Venous air in the bypass circuit: a source of arterial line emboli exacerbated by vacuum-assisted drainage. *Ann Thorac Surg.* 1999; 68(4):1285-1289.
68. Jones TJ, Deal DD, Vernon JC, Blackburn N, Stump DA. Does vacuum-assisted venous drainage increase gaseous microemboli during cardiopulmonary bypass? *Ann Thorac Surg.* 2002;74(6):2132-2137.
69. Norman MJ, Sistino JJ, Acsell JR. The effectiveness of low-prime cardiopulmonary bypass circuits at removing gaseous emboli. *J Extra-Corp Technol.* Dec 2004;36(4):336-342.
70. Young JA, Kisker CT, Doty DB. Adequate anticoagulation during cardiopulmonary bypass determined by activated clotting time and the appearance of fibrin monomer. *Ann Thorac Surg.* 1978;26(3):231-240.
71. Esposito RA, Culliford AT, Colvin SB, Thomas SJ, Lackner H, Spencer FC. The role of the activated clotting time in heparin administration and neutralization for cardiopulmonary bypass. *J Thorac Cardiovasc Surg.* 1983;85(2): 174-185.
72. Radegran K, Aren C, Teger-Nilsson A. Prostacyclin infusion during extracorporeal circulation for coronary bypass. *J Thorac Cardiovasc Surg.* 1982;83:205-211.
73. Longmore DB, Bennett G, Gueirrara D, et al. Prostacyclin: a solution to some problems of extracorporeal circulation. *Lancet.* 1979;1:1002-1005.
74. Slogoff S, Girgis KZ, Keats AS. Etiologic factors in neuropsychiatric complications associated with cardiopulmonary bypass. *Anesth Analgesia.* 1982;61:903-911.
75. Nussmeier NA, Arlund C, Slogoff S. Neuropsychiatric complications after cardiopulmonary bypass: cerebral protection by a barbiturate. *Anesthesiology.* 1986;64(2):165-170.
76. Newberg LA, Michenfelder JD. Cerebral protection by isoflurane during hypoxemia or ischemia. *Anesthesiology.* 1983;59:29-35.
77. Bashein G, Townes BD, Nessly ML, Bledsoe SW, Hornbein TF. Carbon dioxide management during hypothermic cardiopulmonary bypass. *Anesthesiology.* 1989;71(Suppl 3A):A35.
78. Patel RL, Turtle MR, Chambers DJ, James DN, Newman S, Venn GE. Alpha-stat acid-base regulation during cardiopulmonary bypass improves neuropsychologic outcome in patients undergoing coronary artery bypass grafting [see comments]. *J Thorac Cardiovasc Surg.* 1996;111(6): 1267-1279.
79. Henriksen L, Hjelms E, Lindeburgh T. Brain hyperperfusion during cardiac operations. *J Thorac Cardiovasc Surg.* 1983;86:202-208.
80. Davila-Roman VG, Barzilai B, Wareing TH, Murphy SF, Schechtman KB, Kouchoukos NT. Atherosclerosis of the ascending aorta. Prevalence and role as an independent predictor of cerebrovascular events in cardiac patients. *Stroke.* 1994;25(10):2010-2016.
81. Wareing TH, Davila-Roman VG, Barzilai B, Murphy SF, Kouchoukos NT. Management of the severely atherosclerotic ascending aorta during cardiac operations. A strategy for detection and treatment. *J Thorac Cardiovasc Surg.* 1992;103(3):453-462.
82. Davila-Roman VG, Phillips KJ, Daily BB, Davila RM, Kouchoukos NT, Barzilai B. Intraoperative transesophageal echocardiography and epiaortic ultrasound for assessment of atherosclerosis of the thoracic aorta. *J Am Coll Cardiol.* 1996;28(4):942-947.
83. Culliford AT, Colvin SB, Rohrer K, Baumann FG, Spencer FC. The atherosclerotic ascending aorta and transverse arch: a new technique to prevent cerebral injury during bypass: experience with 13 patients. *Ann Thorac Surg.* 1986;41(1): 27-35.
84. Borger MA, Taylor RL, Weisel RD, et al. Decreased cerebral emboli during distal aortic arch cannulation: a randomized clinical trial. *J Thorac Cardiovasc Surg.* 1999;118(4): 740-745.
85. Hammon JW, Stump DA, Butterworth JF, et al. Coronary artery bypass grafting with single cross clamp results in fewer persistent neuropsychological deficits than multiple clamp or off-pump coronary artery bypass grafting. *Ann Thorac Surg.* Oct 2007;84(4):1174-1178. discussion 1178-1179.
86. Brooker RF, Brown WR, Moody DM, et al. Cardiotomy suction: a major source of brain lipid emboli during cardiopulmonary bypass. *Ann Thorac Surg.* 1998;65(6):1651-1655.
87. Kincaid EH, Jones TJ, Stump DA, et al. Processing scavenged blood with a cell saver reduces cerebral lipid microembolization. *Ann Thorac Surg.* 2000;70(4):1296-1300.
88. Djaiani G, Fedorko L, Borger MA, et al. Continuous-flow cell saver reduces cognitive decline in elderly patients after coronary bypass surgery [see comment]. *Circulation.* Oct 23 2007;116(17):1888-1895.
89. Rubens FD, Boodhwani M, Mesana T, et al. The cardiotomy trial: a randomized, double-blind study to assess the effect of processing of shed blood during cardiopulmonary bypass on transfusion and neurocognitive function. *Circulation.* Sep 11 2007;116(11):I89-97.
90. Walpoth BH, Eggensperger N, Hauser SP, et al. Effects of unprocessed and processed cardiopulmonary bypass blood retransfused into patients after cardiac surgery. *Int J Art Organs.* 1999;22(4):210-216.
91. Boodhwani M, Nathan HJ, Mesana TG, Rubens FD, Cardiotomy I. Effects of shed mediastinal blood on cardiovascular and pulmonary function: a randomized, double-blind study. *Ann Thorac Surg.* October 1, 2008;86(4): 1167-1173.

Intraoperative Brain Monitoring in Cardiac Surgery

10

Joseph E. Arrowsmith and Maruthi S.S.R. Ganugapenta

"If the brain was simple enough to understand, we would be too simple to understand it!"

10.1 Introduction

In most centers, continuous monitoring of clinical variables (Table 10.1) during cardiac surgical procedures is considered sufficient to ensure the well-being of the central nervous system and, by logical extension, minimize the risk of perioperative neurological complications. An overwhelming body of evidence, however, indicates that neurological injury may occur following technically successful and seemingly uneventful surgery.[1–3]

Although a variety of monitors of brain substrate delivery and neurological function have been commercially available for many years, they have yet to be universally adopted as "standard of care"[4] and their use remains largely confined to specialist centers, researchers, and enthusiasts. Although the capital cost of equipment is often cited as a deterrent to the more widespread use of neurological monitoring in the setting of cardiac surgery, the most significant barrier is undoubtedly the paucity of incontrovertible (i.e., level 1A) evidence of outcome benefit. It should be borne in mind, however, that the current intraoperative "standard of care" (i.e., monitoring the electrocardiograph, blood pressure, and arterial oxygen saturation) is not supported by the level of evidence demanded of neurological monitoring!

J.E. Arrowsmith (✉)
Department of Anaesthesia and Intensive Care, Papworth Hospital, Papworth Everard, Cambridgeshire, UK
e-mail: jea@nhs.net

A secondary issue when considering the efficacy of a new neurological monitoring device is the failure to make an explicit distinction between *outcome prediction* and *outcome modification* (Fig. 10.1).

A monitor that offers no "window of opportunity" to modify outcome, despite being capable of predicting an adverse neurological outcome with a high degree of specificity and sensitivity, is arguably of no clinical use. The characteristics of an ideal neurological monitor can be summarized as follows:

(a) Safety (i.e., non-invasive or minimally invasive) and physical practicability
(b) High sensitivity and specificity for *reversible* injury
(c) An unambiguous threshold for intervention
(d) Resistance to the effects of anesthetic agents, temperature, and existing neurological dysfunction
(e) Imperviousness to radiofrequency interference
(f) Low cost (disposables, storage media, operator time, and training)
(g) Approved by the operating surgeon
(h) Unambiguous neurological and neuropsychological outcome prediction

This last characteristic would be particularly useful. The declining incidence of clinically obvious focal neurological injury (i.e., stroke) after cardiac surgery has prompted investigators to focus instead on cognitive dysfunction, which is reported to be far more common.[1–3] Unfortunately, formal cognitive function testing is time-consuming and costly and the choice, timing of administration, and scoring of tests remain the subjects of international debate.[5]

The purpose of this chapter is to review the underlying principles and clinical uses of neurological monitoring devices currently available.

R.S. Bonser et al. (eds.), *Brain Protection in Cardiac Surgery*,
DOI: 10.1007/978-1-84996-293-3_10, © Springer-Verlag London Limited 2011

Table 10.1 Neurological monitoring during cardiac surgery

Clinical	Arterial pressure
	Central venous pressure
	CPB pump flow rate
	Arterial oxygen saturation
	Temperature
	Hemoglobin concentration
	Pupil size
	Arterial PCO_2
Substrate delivery	Transcranial Doppler sonography
	Near-infrared spectroscopy
	Jugular venous oxygen saturation
Cerebral activity	Electroencephalography
	Somatosensory-evoked potentials
	Auditory-evoked potentials
	Motor-evoked potentials
Other	Epiaortic ultrasound
	Transesophageal echocardiography

CPB cardiopulmonary bypass

10.2 Routine Clinical Monitoring

Specialized neurological monitoring devices should be regarded as an adjunct to, rather than a replacement for, standard clinical monitoring. The risk of neurological injury may be reduced by early detection of aortic cannula displacement and venous air entrainment, as well as the avoidance of hypoxia, hypoglycemia, acidosis, gross anemia, prolonged cerebral hypoperfusion, and cerebral hyperthermia.

Continuous invasive hemodynamic monitoring is a key component of the management of cardiac anesthesia. The function of pressure transducers, which are traditionally sited at the level of the left atrium, and manometer tubing, should be critically assessed at regular intervals. Cerebral perfusion pressure (CPP) is dependent upon mean arterial pressure (MAP), intracranial pressure (ICP), and central venous pressure (CVP); CPP = MAP − (ICP + CVP). A marked elevation in CVP during displacement of the heart, even in the presence of a seemingly adequate MAP, may result in significant cerebral hypoperfusion. Quite what represents optimal CPP during CPB remains the subject of considerable debate.[6–9] Indeed, a recent evidence-based appraisal[10] suggests that the level of evidence supporting most "neuroprotective" CPB management strategies, regarded as "standard of care," is low to intermediate (i.e., class IIb).

At temperatures >30°C cerebral autoregulation (flow–metabolism coupling) is essentially preserved so that cerebral blood flow (CBF) across a wide range of MAP is governed by $PaCO_2$.[11] At $PaCO_2$ <3.0 kPa (22 mmHg) CBF may be reduced by more than half leading to cerebral ischemia, whereas at $PaCO_2$ >9 kPa (67 mmHg) CBF may be more than doubled, resulting in the delivery of greater numbers of microemboli to

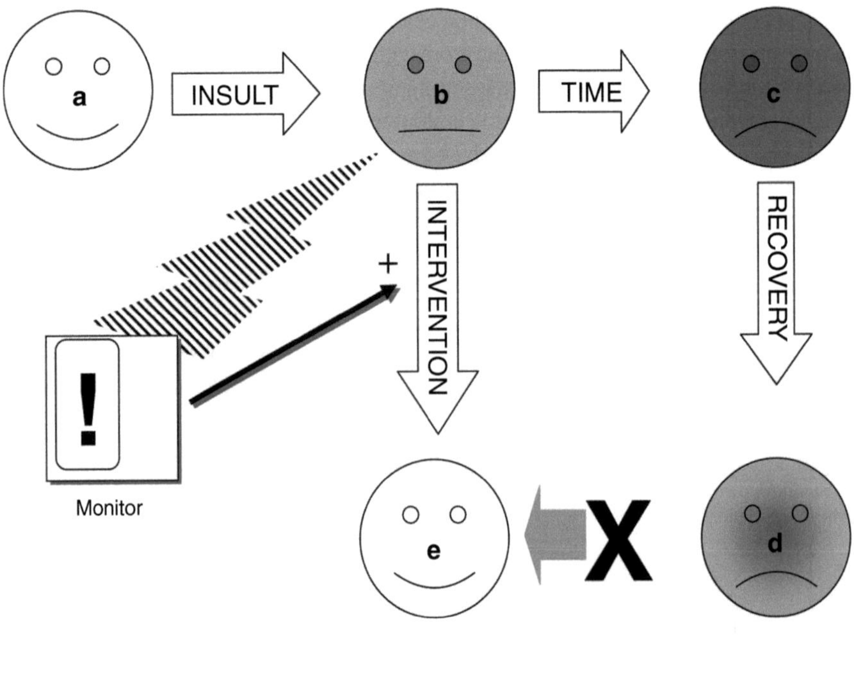

Fig. 10.1 A theoretical model for neurological monitoring. *Outcome prediction:* In response to a physiological insult, a normally functioning brain (**a**) displays evidence of dysfunction (**b**) that is detected by a neurological monitor. In time the dysfunction becomes more severe (**c**) and when the physiological insult is removed functional recovery is incomplete (**d**). *Outcome modification:* Intervention to remove the physiological insult at the point at which dysfunction is detected (**b**) leads to complete functional recovery (**e**)

the cerebral circulation. At lower temperatures, autoregulation and CO_2 reactivity are gradually lost and progressive cerebral "vasoparesis" renders CBF pressure passive.[12]

A tympanic membrane sensor or thermistor placed in the nasopharynx or bladder is the most common method of monitoring core body temperature during cardiac surgery. While these devices are accurate to within a few tenths of 1°C at steady state, evidence suggests that they are subject to hysteresis during periods of temperature change and, as a consequence, may significantly underestimate jugular venous (brain) temperature during rewarming.[13–15]

10.3 Jugular Venous Oximetry

In much the same way that mixed venous oxygen saturation (SvO_2) monitoring provides a measure of the adequacy of total body perfusion, jugular venous oxygen saturation (SjO_2) monitoring provides a measure of the global balance between cerebral oxygen supply and demand. Cerebral metabolic rate ($CMRO_2$) approximately equals CBF x (SaO_2 – SjO_2). The normal range for SvO_2 is quoted to be 55–75%, but may be as high as 85% in some normal individuals.[16] An SvO_2 <50% is regarded as being indicative of inadequate cerebral oxygenation. A normal or near-normal SjO_2 value may, however, mask regional cerebral ischemia; thus SjO_2 monitoring has high specificity but low sensitivity for the detection of cerebral ischemia.

Historically, SjO_2 was determined by analysis of samples of blood drawn from the jugular bulb. Sampling at this level is required to avoid or minimize contamination from extracranial veins – the occipital, pharyngeal, facial, lingual, and thyroid veins. Retrograde cannulation of the internal jugular vein (IJV) using the Seldinger technique, as used by Gejrot and Lauren[17] to facilitate venography, remains the technique of choice. Radiographic confirmation of catheter tip position is recommended. The tip should lie above the level of C_2 on a lateral radiograph, and should lie cranial to a line crossing the C_1–C_2 interspace, cranial to a line joining the tips of the mastoid processes and caudal to the lower margin of the orbit.[18, 19] Complications associated with catheter insertion (hemorrhage, arterial puncture, nerve injury, pneumothorax) are remarkably rare, although prolonged monitoring may be associated with infective and thrombotic complications.[20] Despite correct catheter placement, jugular bulb samples may become contaminated if blood is withdrawn rapidly. Values for SjO_2 may be as much as 25% higher if the withdrawal rate exceeds 2 mL/min.[21] Problems associated with intermittent blood sampling are largely avoided by the use of fiberoptic oximetry catheters, which permit continuous SjO_2 monitoring. Currently available devices emit two[22, 23] or three wavelengths of light, the latter being capable of compensating for changes in hemoglobin concentration.

In normal subjects, left and right SjO_2 are said to be similar. On the assumption that blood from the cerebral hemispheres drains into the ipsilateral IJV it would seem reasonable to use ipsilateral SjO_2 monitoring in a patient with a focal cerebral lesion. Interestingly, when Stocchetti and colleagues[24] performed bilateral SjO_2 monitoring in 32 head-injured patients, they were unable to demonstrate any relationship between SjO_2 and the anatomic site of injury. The optimal site for monitoring appears to be the larger or dominant IJV, which can be determined by ultrasound or computed tomography.

10.3.1 *Intraoperative SjO_2 Monitoring*

The principle uses of SjO_2 monitoring during cardiac surgery have been to assess the adequacy of cerebral oxygenation during CPB and to monitor the impact of rewarming on cerebral oxygen balance. Cook and colleagues[25] measured CBF, cerebral oxygen delivery (CDO_2), and cerebral metabolic rate ($CMRO_2$) in 60 patients randomized to either normothermic (37°C) or hypothermic (27°C) CPB. In normothermic patients, CBF was increased secondary to hemodilution and a fall in cerebral vascular resistance (CVR); and cerebral flow/metabolism coupling remained intact (i.e., $CDO_2 \propto CMRO_2$). In hypothermic patients, both CDO_2 and $CMRO_2$ fell with evidence of flow/metabolism uncoupling (i.e., $CDO_2 \propto CMRO_2$); and CBF and CVR did not change from pre-CPB levels.

Because traditional measures of core temperature may not accurately track brain temperature, SvO_2 monitoring has been postulated as a means of ensuring the adequacy of cerebral cooling prior to deep hypothermic circulatory arrest (DHCA). Low SjO_2 prior to the onset of DHCA is associated with adverse neurological outcome.[26] In a study of 17 infants undergoing cardiac surgery at <15°C, Kern and colleagues[27] found that six (29%) had significantly lower SjO_2 at a tympanic membrane temperature of 15 °C (87±6% vs. 98±1%). It was concluded that this observation represented potentially deleterious inadequate cerebral cooling that could not be predicted by conventional monitoring. In a subsequent study, the same group[28] demonstrated that a more aggressive CPB cooling strategy significantly improved SjO_2-monitored brain cooling.

The impact of rewarming on SjO_2 and cerebral lactate production was studied by Sapire and colleagues[29] in 19 patients undergoing moderate hypothermic CPB. During stable hypothermic CPB (~26°C), the rise in SjO_2 (61±8%→80±7%) was found to be directly related to temperature and $PaCO_2$. During rewarming SjO_2 fell to 43±13%. Sixteen patients had a reduction in SjO_2 <50% for an average duration of 32 min, and increased anaerobic cerebral metabolism developed in 11 patients. Changes in SjO_2 were dependent on MAP hematocrit, and rate of rewarming. The observation that SjO_2 falls during rewarming, which has been demonstrated by others,[30] suggests that reducing the rate of rewarming might be of benefit. Interestingly, Von Knobelsdorff and colleagues[31] could not confirm the putative benefit of slower rewarming on SjO_2 and concluded that changes in SjO_2 were related to temperature rather than rewarming rate. The following year, the same group[32] demonstrated that deliberate, modest hypercapnia ($PaCO_2 \geq 6$ kPa; 45 mmHg) significantly reduced jugular bulb desaturation during rewarming.

Diabetics are known to have impaired cerebral autoregulation, characterized by increased oxygen extraction, during CPB.[33] Similarly, it has long been known that patients with existing cerebrovascular disease are at greater risk of neurological injury during cardiac surgery.[34, 35] In a study of patients undergoing coronary artery bypass graft (CABG) surgery, Kadoi and colleagues[36] compared SjO_2 during normothermic CPB in ten diabetic patients and nine patients with preexisting stroke with 19 control patients matched for age, height and weight. Arterial pressure, $PaCO_2$ and hematocrit were maintained at similar levels in all groups. At 20 and 40 min after the onset of CPB there were significant differences in SjO_2 (at 20 min: stroke 46±9%, diabetics 48±5%, controls 62±7%; at 40 min: stroke 49±4%, diabetics 47±5%, controls 63±5%; $p<0.05$). There were no significant differences in SjO_2 at other study time points. In a small follow-up study[37] hypothermic CPB was not associated with cerebral desaturation in diabetic patients. The same group[38] then examined the impact of deliberately increasing MAP to baseline levels during CPB in a cohort of 20 diabetics and 20 matched controls undergoing tepid (34.5–36°C) CPB. In insulin-dependent diabetics, increasing MAP was found to have no impact on SjO_2.

Goto and colleagues,[27] in a study of 121 elderly patients undergoing CABG surgery with hypothermic CPB, investigated the impact of cerebrovascular disease on cerebral oxygenation during CPB. The 65 (54%) patients found to have small cerebral infarcts on preoperative magnetic resonance imaging had significantly lower SjO_2 values at initiation of CPB and during rewarming.

DHCA has long been used for cerebral protection during aortic arch surgery. An alternative strategy is selective antegrade cerebral perfusion (SACP), which is purported to provide superior cerebral protection and to increase the period of "safe" circulatory arrest. SjO_2 monitoring in the setting of SACP suggests that the technique provides adequate cerebral oxygenation during both deep and moderate hypothermia.[39, 40]

10.3.2 Neurological Outcome

The critical level at which SjO_2 is predictive of neurological injury following cardiac surgery is unknown. In the setting of the neurosurgical ICU, episodes of SjO_2 <50% lasting more than 10 min have been shown to be associated with poorer outcome after head trauma. In one study,[41] a single desaturation episode increased the probability of poorer outcome from 55% to 74%, whereas multiple episodes resulted in a 90% probability of poorer outcome.

In a study of 255 patients undergoing cardiac surgery under hypothermic CPB, Croughwell and colleagues[42] tested the hypothesis that cerebral desaturation contributes to postoperative cognitive dysfunction. Cognitive impairment (defined as ≥1 SD fall in test performance in ≥20% tests) was found in 96 (38%) patients at discharge. Using two multiple logistic regression models, predictors of cognitive impairment were: baseline cognitive function, educational level, SjO_2, and maximum cerebral arterial–venous oxygen content difference ($C[a\text{-}v]O_2$) (Fig. 10.2).

The rate of rewarming seems to have its greatest impact on elderly patients.[43] A subsequent study of

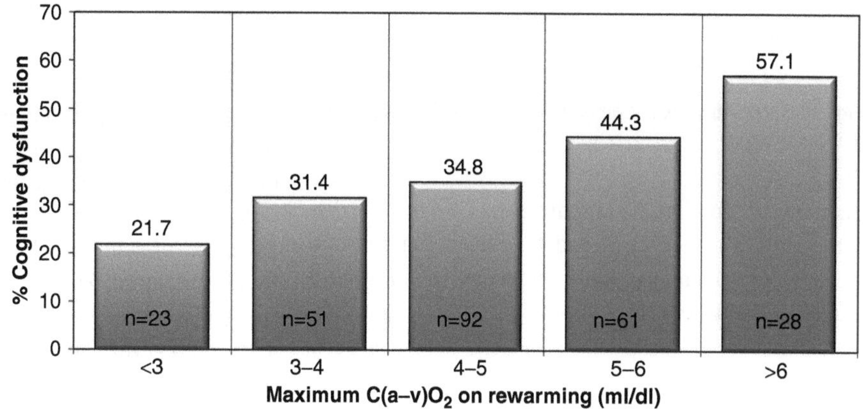

Fig. 10.2 The frequency of cognitive dysfunction in relation to maximum cerebral arterial–venous oxygen content difference at normothermia in 96 patients with postoperative cognitive dysfunction. (Reproduced from Croughwell et al.[42] With permission)

165 patients undergoing CABG surgery at the same institution[44] confirmed the association between rate of rewarming and cognitive dysfunction.

10.4 Near Infrared Spectroscopy

When transilluminated, colored compounds (chromophores) in solution absorb incident light and reduce the intensity of emerging light. The intensity of emergent light decreases exponentially as chromophore concentration and optical path length increase. When light of a known wavelength passes through a chromophore in solution, the chromophore concentration can be derived from the optical path length and degree of light absorption (the extinction coefficient) using the Beer–Lambert law: $I = I_0.10^{-\epsilon CD}$, where I is the intensity of emergent light; I_0 is intensity of the incident light; ϵ is the chromophore extinction coefficient; D is the optical path length; and C is the chromophore concentration. The Beer–Lambert law applies equally to both reflected (back scattered) and transmitted light.[45]

Light in the visible spectrum (450–700 nm) penetrates biological tissue to a depth of only 10 mm due to attenuation (i.e., absorption and scattering). By contrast, tissue is relatively translucent to light in the infrared spectrum (650–1100 nm).[46] Chromophores such as oxyhemoglobin (HbO_2), deoxyhemoglobin (Hb), and the enzyme cytochrome aa_3 (Caa_3) have distinct infrared absorbance spectra. The absorption of infrared light by HbO_2 and Hb is similar at 810 nm – the so-called isobestic point. Hb has greater absorption at shorter wavelengths, whereas HbO_2 has greater absorption at longer wavelengths. Caa_3 has broad absorbance centered around 830 nm, although its extinction coefficient is <10% that of Hb. Because HbO_2 is the source of oxygen and Caa_3 is the terminal member of the respiratory chain in mitochondria, monitoring brain HbO_2 and Caa_3 should, at least in theory, provide a complete picture of oxygen demand and supply. As early as 1977, Jöbsis[46] used transcranial near-infrared light to noninvasively measure brain oxygenation in cats. These findings were subsequently reproduced by Ferrari and colleagues[47] and Kerth and colleagues.[48]

In addition to absorption, near-infrared light is subject to refraction, reflection, and scattering while passing through the biological tissues making the optical path length unpredictable. This "ambiguity" about optical path length is compounded by changes in the optical density and geometry of biological tissue. The increase in the distance travelled by each photon because of scattering is expressed in terms of the differential path-length factor (DPF), which describes the actual distance travelled by the light.[49] DPF is influenced by wavelength of light and tissue geometry, i.e., water content of tissue. Duncan and colleagues[50] have shown that the DPF in adults is 6.3, i.e., photons travel 6.3 times more than the straight-line path.

Near-infrared spectroscopy (NIRS) therefore employs a modified version of the Beer–Lambert equation[49] (Fig. 10.3), where OD is optical density, I_0 is the intensity of incident light, I is the intensity of detected light, α is the absorption coefficient of the chromophore (in mmol/cm), C is the concentration of chromophore (in mmol/l), L is the physical distance between the point of entry to exit in the tissue (in cm), B is the path-length factor, and G is a factor related to tissue

$$\text{Attenuation } (OD) = \log \frac{I_O}{I} = \alpha CLB + G$$

Fig. 10.3 Modified Beer-Lambert equation used in near-infrared spectroscopy

geometry. If continuous measurements are made in the same area of tissue; *L, B,* and *G* will remain constant and changes in chromophore concentration in mmol/l can be derived from the following formula (Fig. 10.4).

10.4.1 Types of Cerebral Oximeter

Clinical cerebral NIRS devices employ either the transmission or reflection of two, three, or four frequencies of light. The small size and thinness of the neonatal skull permit the *transmission* of near-infrared light from laser photodiodes to detectors fixed to the opposite side of the head. By contrast, the size and thickness of the adult skull effectively prevent near-infrared transmission. For this reason, partial transmission or *reflectance spectroscopy* is performed with the near-infrared source and detector being placed 4-5 cm apart on the same side of the forehead (Fig. 10.5).

There are currently three types of oximeters: continuous wave spectrometers (CWS), time-resolved/domain spectrometers (TRS), and frequency domain or phase-modulation spectrometers (PMS). Continuous wave spectrometers cannot be used to independently calculate optical path-length and thus only provide trends in cerebral oxygen supply and demand. However, substantial errors occur when CWS algorithms are applied to different subjects, presumably because of individual variations in optical path-length and scattering.[48] Both TRS and PMS were developed in an attempt to measure optical path-length. In TRS the optical path-length is related to the time taken for a picosecond duration pulse of light to reach a detector. In PMS the intensity of the emitted light is sinusoidally modulated (>200 MHz) and optical path-length related to the phase-shift of the detected light.[45] A more detailed description of the technical aspects of cerebral NIRS is beyond the scope of this chapter and can be found elsewhere.[51, 52]

$$\Delta C = \frac{\Delta OD}{\alpha LB}$$

Fig. 10.4 Change in chromophore concentration (*ΔC*) can be calculated from the physical distance between the point of entry to exit in the tissue (*L*), the path-length factor (*B*) and a factor to tissue geometry-related factor (*G*)

10.4.2 Regional Cerebral Oxygen Saturation (rSO_2)

In contrast to global cerebral oximetry, which requires measurement of cerebral arterial (SaO_2) and jugular venous (SjO_2) oxygen saturation, NIRS allows monitoring of a region of tissue containing arteries,

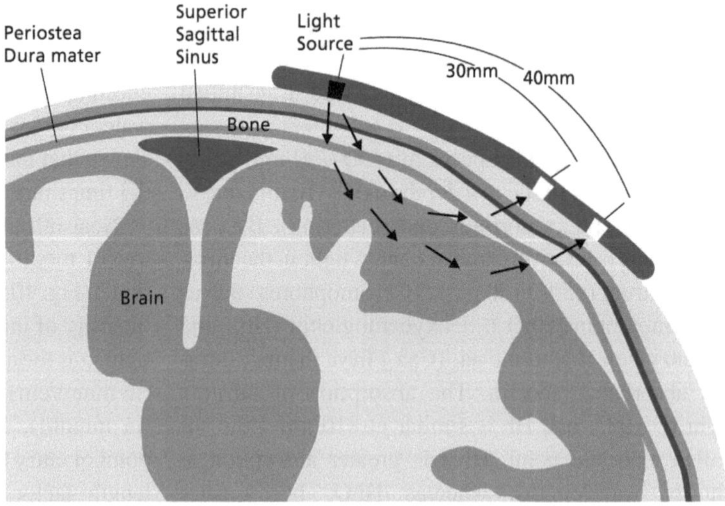

Fig. 10.5 Cerebral near-infrared spectroscopy. (Courtesy of Somanetics Inc.; Reproduced from Arrowsmith, 2004[65]. With permission)

capillaries, and (predominantly) veins. Figure 10.6 although NIRS algorithms are typically based on a fixed ratio of arterial-to-venous blood (e.g., 1:3) in the sample volume, actual arterial-to-venous blood ratios are likely subject to both intra- and interindividual variation.[53] As the value for rSO_2 measured by NIRS represents an average how can we be certain that this value accurately represents actual tissue oxygenation?

Of necessity, the region of interest will also include extracranial blood which may significantly "contaminate" the rSO_2 obtained.[54,55] In a study of 14 adults who had indocyanine green injected into a carotid artery during cerebral angiography, however, Hongo and colleagues[56] showed that spatially resolved NIRS could differentiate between photons reflected from intracranial and extracranial tissues. Similarly, Kaminogo and colleagues[57] compared simultaneous 99mTc-hexamethyl propyleneamine oxime (HMPAO) single photon emission computed tomography (SPECT) and NIRS monitoring in a study of 16 patients during balloon occlusion of a carotid artery. An asymmetrical SPECT pattern was always found to accompany a marked fall in rSO_2. In cases exhibiting a symmetrical SPECT pattern, rSO_2 paralleled a fall in carotid artery stump pressure. In a study of ten patients with severe head injury, Holzschuh and colleagues[58] compared forehead NIRS with invasive measurement of frontal white matter oxygenation. In seven patients, there was a good correlation (r=0.7) between rSO_2 and tissue oxygenation.

In a study of 94 randomly selected subjects from a diverse population of adults, Misra and colleagues[59] reported mean ± SD rSO_2 to be 67.14 ±8.84%. There was no obvious relationship between age and rSO_2. In a study of 42 subjects, Kim and colleagues[60] compared bilateral forehead NIRS rSO_2 with SaO_2 and SjO_2 at end-tidal oxygen concentrations ranging from 41 to 80 mmHg (5.5 – 10.8 kPa). The mean value for rSO_2 was 71 ±6% and there was a close correlation (bias of 5.2%; precision of 10.7%) between rSO_2 and SjO_2. In a study of 111 patients undergoing sevoflurane anesthesia, Kishi and colleagues[61] demonstrated a significant positive correlation between rSO_2 and Hb concentration and a significant negative relationship between rSO_2 and age. Normal values of rSO_2 were unrelated to weight, height, sex, or head size.

During cardiac surgery with CPB, cerebral blood flow – and, by extension, cerebral oxygenation – may be profoundly affected by anesthetic drugs, hypothermia, pH, PaO_2, $PaCO_2$, Hb concentration, and cerebral perfusion pressure. Edmonds and colleagues[62] recorded rSO_2 in 1,000 patients (age 21 – 91 years, 68% male) before CABG, mitral valve, or aortic valve surgery. The mean rSO_2 was 67 ± 10%, significantly lower than the 71 ± 6% reported in healthy adult volunteers aged 20–36 years[60].

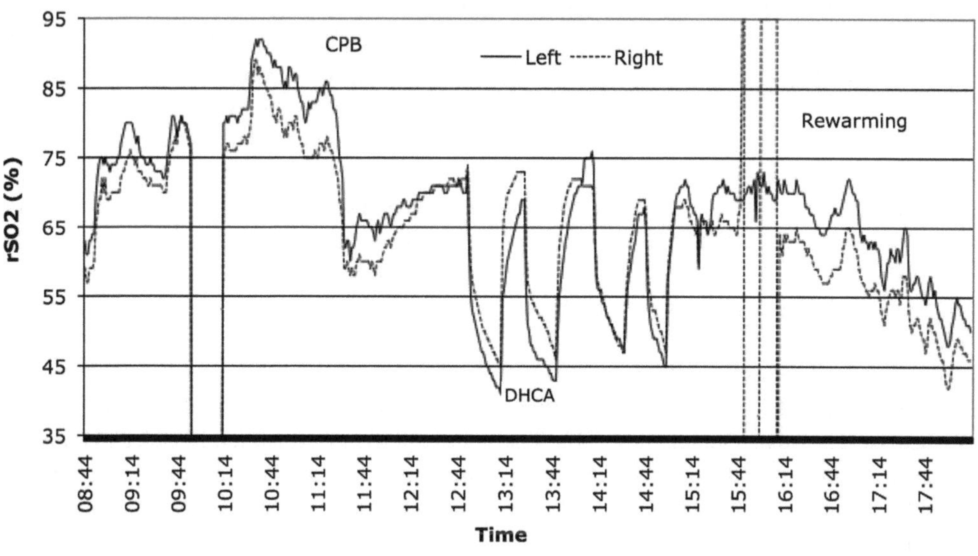

Fig. 10.6 Near-infrared spectroscopy monitoring during pulmonary thromboendarterectomy. Significant cerebral desaturation is seen at the onset of CPB, during four periods of hypothermic circulatory arrest (*DHCA*), and during rewarming

10.5 Clinical Applications of NIRS

Cerebral NIRS has found a number of clinical applications: detection of cerebral ischemia; assessment of selective cerebral perfusion; and the prediction of perioperative neurological injury, postoperative cognitive dysfunction, and duration of intensive care unit and hospital stay.

Deliberately inducing cerebral hypoxia in human volunteers to assess the efficacy of cerebral NIRS is fraught with ethical issues. In 1996, however, Pollard and colleagues[63] reported the use of cerebral NIRS (Invos 3100) in 22 human volunteers. An algorithm for calculating brain Hb oxygen saturation was first derived from measurements of rSO_2, SaO_2, and SjO_2 in 12 subjects. The algorithm was then validated in the remaining ten subjects who were exposed to a progressively hypoxic air mixture. Alveolar hypoxia was shown to correlate with a fall in rSO_2. As rSO_2 fell, the specificity of NIRS for hypoxia increased (88% at rSO_2 60%, 94.7% at rSO_2 50%) whereas the sensitivity decreased (91.7% at rSO_2 60%, 47.8% at rSO_2 50%).

NIRS monitoring during cardiac surgery is further discussed in Chapter 11.

10.6 Transcranial Doppler Sonography

Sound above the audible range (i.e., >20 kHz) is termed ultrasound. Sound waves behave very much like light waves – they can be focused, they are absorbed as they pass through a propagating medium, and they undergo reflection, refraction, and scattering at interfaces between media of differing acoustic density. The degree of reflection is a function of the difference in acoustic density of adjacent media. For this reason, the propagation of ultrasound through tissue–air interfaces is extremely poor.

The detection of reflected sound waves forms the basis of ultrasound imaging. When sound waves are reflected from a moving object, the frequency of the reflected sound is changed or "shifted" – a phenomenon described by Christian Doppler in 1842. The difference in transmitted and received frequency (the Doppler frequency) is dependent upon both the speed of the moving object and the angle at which the incident sound impinges on the object's direction of travel (Fig. 10.7). Knowledge of the speed of sound in the propagating medium permits calculation of the speed of the object – a fact known to every motorist! Ultrasound scattered by erythrocytes and other material moving in blood vessels forms the basis of clinical Doppler ultrasound systems.

$$V = \frac{(f_r - f_t)\, c}{2 f_t\, Cos\theta} \qquad Vm = \frac{c^2}{8 f_t\, R}$$

Fig. 10.7 *Left*: The Doppler equation permits calculation of velocity (*V*) from received frequency (*fr*), transmitted frequency (*ft*), the angle between the direction of the moving target and the path of the sound beam (θ), and the speed of sound in the propagating medium (*c*). For tissue c = 1,540 m/s. *Right*: The maximum velocity (*Vmax*) in meters per second detectable by pulsed-wave Doppler is dictated by the transmitted frequency and the distance of the object (*R*) in centimeters from the sound source/detector. High velocities are best detected with lower frequency ultrasound

Clinical Doppler ultrasound systems measure blood flow velocity. In continuous wave Doppler (CWD) ultrasound is simultaneously transmitted and received. This provides velocity information about *all* moving objects on the *entire* ultrasound path but gives no information about the distance of moving objects from the ultrasound source. In pulsed-wave Doppler (PWD), discrete "pulses" of ultrasound are transmitted at a frequency known as the pulse repetition frequency (PRF). Because only sound reflected from an area (gate) a predefined distance from the source is detected, PWD provides velocity information at a specific distance from the ultrasound source.[64]

High-frequency (10–20 MHz) medical ultrasound provides excellent spatial resolution but has low tissue penetration. By contrast, low-frequency (1–2 MHz) ultrasound offers good tissue penetration at the expense of spatial resolution. The trade-off between penetration and resolution has an impact on the maximum velocity that can be detected using pulsed-wave Doppler (PWD) (Fig. 10.7). When the velocity of the moving object produces a shift in frequency that exceeds half the PRF, the phenomenon of aliasing prevents accurate measurement of velocity.

Sound returning to the transducer is demodulated and filtered to extract the Doppler frequencies, which then undergo fast Fourier transformation in overlapping 4–12 mS epochs. The resulting data are then typically presented as a density spectral array – a moving display with time of the x-axis, velocity on the y-axis, and the amplitude or intensity of specific Doppler frequencies – a measure of the number of erythrocytes traveling at a particular velocity–presented using a color or gray scale.

Although low-frequency ultrasound can easily penetrate, and indeed traverse, the neonatal skull, the cancellous tissue between the inner and outer tables of the adult skull (diploë) acts as an effective barrier to ultrasound. Fortunately, the temporal and occipital bones have little in the way of diploë and these areas can be used as "windows" to insonate the basal cerebral arteries with transcranial Doppler (TCD) ultrasound (Fig. 10.8).[65] The first description of the use of PWD to measure the velocity of blood flow in the basal cerebral arteries was published in 1982.[66] Nowadays, clinical TCD systems permit simultaneous recording from two, four, or more sites and typically have the following characteristics: transmitted frequency, 2–2.5 MHz ($\lambda = 780\ \mu m$); PRF, 4–12 kHz; pulse duration, 10 μS. A more detailed description of the physics and limitations of PWD can be found in any primer on medical ultrasound.[67] The principles of embolus detection, including the differentiation of gaseous and particulate matter, are discussed further in Chapter 4.

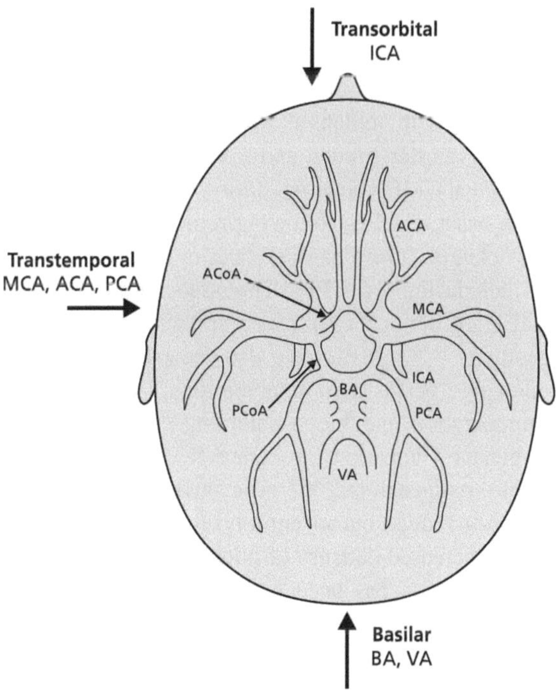

Fig. 10.8 TCD ultrasound windows for examination of the basal cerebral arteries (the Circle of Willis) – submandibular approach not shown. *ACA* anterior cerebral artery; *ACoA* anterior communicating artery; *MCA* middle cerebral artery; *ICA* internal carotid artery; *PCoA* posterior communicating artery; *BA* basilar artery; *PCA* posterior cerebral artery; *VA* vertebral arteries. (Reproduced from Arrowsmith.[65] With permission)

In most applications, unobtrusive low-profile transducers are used to insonate the middle cerebral artery (MCA) via the temporal window. An elasticated fixation harness with lockable gimbals ensures that the transducers remain in position and facilitates small adjustments in their position. Locating the MCA and obtaining an adequate Doppler signal can be time consuming. Vessel location is significantly improved by TCD systems that incorporate two-dimensional imaging and color-flow Doppler modalities. In some groups of patients, however, anatomical variations in skull anatomy make vessel identification extremely difficult or impossible.

10.7 TCD in Cardiac Surgery

In the setting of cardiac surgery, TCD has been mainly used to measure cerebral blood flow velocity (CBFV; a surrogate measure of CBF) and for detecting microemboli. The fact that wide inter-patient variability prevents TCD from being used as an absolute measure of CBF was demonstrated by Bishop and colleagues[68] in a study of 17 patients with symptomatic cerebrovascular disease. Although there was poor correlation between MCA blood flow velocity measured by TCD and ipsilateral hemispheric blood flow measured by $Xenon^{133}$ clearance at rest, there was a good correlation in CBF responses to hypercapnia. Although the lack of correlation between TCD and Xe^{133} clearance was confirmed by Grocott and colleagues,[69] correlation between relative changes in CBF measured by TCD and Xe^{133} clearance was confirmed by Trivedi and colleagues[70] in a study of patients undergoing hypothermic CPB with both α-stat and pH-stat blood gas management.

TCD has been extensively used to both characterize and assess the adequacy of CBF during and after cardiac surgery.[64] TCD is particularly useful for detecting venous air entrainment[71] and abrupt changes in CBF secondary to aortic cannula[71] displacement, occlusion of the superior vena cava,[72] aortic endo clamp migration,[73,74] and inadvertent ventilator disconnection (Arrowsmith JE. Unpublished observation) that might otherwise go undetected.

Taylor and colleagues[11] examined the effects of temperature on the relationship between CPP and

CBFV in a study of 25 neonates and infants undergoing hypothermic CPB. As expected, CBF became progressively pressure-passive with decreasing temperature. Irrespective of pump flow rate, CBFV became undetectable at CPP <9 mmHg. In a study of ten infants subjected to DHCA or mild hypothermic CPB, O'Hare and colleagues[75] demonstrated that, despite seemingly adequate perfusion pressure, CBFV was significantly lower in the DHCA group in the first 4 h after surgery. Astudillo and colleagues[76] demonstrated that low CBF following DHCA in infants was characterized by prolonged periods of absent diastolic CBF in the MCA. Interestingly, infants managed with continuous low-flow cerebral perfusion during DHCA had CBFV values close to baseline at the end of surgery.

Zimmerman and colleagues,[77] in a study of 28 neonates undergoing the arterial switch procedure with deep hypothermic low-flow CPB, evaluated the limits of CBF detection using TCD. At the initiation of CPB, pump flow rates were decreased in steps from 50 to 10 mL/kg/min. At a flow rate of 10 mL/kg/min CBF could not be detected in eight (29%) patients, whereas at 30 mL/kg/min CBF was detected in all patients.

Changes in cerebral autoregulation following DHCA have also been demonstrated in adults. In a study of 67 patients undergoing aortic arch surgery, Neri and colleagues[78] compared the influence of intraoperative DHCA ($n=23$) SACP ($n=25$) and retrograde cerebral perfusion (RCP; $n=19$). Dynamic cerebral autoregulation was assessed using bilateral thigh compression to produce a step decrease in arterial pressure. Autoregulation was preserved only in patients managed with SACP. In some of the patients in the other two groups, impaired autoregulation persisted until the seventh postoperative day.

In a study of 32 consecutive adults undergoing thoracic aortic aneurysm repair, Tanoue and colleagues[79] used TCD to monitor low-flow cerebral perfusion during DHCA. MCA blood flow could only be detected in 3/15 patients managed with RCP (15-25 mmHg), whereas flow was detected in 16/17 patients managed with SACP (500 mL/min). Patients managed with RCP had significant cerebral hyperemia in the early postoperative period. It is suggested that the use of RCP pressures higher than those usually recommended (≥40 mmHg) may improve cerebral protection.[80]

A fifth of individuals have an intact Circle of Willis. The absence of an anterior cerebral collateral circulation may expose as many as 25% patients to left-hemisphere ischemia during unilateral SACP.[81] The posterior communicating circulation appears to contribute little contralateral perfusion in patients with carotid artery occlusion.[82] For this reason, bilateral TCD monitoring should be considered and it is recommended that contralateral MCA velocity be maintained at ≥ 50% ipsilateral MCA velocity.

10.8 Embolus Detection

Cerebral microembolic events (CMEE) have been detected in a wide variety of clinical settings, such as stroke, atrial fibrillation, and amaurosis fugax[83–93] and during medical interventions, such as angiography, cardiac surgery, carotid surgery, major joint replacement, and percutaneous atrial septal defect closure.[94–102]

During cardiac surgery, CMEE can be detected in virtually every patient regardless of whether CPB is used or not. Although CMEE may occur during stable CPB, they are more frequently associated with distinct surgical and perfusion events. In a study of ten patients monitored with unilateral MCA TCD during valve surgery, van der Linden and Casimir-Ahn[103] demonstrated that CMEE occurred during aortic cannulation, at the onset of CPB, following removal of the aortic cross-clamp, during cardiac ejection on CPB and at the conclusion of CPB. The association between CMEE and surgical events has been widely confirmed by others.[104–106] CMEE have also been shown to occur following "perfusionist interventions," such as drug administration and blood sampling.[107,108] Membrane oxygenators appear to generate fewer CMEE than bubble oxygenators.[109–112] The avoidance of CPB appears to reduce, but not entirely eliminate, CMEE.[113–115] The increased delivery of microemboli to the cerebral circulation has been postulated as a reason for worse neuropsychological outcome following pH-stat arterial blood gas management during CPB[116,117] (Fig. 10.9).

The importance of CMEE during cardiac surgery is highlighted by studies demonstrating a relationship between microembolic load and neurological outcome.[118–120] It is clear from studies of patients undergoing off-pump surgery, however, that CMEE are but one of many factors that contribute to postoperative

Fig. 10.9 Transcranial Doppler (*TCD*) examination of the middle cerebral artery (*MCA*) during coronary artery bypass graft (*CABG*) surgery; before (*left*), during (*center*), and immediately after (*right*) CPB. The high-amplitude signals (*center* and *right*) represent cerebral microemboli. (Reproduced from Arrowsmith et al.[65] with permission)

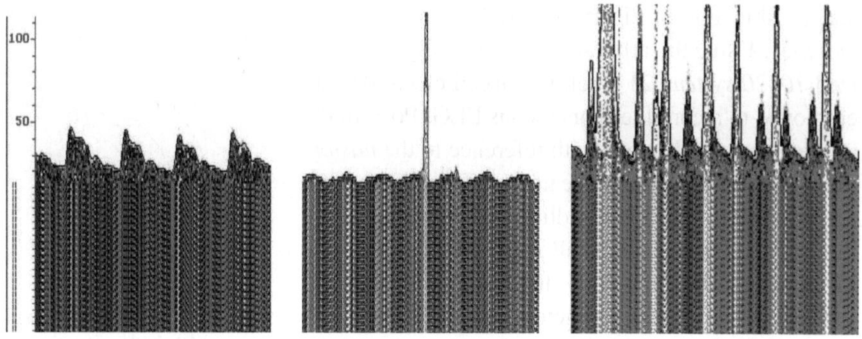

neurological dysfunction.[121,122] The etiological significance of atheroma of the proximal aorta[1, 123] has been confirmed by observation of the relationship between burden of atheroma – determined by transesophageal echocardiography – and CMEE.[124]

One of the most useful applications of TCD in cardiac surgery has been the evaluation of procedure modifications, perfusion techniques, and novel devices that may reduce CMEE. Pugsley and colleagues[125] demonstrated that use of a 40 μm arterial line filter significantly reduced CMEE during CABG surgery. In a later study of 100 patients undergoing CABG surgery, the same group[118] confirmed the efficacy of arterial line filtration and demonstrated that filtration was associated with improved postoperative neuropsychological test performance. The use of a "suture-less" proximal aorto-coronary anastomosis device, which obviates the need for application of an aortic cross clamp, has been shown to reduce CMEE.[126] The choice of site for aortic cannulation has an influence on CMEE.[127] In a study of 34 patients undergoing CABG surgery, Borger and colleagues[128] showed that cannulation of the distal aorta was associated with significantly fewer CMEE.

10.9 Electroencephalography

The detection of electrical activity at the surface of the brain of animals was first described in 1875 by Richard Caton.[129, 130] The term *elektroenkephalogram* (electroencephalogram; EEG) was coined by the German psychiatrist Hans Berger who, in 1924, was the first to record the electrical activity of the human brain.[130–132] The electrical activity measured by the EEG is thought to represent the summation of excitatory and inhibitory postsynaptic potentials in neuronal pathways running from the thalamic nuclei to pyramidal cells in laminae I, II, and IV of the cerebral cortex.[132–134] The EEG has a bandwidth of <1 to 50 Hz and an amplitude of ~100 μV when measured on the scalp, and 1–2 mV when measured on the surface of the brain. The components of the EEG signal are classified according to their frequency and amplitude (Table 10.2).

In clinical practice, the EEG is a time-domain representation of electrical activity recorded *between* pairs (i.e., bipolar EEG) of silver chloride or platinum needle scalp electrodes. In the unipolar EEG, the potential at each electrode is compared to either a neutral electrode or to the average of all electrodes. The placement

Table 10.2 EEG waveforms

Waveform	Frequency (Hz)	Amplitude (μV)	Comments
Delta (δ)	1.5–3.5	>50	Normal during sleep and deep anesthesia, indication of neuronal dysfunction.
Theta (θ)	3.6–7.5	20–50	Normal in children and elderly, normal adults during sleep, produced by hypothermia
Alpha (α)	7.6–12.5	20–50	Awake, relaxed, eyes open, mainly over occiput
Beta (β)	12.6–25	<20	Awake, alert, eyes open, mainly in parietal cortex, produced by barbiturates, benzodiazepines, phenytoin, alcohol
Gamma (γ)	25.1–50	<20	

and combination of electrodes used is known as the *montage*. Using the arbitrary internationally standardized *10–20 system*, 21 carefully placed electrodes are employed to record the spontaneous EEG. Positioning of the electrodes is made with reference to the *nasion*, the concavity at the top of the nose, level with the eyes; and the *inion*, the bony midline protuberance at the base of the back of the skull (Fig. 10.10). Electrode locations are determined by dividing the median and traverse nasion–inion perimeters into 10% and 20% intervals.[135, 136] In addition to the 21 electrodes of the international 10–20 system, intermediate 10% electrode positions are also used. Somewhat confusingly, the T_7, T_8, P_7, and P_8 electrodes have different names in the more complex 10–10 system.

Investigational and diagnostic quality EEG acquisition using the 10–20 system typically requires simultaneous recording from 16 or more electrode pairs or channels. This degree of complexity is regarded as being too cumbersome for monitoring in the setting of the operating room or the intensive care unit, where two- or four-channel systems are more commonly used.

In order to be of use, the electrical signals detected at the scalp must first be amplified and separated from extraneous sources of electrical activity. Differential amplifiers and band-pass filters are used to reduce electromyographic (EMG; scalp and ocular muscles), electrooculographic (dipoles within the globes), electrocardiographic (principally the R-wave), and radiofrequency interference. (RFI; power lines, other electrical equipment, unipolar diathermy). The resulting "raw" waveforms are then available for transcription or signal processing. Historically, the raw EEG was recorded on continuous "fan-folding" paper using a multichannel printer – the author recalls the seemingly endless and impenetrable documents produced in this way. The term *signal processing* encompasses a number of techniques ostensibly designed to make the information contained within the raw EEG more accessible to clinicians. The advent of fast multi-bit analog-to-digital converters (ADCs), digital computers, and "very large-scale integration" (VLSI) hybrid devices, such as programmable fast Fourier transform (FFT) processors, has brought real-time digital signal processing (DSP) to the bedside. Paradoxically, the application of rapidly evolving technology and mathematical modeling (e.g., stochastic vs. deterministic, Gaussianity, stationary, linear vs. nonlinear) has yielded an array of complex processing techniques, descriptions of which are far

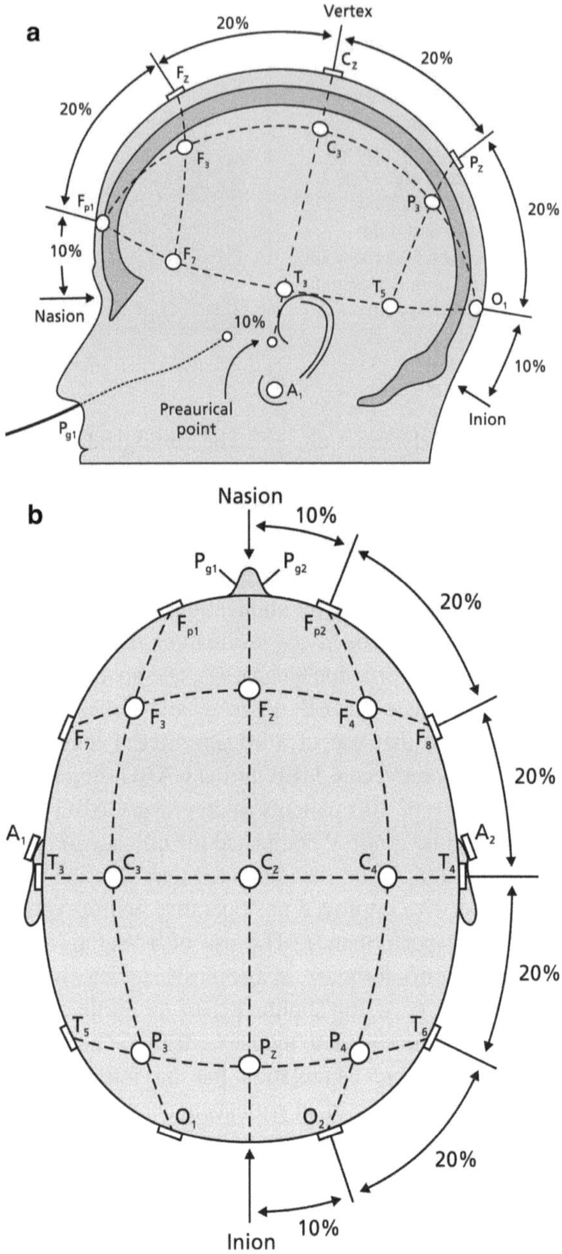

Fig. 10.10 (**a**) left lateral view, (**b**) aerial view, The internationally standardized *10–20 system* of EEG electrode placement.[136] *F* frontal; *Fp* frontal polar; *C* central; *O* occipital; *P* parietal; *T* temporal; *A* ear lobe; *Pg* nasopharyngeal. Right-sided placements are indicated by even numbers, left-sided placements by odd numbers, and midline placements by Z. In addition, intermediate electrodes located at 10% positions may also be used. The location and nomenclature of these electrodes is standardized by the American Clinical Neurophysiology Society formerly the American Electroencephalographic Society[135] (Adapted with permission from Malmivuo, Plonsey)[234]

Table 10.3 Terms commonly used in EEG analysis and representation

Term	Description
Compressed spectral array (CSA)	Linear plots of consecutive epochs of time are superimposed on each other, generating a three-dimensional "hill and valley" display of the power amplitude vertically (y-axis), frequency horizontally (x-axis), and time (z-axis). As successive epochs are added, information can become hidden behind "hills" of increased power at particular frequencies
Density spectral array (DSA)	Lines running from low to high frequency represent consecutive epochs of time. The EEG power at each frequency is represented by either a color-map or gray-scale intensity
Median power frequency (MPF)	The frequency below which 50% of the global EEG power is contained
Spectral edge frequency (SEF)	The highest significant frequency present in the recorded EEG spectrum for each epoch. SEF-90 represents the frequency below which 90% of the entire EEG power is located
Fourier transform	Decomposition of a complex function into sinusoidal functions of different frequency, phase, and amplitude that can be recombined to obtain the original function. The transform is described in terms of domains (time vs. frequency) and the properties of the domain (continuous vs. discrete) and the transform function (periodic vs. aperiodic)
Discrete Fourier transform	The frequency domain representation of the original function
Fast Fourier transform	An efficient algorithm for computing the discrete Fourier transform (DFT). The most commonly used algorithm (the Cooley-Tukey algorithm[137]) recursively divides the DFT into smaller DFTs
Cerebral function monitor (CFM)	An EEG signal obtained from one (biparietal) or two (bitemporal) electrodes is filtered, semi-logarithmically compressed, and rectified providing a representation of the overall EEG activity
Cerebral function analyzing monitor (CFAM)	A two-channel EEG signal is displayed as (i) log-weighted-mean amplitude, and (ii) the percentage of overall power within each frequency band[138]
Quantitative EEG (QEEG)	An EEG epoch, typically 60–120 S in duration, is analyzed using a FFT to quantify the power at each frequency (power spectrum) of the EEG averaged across the entire sample. The power spectrum of clinical interest lies in the 1–20 Hz range
Burst suppression	Alternating periods of normal to high voltage activity changing to low or isoelectric voltage
Bispectral index (BSI)	A complex parameter, composed of a combination of time domain, frequency domain, and high-order spectral subparameters incorporating both phase and power information of two primary EEG frequencies[133]
Patient state index (PSI)	Quantitative multivariate EEG-based measure of hypnosis[139]
Spectral entropy	A measure of time-frequency balanced spectral "randomness" off the EEG and frontal electromyogram from which two parameters, response entropy and state entropy, are derived. Entropy decreases with increasing hypnosis

beyond the scope of this contribution. For the purposes of this description, the reader should be aware of the number of terms used (Table 10.3)[137–139] (Fig. 10.11).

10.10 Pre- and Postoperative Monitoring

In the earliest application of perioperative EEG, Sachdev and colleagues[140] examined the relationship between postoperative neurological dysfunction and EEG abnormalities in ten patients undergoing cardiac valve replacement. CPB times were long by contemporary standards (168 ± 47 min) and all patients developed clinically demonstrable neurological signs and bilateral, generalized EEG slowing. In 8/10 patients, the EEG abnormalities were more pronounced in the early postoperative period. At follow-up, 6/9 survivors were found to have made a full neurological recovery.

In one of the first long-term follow-up studies, Sotaniemi and colleagues[141,142] performed pre- and postoperative 16-channel EEG and QEEG recording in 65 consecutive patients undergoing valve replacement

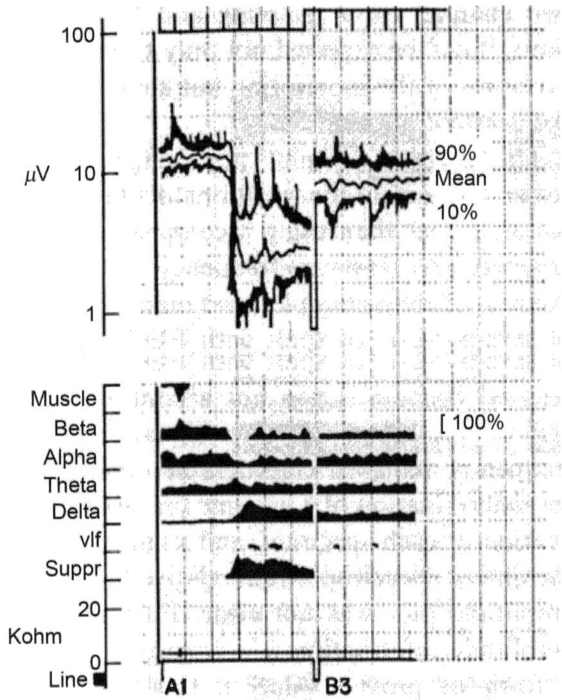

Fig. 10.11 Typical CFAM tracing. The upper trace displays the log-weighted-mean raw EEG amplitude distribution in mV, 10th and 90th centiles, and maximum and minimum amplitudes. The lower trace displays; electromyography ("Muscle"), percentage α, β δ, θ, and very low frequency ("vlf"<1) activity, percentage of suppression ("Suppr.")<1 peak-to-peak, and electrode impedance in kOhm (Reproduced with permission from Arrowsmith[67])

surgery. Three patients died within 8 days of surgery – two from brain injury. Neurological injury was found in 31 patients – hemiparesis in 19 and either aphasia, confusion, brain stem, or cerebellar signs in the remainder. Preoperative EEG abnormalities (decreased α amplitude, increased δ and θ amplitude) were found in ~50% cases. The incidence of EEG abnormalities 10 days after surgery was 97% in patients with neurological complications and 67% in patients without such complications. The incidence of EEG abnormalities was seen to decline in both groups at 2, 5, 8, and 12-month follow-up. Neurological signs were still present in 5/31 patients 1 year after surgery. At 5-year follow-up[143], the prevalence of EEG abnormalities in the 55 (89%) survivors was 25%, and was greater in patients who had sustained a neurological injury (32% vs. 20%). Interestingly, the prevalence of EEG abnormalities was greater in patients subjected to more than 120 min of CPB.

10.11 Intraoperative Monitoring

The rationale for intraoperative EEG monitoring is that changes in neuronal perfusion and oxygen delivery lead to changes in the EEG. The use of EEG monitoring during surgery is complicated by the fact that hypothermia[144] and virtually all anesthetic drugs[145–148] have direct and profound effects on neuroelectrophysiology. These effects have been harnessed in burst suppression monitoring[149] prior to DHCA and form the basis of several "depth of anesthesia" monitors.[150–154]

The EEG has long been regarded as the "gold standard" for the detection of cerebral ischemia. At constant temperature and depth of anesthesia, progressive ischemia produces a reduction in total power and slowing – decreased α and β power and increased δ and θ power – that may show hemispheric asymmetry.[155] However, these changes typically only become apparent when CBF falls below half the normal value of 50 mL/100 g/min. EEG amplitude attenuation of <50% or increased δ power is regarded as being indicative of mild ischemia, whereas >50% attenuation or a doubling in δ power is regarded as being indicative of severe ischemia. An isoelectric or "silent" EEG is seen when CBF falls below 7–15 mL/100g/min. While the EEG is sensitive to subtle changes in neuronal electrophysiology, it should be borne in mind that it is not specific for pathology.[156]

10.11.1 Carotid Artery Surgery

In the setting of carotid endarterectomy (CEA), the EEG has been used to monitor the effects of carotid clamping and assess the need for a temporary intraluminal vascular shunt. In a study of 30 patients undergoing CEA, Schwartz and colleagues[157] performed preoperative cerebral angiography to assess collateral circulation. Intraoperative EEG monitoring was used to assess the adequacy of collateral circulation during carotid clamping. Only 1/15 patients with a demonstrable collateral circulation required a shunt, whereas a shunt was required in all 15 patients in whom no collateral flow was shown.

In a study of 19 patients, Hanowell and colleagues[158] used EEG power and spectral edge frequency (SEF) monitoring during CEA. Nine patients had EEG changes suggestive of ischemia, defined as >40% fall in EEG power or ≥ 3 Hz fall in spectral edge frequency and later confirmed by raw EEG analysis. Eight of these episodes occurred at the time of carotid clamping. While power band analysis detected all nine episodes of suspected ischemia, alteration in SEF detected only two episodes. The authors concluded that EEG power monitoring was a more sensitive indicator of cerebral ischemia than SEF alteration. More recently, Hans and Jareunpoon[159] reported on the utility of continuous EEG and carotid stump pressure monitoring in a consecutive series of 314 awake patients undergoing CEA under cervical block anesthesia. Ischemic EEG changes were observed in 19 (59.4%) of the 32 patients who had neurological impairment following carotid clamping (false-negative rate, 40.6%). Three patients had false-positive EEG results and did not require shunt placement (false-positive rate, 1.0%). This finding supports the notion that the awake patient is the "best" ischemia monitor!

10.11.2 EEG Monitoring During Cardiac Surgery

Despite the fact that EEG monitoring has been used in the setting of cardiac surgery for more than 5 decades,[141–143, 148, 160–170] a consistent and reproducible descriptor of reversible cerebral injury remains frustratingly elusive.

During cardiac surgery there is invariably a fall in core temperature. Mild hypothermia (34–36°C) is characterized by a modest fall in predominant EEG frequencies without significant amplitude changes.[171] Moderate hypothermia (28–34°C) is characterized by a gradual loss of absolute spectral power across all frequency bands.[166, 172] Below 28°C there is progressive slowing until the EEG becomes isoelectric – a phenomenon that is used as measure of adequacy of cooling prior to DHCA.[173, 174] The temperature at which EEG activity is lost is subject to considerable interpatient variation and is typically *higher* during the cooling phase than during rewarming.[174] In a study of 109 patients undergoing aortic arch surgery with DHCA,[175] the risk for postoperative neurological impairment increased by a factor of 1.56 for every 1°C increase in temperature at which EEG activity first became continuous during rewarming.

In a study of two nonconcurrent groups of cardiac surgery patients, Arom and colleagues[165] first examined neurological outcome in 50 patients. Changes in the EEG were described using a derived power drop index (PDI) and banded-average-frequency value (AFV). Abnormal neurological findings were found in 32 (64%) patients on the first postoperative day. When compared to neurologically intact patients, those with global neurological impairment were subjected to significantly longer CPB and had a significantly greater mean PDI. In the second half of the investigation, the period of CPB in 41 patients was managed according to an EEG-driven intervention algorithm designed to increase cerebral perfusion. Although the mean duration of CPB was significantly greater in the intervention group, the mean PDI was significantly lower (71 vs. 143, $p<0.01$). Abnormal neurological findings were found in 10 (24%) patients on the first postoperative day. The number of patients with global neurological impairment on the first postoperative day was significantly lower in the intervention group (2 vs. 22, $p<0.001$). Hospital length of stay was shorter in the intervention group (10.1 ± 2.4 vs. 12.8 days, $p=$NS).

In a similarly designed study, Edmonds and colleagues[167] used changes in low-frequency (1.5–3.5 Hz) QEEG power to guide interventions in 96 patients undergoing myocardial revascularization using hypothermic CPB. The pre-sternotomy value served as a reference value for each patient. Prolonged (>5 min) and statistically significant (>3 SD) focal increases in relative low-frequency power were temperature-corrected to determine a standardized cerebrocortical dysfunction time at 37°C (CDT37). In the observation group ($n=48$), episodes of CDT37 >5 min occurred on 38 occasions in 19 patients and were frequently associated with systemic hypotension (<50 mmHg). The QEEG descriptor predicted postoperative disorientation in 14/48 (29%) patients (false-positive rate, 68%; false-negative rate, 8%). In the subsequent intervention study ($n=48$), putative ischemic events prompted interventions to improve cerebral perfusion. The incidence of disorientation in this group was significantly lower (4%, $p<0.002$). The authors concluded that EEG monitoring offered an opportunity for the timely correction of perfusion abnormalities or the administration of cerebro-protectant compounds.

In the same year, Bashien and colleagues[166] reported the findings of two-channel EEG monitoring in 78 patients undergoing hypothermic CPB. More than a third of recordings were corrupted by electrical noise. Changes in total and θ band power were weakly associated with short-term (but not long-term) neuropsychological outcome. Despite exhaustive analysis, no consistent variation in EEG descriptor could be associated with hypothermia. The authors concluded that EEG had little value for detecting "the harbingers of brain injury." These findings may, at least in part, be attributable to the small number of EEG channels used –the previous two studies[165,167] used 16-channel EEG. Although the optimal number of EEG channels required remains unclear, as few as four may be sufficient to reliably detect ischemic episodes.[156]

Using pre- and postoperative QEEG and neuropsychological testing in a small group of cardiac surgical patients ($n=32$), Gugino and colleagues[169,170,172] found that two in five patients had evidence of abnormal cerebral function before surgery. Preoperative QEEG and neuropsychological abnormalities were predictive of outcome 2–3 months after surgery.

Pharmacological EEG suppression with drugs such as isoflurane,[176,177] thiopental,[178–180] and propofol[181] has long been postulated as a means of reducing cerebral metabolic rate and protecting the brain during cardiac surgery. Despite the fact that these agents have profound and potentially beneficial effects on cerebral blood flow and metabolism,[149,182] the weight of accumulated evidence suggests that they have little impact on neurological outcome.[183] Nevertheless, thiopental has been shown to reduce mortality in patients undergoing CABG surgery[180] and its administration prior to DHCA remains a standard of care in many institutions.

10.11.3 Depth of Anesthesia Monitoring

The search for the "Holy Grail" – a reliable monitor of depth of anesthesia that ensures adequate anesthesia and permits rapid emergence – has led to the development of a number of EEG-based technologies. As all rely on complex EEG signal processing algorithms, it is logical to assume that conditions such as ischemia that affect the EEG will be reflected in the output of these devices. Despite the obvious difficulty of separating changes secondary to ischemia from changes in depth of anesthesia, bispectral index monitoring has been shown to be capable of detecting cerebral ischemia during cardiac surgery.[184,185] At the very least, this type of monitoring might ameliorate cerebral hypoperfusion secondary to the cardiovascular depression associated with inappropriately deep anesthesia.[186] To date, there has been no systematic evaluation of these devices as monitors of cerebral "well-being" during cardiac surgery.

10.12 Evoked Potential Monitoring

Evoked potential monitoring refers to a number of techniques that measure the response of the nervous system to external stimulation. Sensory evoked potential monitoring techniques measure the cortical or brain stem responses to auditory, visual, spinal cord, or somatic stimulation. Motor evoked potential (MEP) monitoring techniques measure the spinal cord or compound muscle action potential response to cortical stimulation.

10.12.1 Somatosensory-Evoked Potential Monitoring

Somatosensory-evoked potentials (SSEPs) are typically generated by transcutaneous or subdermal electrical stimulation of a peripheral mixed motor and sensory nerve. Although SSEPs can be measured in peripheral nerve, nerve plexus, nerve root, and spinal cord, they are frequently monitored over the sensory cortex using adhesive Ag/AgCl electrodes. Monophasic square wave pulses, 100–300 μS in duration and of sufficient amplitude to produce a consistent muscle twitch, are delivered at a rate of 2–10 Hz using a constant voltage or constant current source.[187] Upper-limb SSEP can be generated in either the ulnar (C8–T1) or median (C6–T1) nerve. Lower-limb SSEP can be generated in the posterior tibial or common peroneal nerves. (Table 10.4)

In addition to scalp electrodes,[135, 136] the minimum montages recommended by the American Clinical Neurophysiology Society include recording electrodes placed on the neck at Erb's point (brachial plexus), in the midline over the spine, and over the iliac crest.[188–190] The amplitude of the signals detected

Table 10.4 Stimulating electrode placement for upper and lower SSEP monitoring. SSEPs from the upper limb primarily represent activity in the posterior columns (i.e., vibration and proprioception), those from the lower limb include components that travel in spinocerebellar pathways.

Upper limb	Ulnar nerve	Anode placed between wrist creases at base of hypothenar eminence Cathode placed 3 cm proximal over tendon of flexor digitorum ulnaris
	Median nerve	Anode placed just proximal to palmar crease Cathode placed 3 cm proximal between tendons of palmaris longus
Lower limb	Posterior tibial nerve	Cathode placed midway between Achilles' tendon and medical malleolus Anode placed 3 cm distal to cathode
	Peroneal nerve	Cathode placed in popliteal fossa below skin crease just medial to tendon of biceps femoris Anode placed 3 cm distal to cathode

is typically in the μV or nV range. Signal averaging over several tens or hundreds of responses may be required to extract the SSEP from background EEG and scalp EMG noise, and external RFI. Short-latency SSEPs (25–50 mS in duration; thought to originate in the thalamus, parietal sensory cortex, medial lemniscus, and dorsal column nucleus cuneatus) are most commonly studied during surgery because they are influenced to a lesser degree by factors such as depth of anesthesia (Fig. 10.12).

As temperature falls, axonal conduction velocity decreases[191] and SSEP latency increases.[192] The consequent increase in neuronal refractoriness dictates lower peripheral nerve stimulation frequencies and longer SSEP averaging cycles. At moderate levels of hypothermia (>34°C), SSEP amplitude remains relatively unchanged, whereas more profound hypothermia is associated with a progressive fall in amplitude, such that SSEP components disappear between 17°C and 24°C. The relationship between SSEP amplitude and latency at any given temperature is subject to considerable variability and hysteresis so that during rewarming certain SSEP components reappear at temperatures lower than that at which they disappeared during cooling.[175, 193, 194]

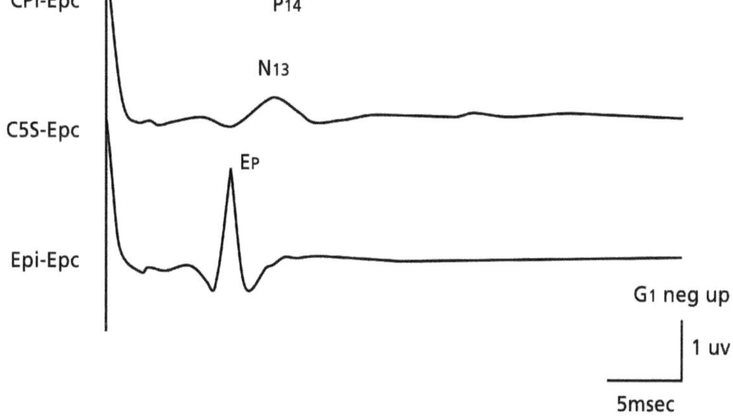

Fig. 10.12 Normal median nerve SSEPs using minimum recommended montage. Electrode CPi denotes either CP3 or CP4, whichever is ipsilateral to the stimulated limb; CPc is the contralateral centroparietal scalp electrode. Epi and Epc refer to electrodes sited at Erb's point on the ipsilateral and contralateral sides, respectively. The C5S electrode is placed over the body of the fifth cervical vertebra

Anesthetic drugs have direct actions on axonal membranes and have significant actions at synapses.[195] Short latency evoked potentials, which typically involve a small number of synapses, are influenced by anesthetic drugs to a far less extent, than multi-synaptic long latency evoked potentials. The influence of inhalational agents (e.g., isoflurane) on SSEP is greater than that of intravenous agents (e.g., propofol, etomidate, ketamine, thiopental) and is significantly potentiated by hypothermia.[196, 197] By contrast, opioids and benzodiazepines have minimal effects on SSEPs.

A disturbance at any point in the afferent pathway may cause SSEP modification or extinction. For this reason SSEP monitoring has been used to assess the functional integrity of sensory pathways rendered vulnerable to injury during surgery.[187] While direct nerve or plexus injury may cause SSEP degradation, ischemia is by far the most important pathophysiological factor in the context of cardiac surgery. The effects of ischemia on SSEP can usually be distinguished from the effects of hypothermia and anesthesia on the grounds that ischemic changes tend to be abrupt, unilateral, and demonstrate a different response to a variation in interstimulus interval.[198]

10.12.1.1 Clinical Applications

In the setting of cardiac surgery, SSEP monitoring has been used for the detection of cerebral ischemia during CPB, temperature management prior to DHCA, cerebral function monitoring during SACP, and detection of brachial plexopathy.

In a study of 25 adults undergoing cardiac surgery with hypothermic CPB (18–32°C), Stecker et al.[199] supplemented detailed preoperative and postoperative neurological evaluation with intraoperative bilateral upper limb SSEP monitoring. A significant change in SSEP was defined as acute, unilateral extinction of one or more SSEP waves for >3 min. Changes in SSEP amplitude during surgery were detected in two patients who had intraoperative strokes ($P<0.004$). In a case report, Cheung et al.[200] reported the use of SSEP monitoring to detect cerebral ischemia in an elderly patient undergoing mitral valve surgery. Following removal of the aortic cross-clamp there was abolition of the right N20 and P22 components that could only be partially reversed by increasing cerebral oxygen delivery. The patient emerged from anesthesia with a dense left hemiparesis. Computed tomography revealed a small, watershed infarct in the right frontal periventricular region.

In a study of 32 patients undergoing surgery with DHCA, Guerit et al.[201] used disappearance of the P14 SSEP component as a measure of adequate brain cooling. At a mean temperature of 16.9°C, no patient in whom P14 was absent suffered any neurological sequelae. Stecker and colleagues[175] demonstrated that the risk of neurological injury following DHCA and RCP was dependent on the temperature at which the N20–P22 complex reappeared. The temperature at which N20–P22 complexes appeared was different from the temperature at which continuous EEG activity returned. The time taken for SSEP components to return during rewarming appears, at least in part, to be related to the duration of circulatory arrest.[202]

SSEP monitoring has been used to detect brachial plexus injury; a complication that may occur in up to 15% cardiac surgery patients. Hickey and colleagues[203] used the amplitude of the cortical component of the upper-limb SSEP (N19–P22) to study 30 patients. Significant changes were noted during central venous cannulation (13%) and with use of the Favoloro retractor (70%). SSEP changes persisted until the end of surgery in the five patients who developed a neurological deficit. Jellish and colleagues[204,205] have used the Erb point potential, subcortical far-field potential (N13), and cortical (N20) potentials to compare the impact of different types of sternal retractor on SSEPs. The Rultract and Pittman retractors were associated with significantly more episodes of ≥ 50% decrease in cortical SSEP amplitude (45% and 25% respectively) than the Delacroix-Chevalier retractor (5%). Although, the adverse impact of sternal retractor on SSEPs has been confirmed in other studies,[206] some investigators have found no significant changes.[207]

10.12.2 Auditory Evoked Potential Monitoring

Auditory evoked potential (AEP) monitoring is used to assess the brain stem, mid brain, and auditory cortices (Fig. 10.13). Electrodes are typically placed near or in the ear (recording), at the vertex (Cz; reference) and on the forehead (Fz; ground). An auditory stimulus, consisting of "clicks" or tone bursts (1–10 kHz) of alternating polarity, 40–500 μS in duration, is repeated at regular

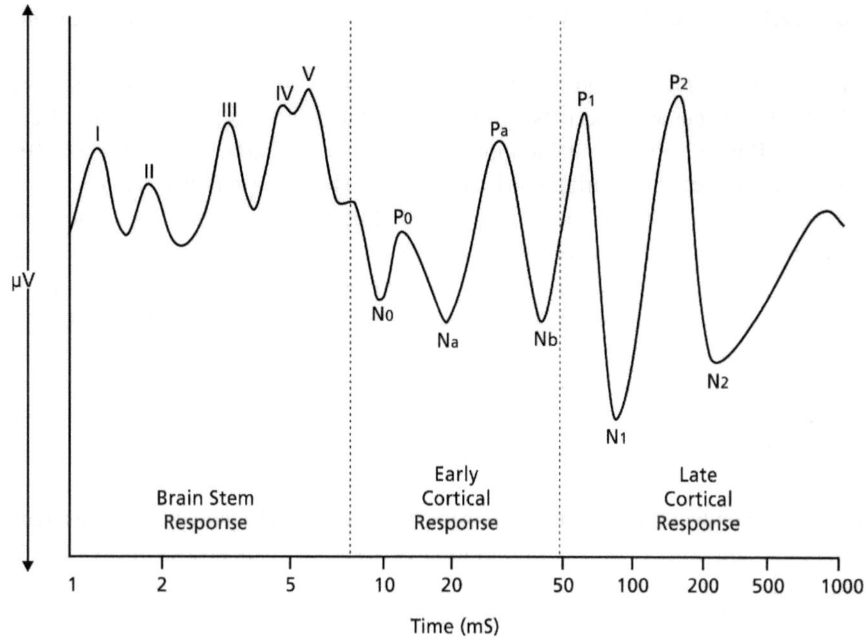

Fig. 10.13 Auditory evoked potentials (*AEPs*) and standard electrophysiological nomenclature. The P3 or event-related P300 component (not shown) is a positive potential occurring 250–500 mS after stimulation. (Reproduced from Arrowsmith.[65] with permission)

intervals and signal averaging over several cycles used to extract the AEP from background EEG activity.[187,208] The amplitude of the evoked response increases with increasing click frequency, to a maximum at ~40 Hz. This so-called auditory steady-state response (ASSR), thought to occur as a result of the superimposition of the Pa and Pb waves from overlapping AEPs, has been used to assess the level of consciousness.[150]

Short-latency (<10 mS) brain stem auditory evoked responses (BAERs) are characterized by seven waves (I–VII), reflecting neural activity between the acoustic nerve (I), cochlear nucleus (II), superior olivary complex (III), lateral lemniscus (IV), and inferior colliculus (V). The origins of waves VI and VII are not well defined. In neonates and infants, only peaks I, III, and V, with differing amplitude and longer latencies are present. BAERs are generally unaffected by anesthetic drugs (except halothane, enflurane, and isoflurane) but are temperature-sensitive, making them useful for monitoring the effects of cooling and rewarming.

Mid-latency (10–100 mS) AEPs represent polysynaptic activity in the medial geniculate body (midbrain) and primary auditory cortex – necessary for awareness and recall of auditory events.[209] The prominence of Na and Pa increases with age and achieve adult levels by the age of ten years. Both intravenous and inhalational anesthetic drugs affect the amplitude and latency of the Pa and Nb waves in a dose-dependent manner.[187,210] Children exhibit the typical adult Na, Pb, Nb pattern, whereas infants only exhibit a small Pa wave.[211] The benzodiazepines, ketamine, and opioids have little effect on mid-latency AEPs even when explicit memory and response to verbal commands are abolished.

Late cortical responses represent activity in the frontal cortex and associations areas. In humans, this is thought to reflect higher functions such as selective attention and auditory discrimination.[212] This aspect of cognitive function can be tested in conscious subjects using the P300 paradigm,[213–215] and has been used to assess neurological changes after cardiac surgery. P300 event-related potential recording requires electrodes placed at Cz and Pz (active), A1 and A2 (reference), and Fz (ground). Two types of stimuli (1 and 2 kHz) are randomly presented to both ears in a ratio of 4:1 and responses averaged over ~30 cycles. The response to the less frequent or "deviant" stimulus is of interest. Passive techniques have been used in children, comatose patients, and subjects with impaired vigilance.[216,217] An important component of the response to a deviant stimulus is the N2a or mismatch negativity (MMN) wave occurring some 150–250 mS after the stimulus. The MMN, which is thought to originate in the frontal lobes and auditory cortex,[218–220] represents the unconscious mismatch between the sensory memory of the standard stimulus and the deviant sensory input.[221,222]

10.12.2.1 Clinical Applications

The increase in latency and decrease in amplitude of BEARs that occur with decreasing brain temperature make AEP monitoring a suitable monitor for the adequacy of brain cooling during CPB and for assessing brain stem integrity during rewarming.[211] BAER-based temperature monitoring is proposed as being superior to EEG monitoring on the grounds that brain stem temperature is usually higher than cortical temperature during cooling and because brain stem electrical activity may persist when cortical activity has been suppressed.

The close anatomical correlation with components of the AEP may be useful in determining the location of specific conduction anomalies within the brain stem, midbrain, and cortex. If the concentration of volatile anesthetic agents is kept low and constant, changes in BAERs may indicate the presence of structural pathology in the auditory pathway. Lesions of the higher auditory pathways require mid-latency AEP monitoring.[223] The use of steady-state anesthesia permits a comparison of responses with those obtained at baseline.[224] Abnormalities in mid-latency AEPs should be regarded as suspicious and evaluated in the context of current hemodynamic status and changes in other electrophysiological monitoring modalities (i.e., BAERs and EEG).[225]

The differentiation between neuronal injury and the effects of anesthetic and sedative drugs is particularly important in patients requiring prolonged mechanical ventilation[226] and in those who fail to awaken from general anesthesia. In a study of 103 AEP-monitored comatose patients, Guerit and colleagues[216] showed that the presence of MMN predicted a good outcome in 75% cases. Furthermore, all patients with a P3a wave recorded within 4 days of the onset of coma eventually regained consciousness. The presence, albeit uncommon, of a clear P3 wave in comatose patients is a good prognostic sign.[217] In propofol-sedated adult patients, increased latency and decreased amplitude of the N1, MMN, and P3a waves correlate with level of sedation assessed by the Ramsey score.[227] The preservation of mid-latency AEPs during general anesthesia appears to indicate that auditory information may be processed and be remembered following emergence by an implicit memory task. In a study of 45 cardiac surgical patients, Pa latency was found to have 100% sensitivity and 77% specificity for distinguishing patients with implicit postoperative memory from those who did not.[228]

Several groups have used binaural discrimination tasks to evaluate the effects of cardiac surgery on P300 latency. In a study of 308 consecutive patients surviving cardiac surgery, Kilo and colleagues[229] reported significant impairment of P300 AEPs (increased peak latencies) seven days after surgery, which in most cases returned to normal within four months of surgery. CPB was the only independent predictor of postoperative cognitive deficit. AEP changes did not correlate with changes in performance on two cognitive function tests, possibly because they examined different aspects of cognitive function. The same group went on to examine 40 patients undergoing mitral valve surgery.[230] Despite the obvious fact that CPB was used in all patients, the incidence of P300 changes and impaired cognitive function test performance was significantly lower in those undergoing valve repair, compared to those undergoing valve replacement. Changes in AEP correlated with performance on the Trailmaking-A test but not the Mini Mental State Examination.

Zimpfer and colleagues[231] examined the impact of age on recovery of P300 latency after cardiac surgery in a study of 82 consecutive patients undergoing aortic valve replacement. Preoperative peak P300 latency was found to increase with age. In contrast to younger patients, who typically had a mechanical valve implanted, more elderly patients, who typically had a biological valve implanted, showed little recovery in P300 latency 4-months after surgery.

The clinical significance of prolonged P300 latency following cardiac surgery is uncertain and may correlate with neither the anatomical location nor the severity of brain injury. In a study of 38 patients with minor ischemic stroke, Korpelainen and colleagues[232] found that changes in age-related P300 latency were more indicative of post-stroke depression than severity of stroke.

10.13 Multimodal Brain Monitoring

The rationale for using two or more brain-monitoring modalities is increased sensitivity to ischemic cerebral dysfunction and widening of the window of opportunity in which remedial interventions can be initiated. Despite the paucity of large, prospective randomized studies, evidence from a small number of studies is suggestive of benefit.

The utility of multimodal monitoring (MMM) was assessed by Edmonds[156] in a retrospective, single-surgeon case-control study, of 78 patients undergoing CABG surgery. An intervention algorithm (Table 10.5) was developed on the basis of changes in four-channel EEG, bilateral cerebral NIRS, and unilateral TCD monitoring. Outcomes were compared to a historical control group of 386 patients in whom single-channel EEG and bispectral index monitoring was used without intervention. The incidence of neurological complications in the nonintervention group was 6.2% compared to 0% ($p=0.05$) in the intervention group. Fewer patients in the intervention group required ventilator support for >24 h and patients in this group were discharged home an average of 2.4 days earlier.

In a similar study, Novitsky and Boswell[113] monitored 550 patients undergoing off-pump CABG surgery with 2-channel EEG (compressed spectral array) and NIRS. Hemodynamic changes accompanied by ≥ 20% in peak EEG frequency amplitude or ≥ 20% fall in rSO_2 from baseline were treated with a vasoconstrictor. Significant NIRS and EEG changes were seen in 33 (6%) and 82 (15%) patients, respectively. No patient suffered a perioperative stroke. This, the authors concluded, compared very favorably with outcomes in a historical sample of 409 patients undergoing CABG surgery with or without CPB at the same institution. The lack of randomization to monitor-based intervention makes an efficacy analysis rather difficult.

Austin and colleagues[233] used a TCD/EEG/NIRS-based intervention algorithm, similar to that later used by Edmonds, to manage 250 children undergoing cardiac surgery. Significant disturbances in cerebral perfusion (fall in CBFV ≥ 20 cm/s or ≥ 50% from baseline or rise in CBFV ≥ 100% from baseline) or metabolism (fall in $rSO_2 \geq 20\%$ from baseline for ≥ 3 min) were seen in 176 (70%) cases, in which interventions were deemed necessary in 130/176 (74%). Neurologic complications (seizure, movement, vision, or speech disorder) occurred in 5/74 (7%) patients without MMM changes; 7/130 (6%) patients with intervention, and 12/46 (26%) patients without intervention (Table 10.6).

Ganzel and colleagues[80] used EEG, TCD, and NIRS to monitor 30 patients undergoing complex aortic procedures under DHCA. All patients received phenytoin

Table 10.5 Neuromonitoring-based intervention algorithm for cardiac surgery

Stage	EEG	Temp	MAP	mCBFV	rSO_2	Problem	Intervention
Any	↓	↔	↔	↔	+	Anesthesia excess	↓ Anesthesia
	↑	↔	↔ ↑	↔ ↑	↓	Inadequate anesthesia	↑ Anesthesia
	↓	↔	↔	↓	↓	Dysautoregulation	↑ MAP ↑ Flow
Pre-CPB	↓	↔	↔	↓ Sys	↓	Aortic cannula malposition	Reposition cannula
	↓	↔	↔	↓ Dias	↓	Venous cannula malposition	Reposition cannula
Onset CPB	↓	↔	↔ ↓	↔	↓	Pump rime transient	None
CPB	↓	↔	↔	HITS	↓	Embolization	Retrograde brain perfusion
	↓	↓	↔	↓	↔	Flow-metabolism coupling	None
	↓	↑	↔	↔	↓	Flow-metabolism uncoupling	↑ Anesthesia ↑ NMB
Post-CPB	↓	↔	↔	↓ Dias	↓	Cerebral edema	Ultrafiltration
Decannulation	↓	↔	↔	HITS	↓	Particulate embolization	Fosphenytoin ↑ MAP
		↓		HITS		Gas embolization	Hyperbaric chamber
ICU	↓	↔	↔	HITS	↓	Thromboembolization	Anti-platelet therapy
	↓	↑	↔	↔	↓	Hypermetabolism	O_2 supplementation

↑ increase; ↓ decrease; ↔ no change; *Sys* systolic; *Dias* diastolic; *Temp* nasopharyngeal temperature; *MAP* mean arterial pressure; *mCBFV* mean cerebral blood flow velocity; rSO_2 regional cerebral oxygen saturation; *HITS* high-intensity transient TCD signals emboli; *ICU* intensive care unit. (Reproduced and adapted from Austin.[233] With permission)

Table 10.6 Outcomes in 176 children found to have noteworthy changes in cerebral perfusion or metabolism during cardiac surgery. Algorithm-based intervention resulted in fewer neurological complications and a greater likelihood of discharge within 1 week. (Reproduced from Austin.[233] With permission)

	Intervention	No-intervention	p
Neurological complication	7/130 (6%)	12/46 (26%)	0.001
Discharge in <1 week	51%	32%	0.05

15 mg/kg before the institution of CPB and methylprednisolone 3 mg/kg during cooling. Retrograde cerebral perfusion (30–49 mmHg; 0.9–1.6 L/min) was used during DHCA in 22/30 (73%) cases. Neurological monitoring was used to ensure adequate cerebral perfusion prior to CPB, define the optimal temperature for DHCA, guide RCP perfusion pressure and flow, guide rewarming, and ensure adequate depth of anesthesia. The temperature required to produce a flat EEG (amplitude <10 pW) varied from 8°C to 22°C. During rewarming, patients managed with RCP had a more rapid return of EEG activity (21 vs. 55 min). A greater proportion of RCP patients regained consciousness within 12 h (81% vs. 0%), were weaned from mechanical ventilation within 18 h (42% vs. 13%), and were discharged from ICU within 24 h (32% vs. 0%). Neurological complications occurred in 2/22 (9%) RCP patients and 1/8 (12%) DHCA patients. The authors concluded that MMM-guided RCP using relative high pressure and flow was at least as safe as DHCA alone.

10.14 Conclusions

Although a variety of monitors of brain substrate delivery and neurological function have been commercially available for many years, they have yet to be universally adopted as "standard of care" and their use remains largely confined to specialist centers, researchers, and enthusiasts. Advanced neurological monitoring in cardiac surgery appears to offer the opportunity to detect neurological injury; to predict neurological and other outcomes; and, crucially, to modify neurological outcome. The perceived benefits of these monitoring modalities have to be balanced against the increased complexity that attends their use; an inevitable increase in operating-room time and cost; and the risk of unnecessary and potentially harmful monitor-guided intervention. While reserving this technology for high-risk patients and those undergoing procedures with a high incidence of neurological complications, the fact that neurological injury does occur in low-risk patients undergoing low-risk procedures may make this approach unjustifiable. Multimodal monitoring may offer significant advantages over single-modality monitoring, but data from prospective, randomized studies are currently lacking. Regardless of the type or types of monitor used, all should be regarded as an adjunct to, rather than a replacement for, standard clinical monitoring.

References

1. Roach GW, Kanchuger M, Mangano CM, et al. Adverse cerebral outcomes after coronary bypass surgery Multicenter Study of Perioperative Ischemia Research Group and the Ischemia Research and Education Foundation Investigators. *N Engl J Med.* 1996;335(25):1857-1863.
2. Arrowsmith J, Grocott H, Reves J, Newman M. Central nervous system complications of cardiac surgery. *Br J Anaesth.* 2000;84(3):378-393.
3. Newman M, Mathew J, Grocott H, et al. Central nervous system injury associated with cardiac surgery. *Lancet.* 2006; 368(9536):694-703.
4. Hoffman GM. Neurologic monitoring on cardiopulmonary bypass: what are we obligated to do? *Ann Thorac Surg.* 2006;81(6):S2373-S2380.
5. Murkin JM, Newman SP, Stump DA, Blumenthal JA. Statement of consensus on assessment of neurobehavioral outcomes after cardiac surgery. *Ann Thorac Surg.* 1995; 59(5):1289-1295.
6. Keats AS, Slogoff S. Perfusion pressure and coronary bypass. *J Thorac Cardiovasc Surg.* 1996;112(1):204-206.
7. Gold JP, Charlson ME, Williams-Russo P, et al. Improvement of outcomes after coronary artery bypass A randomized trial comparing intraoperative high versus low mean arterial pressure. *J Thorac Cardiovasc Surg.* 1995;110(5):1302-1311.
8. Hill SE, van Wermeskerken GK, Lardenoye JW, et al. Intraoperative physiologic variables and outcome in cardiac surgery: Part I In-hospital mortality. *Ann Thorac Surg.* 2000; 69(4):1070-1075.
9. van Wermeskerken GK, Lardenoye JW, Hill SE, et al. Intraoperative physiologic variables and outcome in cardiac surgery: Part II Neurologic outcome. *Ann Thorac Surg.* 2000;69(4):10771083.
10. Hogue CW Jr, Palin CA, Arrowsmith JE. Cardiopulmonary bypass management and neurologic outcomes: an evidence-based appraisal of current practices. *Anesth Analg.* 2006; 103(1):21-37.
11. Taylor RH, Burrows FA, Bissonnette B. Cerebral pressure-flow velocity relationship during hypothermic cardiopulmonary bypass in neonates and infants. *Anesth Analg.* 1992; 74(5):636-642.

12. Kern FH, Ungerleider RM, Quill TJ, et al. Cerebral blood flow response to changes in arterial carbon dioxide tension during hypothermic cardiopulmonary bypass in children. *J Thorac Cardiovasc Surg*. 1991;101(4):618-622.
13. Stone JG, Young WL, Smith CR, et al. Do standard monitoring sites reflect true brain temperature when profound hypothermia is rapidly induced and reversed? *Anesthesiology*. 1995;82(2):344-351.
14. Grocott HP, Newman MF. Temperature measurement during cardiac surgery. *Can J Anaesth*. 1998;45(11):1133-1134.
15. Grocott HP, Newman MF, Croughwell ND, White WD, Lowry E, Reves JG. Continuous jugular venous versus nasopharyngeal temperature monitoring during hypothermic cardiopulmonary bypass for cardiac surgery. *J Clin Anesth*. 1997;9(4):312-316.
16. Matta B. Advances in monitoring cerebral oxygenation. *Curr Opin Anaesthesiol*. 1996;9:365-370.
17. Gejrot T, Lauren T. Retrograde Venography of the Internal Jugular Veins and Transverse Sinuses; Technique and Roentgen Anatomy. *Acta Otolaryngol*. 1964;57:556-570.
18. Hayman LA, Fahr LM, Taber KH, Hughes CL, Ritter AM, Robertson C. Radiographic assessment of jugular bulb catheters. *Emerg Radiol*. 1995;2(6):331-338.
19. Bankier AA, Fleischmann D, Windisch A, et al. Position of jugular oxygen saturation catheter in patients with head trauma: assessment by use of plain films. *Am J Roentgenol*. 1995;164(2):437-441.
20. Coplin WM, O'Keefe GE, Grady MS, et al. Thrombotic, infectious, and procedural complications of the jugular bulb catheter in the intensive care unit. *Neurosurgery*. 1997;41(1):101-107.
21. Matta BF, Lam AM. The rate of blood withdrawal affects the accuracy of jugular venous bulb Oxygen saturation measurements. *Anesthesiology*. 1997;86(4):806-808.
22. Millar SA, Alston RP, Souter MJ, Andrews PJ. Continuous monitoring of jugular bulb oxyhaemoglobin saturation using the Edslab dual lumen oximetry catheter during and after cardiac surgery. *Br J Anaesth*. 1999;82(4):521-524.
23. Souter MJ, Andrews PJ. Validation of the Edslab dual lumen oximetry catheter for continuous monitoring of jugular bulb oxygen saturation after severe head injury. *Br J Anaesth*. 1996;76(5):744-746.
24. Stocchetti N, Paparella A, Bridelli F, Bacchi M, Piazza P, Zuccoli P. Cerebral venous oxygen saturation studied with bilateral samples in the internal jugular veins. *Neurosurgery*. 1994;34(1):38-43.
25. Cook DJ, Oliver WC Jr, Orszulak TA, Daly RC, Bryce RD. Cardiopulmonary bypass temperature, hematocrit, and cerebral oxygen delivery in humans. *Ann Thorac Surg*. 1995; 60(6):1671-1677.
26. Greeley WJ, Kern FH, Ungerleider RM, et al. The effect of hypothermic cardiopulmonary bypass and total circulatory arrest on cerebral metabolism in neonates, infants, and children. *J Thorac Cardiovasc Surg*. 1991;101(5):783-794.
27. Goto T, Yoshitake A, Baba T, Shibata Y, Sakata R, Uozumi H. Cerebral ischemic disorders and cerebral oxygen balance during cardiopulmonary bypass surgery: preoperative evaluation using magnetic resonance imaging and angiography. *Anesth Analg*. 1997;84(1):5-11.
28. Kern FH, Ungerleider RM, Schulman SR, et al. Comparing two strategies of cardiopulmonary bypass cooling on jugular venous oxygen saturation in neonates and infants. *Ann Thorac Surg*. 1995;60(5):1198-1202.
29. Sapire KJ, Gopinath SP, Farhat G, et al. Cerebral oxygenation during warming after cardiopulmonary bypass. *Crit Care Med*. 1997;25(10):1655-1662.
30. Andropoulos DB, Stayer SA, McKenzie ED, Fraser CD Jr. Novel cerebral physiologic monitoring to guide low-flow cerebral perfusion during neonatal aortic arch reconstruction. *J Thorac Cardiovasc Surg*. 2003;125(3):491-499.
31. von Knobelsdorff G, Tonner PH, Hanel F, Bischoff P, Scholz J, Schulte am Esch J. Prolonged rewarming after hypothermic cardiopulmonary bypass does not attenuate reduction of jugular bulb oxygen saturation. *J Cardiothorac Vasc Anesth*. 1997;11(6):689-693.
32. Hänel F, von Knobelsdorff G, Werner C, Schulte am Esch J. Hypercapnia prevents jugular bulb desaturation during rewarming from hypothermic cardiopulmonary bypass. *Anesthesiology*. 1998;89(1):19-23.
33. Croughwell N, Lyth M, Quill TJ, et al. Diabetic patients have abnormal cerebral autoregulation during cardiopulmonary bypass. *Circulation*. 1990;82(5):IV407-IV412.
34. Schwartz LB, Bridgman AH, Kieffer RW, et al. Asymptomatic carotid artery stenosis and stroke in patients undergoing cardiopulmonary bypass. *J Vasc Surg*. 1995;21(1):146-153.
35. Goto T, Baba T, Yoshitake A, Shibata Y, Ura M, Sakata R. Craniocervical and aortic atherosclerosis as neurologic risk factors in coronary surgery. *Ann Thorac Surg*. 2000;69(3): 834-40.
36. Kadoi Y, Saito S, Kawahara F, Goto F, Owada R, Fujita N. Jugular venous bulb oxygen saturation in patients with preexisting diabetes mellitus or stroke during normothermic cardiopulmonary bypass. *Anesthesiology*. 2000;92(5): 1324-1329.
37. Kadoi Y, Saito S, Goto F, Someya T, Kamiyashiki S, Fujita N. Time course of changes in jugular venous oxygen saturation during hypothermic or normothermic cardiopulmonary bypass in patients with diabetes mellitus. *Acta Anaesthesiol Scand*. 2001;45(7):858-862.
38. Kadoi Y, Saito S, Yoshikawa D, Goto F, Fujita N, Kunimoto F. Increasing mean arterial blood pressure has no effect on jugular venous oxygen saturation in insulin-dependent patients during tepid cardiopulmonary bypass. *Anesth Analg*. 2002;95(2):266-272. table of contents.
39. Kuwabara M, Nakajima N, Yamamoto F, et al. Continuous monitoring of blood oxygen saturation of internal jugular vein as a useful indicator for selective cerebral perfusion during aortic arch replacement. *J Thorac Cardiovasc Surg*. 1992;103(2):355-362.
40. Matsuwaka R, Sakakibara T, Mitsuno M, et al. Improved management of selective cerebral perfusion in aortic arch surgery. *ASAIO J*. 1996;42(5):M794-M796.
41. Gopinath SP, Robertson CS, Contant CF, et al. Jugular venous desaturation and outcome after head injury. *J Neurol Neurosurg Psychiatr*. 1994;57(6):717-723.
42. Croughwell ND, Newman MF, Blumenthal JA, et al. Jugular bulb saturation and cognitive dysfunction after cardiopulmonary bypass. *Ann Thorac Surg*. 1994;58(6):1702-1728.
43. Newman MF, Kramer D, Croughwell ND, et al. Differential age effects of mean arterial pressure and rewarming on cognitive dysfunction after cardiac surgery. *Anesth Analg*. 1995;81(2):236-242.

44. Grigore AM, Grocott HP, Mathew JP, et al. The rewarming rate and increased peak temperature alter neurocognitive outcome after cardiac surgery. *Anesth Analg*. 2002;94(1): 4-10. table of contents.
45. Kurth CD, Steven JM, Swedlow D. New frontiers in oximetry. *Am J Anesthesiol*. 1996;23:169-175.
46. Jöbsis FF. Noninvasive, infrared monitoring of cerebral and myocardial oxygen sufficiency and circulatory parameters. *Science*. 1977;198(4323):1264-1267.
47. Ferrari M, Wilson DA, Hanley DF, Hartmann JF, Rogers MC, Traystman RJ. Noninvasive determination of hemoglobin saturation in dogs by derivative near-infrared spectroscopy. *Am J Physiol*. 1989;256(5 Pt 2):H1493-H1499.
48. Kurth CD, Steven JM, Benaron D, Chance B. Near-infrared monitoring of the cerebral circulation. *J Clin Monit*. 1993; 9(3):163-170.
49. Delpy DT, Cope M, van der Zee P, Arridge S, Wray S, Wyatt J. Estimation of optical pathlength through tissue from direct time of flight measurement. *Phys Med Biol*. 1988;33(12): 1433-1442.
50. Duncan A, Meek JH, Clemence M, et al. Optical pathlength measurements on adult head, calf and forearm and the head of the newborn infant using phase resolved optical spectroscopy. *Phys Med Biol*. 1995;40(2):295-304.
51. Elwell CE, Cope M, Edwards AD, Wyatt JS, Delpy DT, Reynolds EO. Quantification of adult cerebral hemodynamics by near-infrared spectroscopy. *J Appl Physiol*. 1994; 77(6):2753-2760.
52. Elwell CE. *A Practical Users Guide to Near Infrared Spectroscopy*. London: Hamamatsu Ohotonics KK/UCL Reprographics; 1995.
53. Watzman HM, Kurth CD, Montenegro LM, Rome J, Steven JM, Nicolson SC. Arterial and venous contributions to near-infrared cerebral oximetry. *Anesthesiology*. 2000;93(4): 947-953.
54. Germon TJ, Kane NM, Manara AR, Nelson RJ. Near-infrared spectroscopy in adults: effects of extracranial ischemia and intracranial hypoxia on estimation of cerebral oxygenation. *Br J Anaesth*. 1994;73(4):503-506.
55. Grubhofer G, Lassnigg A, Manlik F, Marx E, Trubel W, Hiesmayr M. The contribution of extracranial blood oxygenation on near-infrared spectroscopy during carotid thrombendarterectomy. *Anesthesia*. 1997;52(2):116-120.
56. Hongo K, Kobayashi S, Okudera H, Hokama M, Nakagawa F. Noninvasive cerebral optical spectroscopy: depth-resolved measurements of cerebral haemodynamics using indocyanine green. *Neurol Res*. 1995;17(2):89-93.
57. Kaminogo M, Ochi M, Onizuka M, Takahata H, Shibata S. An additional monitoring of regional cerebral oxygen saturation to HMPAO SPECT study during balloon test occlusion. *Stroke*. 1999;30(2):407-413.
58. Holzschuh M, Woertgen C, Metz C, Brawanski A. Dynamic changes of cerebral oxygenation measured by brain tissue oxygen pressure and near infrared spectroscopy. *Neurol Res*. 1997;19(3):246-248.
59. Misra M, Stark J, Dujovny M, Widman R, Ausman JI. Transcranial cerebral oximetry in random normal subjects. *Neurol Res*. 1998;20(2):137-141.
60. Kim MB, Ward DS, Cartwright CR, Kolano J, Chlebowski S, Henson LC. Estimation of jugular venous O2 saturation from cerebral oximetry or arterial O2 saturation during isocapnic hypoxia. *J Clin Monit Comput*. 2000;16(3): 191-199.
61. Kishi K, Kawaguchi M, Yoshitani K, Nagahata T, Furuya H. Influence of patient variables and sensor location on regional cerebral oxygen saturation measured by INVOS 4100 near-infrared spectrophotometers. *J Neurosurg Anesthesiol*. 2003; 15(4):302-306.
62. Edmonds HL Jr, Ganzel BL, Austin EH 3rd. Cerebral oximetry for cardiac and vascular surgery. *Semin Cardiothorac Vasc Anesth*. 2004;8(2):147-166.
63. Pollard V, Prough DS, DeMelo AE, Deyo DJ, Uchida T, Stoddart HF. Validation in volunteers of a near-infrared spectroscope for monitoring brain oxygenation in vivo. *Anesth Analg*. 1996;82(2):269-277.
64. Doblar DD. Intraoperative transcranial ultrasonic monitoring for cardiac and vascular surgery. *Semin Cardiothorac Vasc Anesth*. 2004;8(2):127-145.
65. Arrowsmith JE. Neurological monitoring. In: Mackay JM, Arrowsmith JE, eds. *Core Topics in Cardiac Anesthesia*. Cambridge: Cambridge University Press; 2004:141-146.
66. Aaslid R, Markwalder TM, Nornes H. Noninvasive transcranial Doppler ultrasound recording of flow velocity in basal cerebral arteries. *J Neurosurg*. 1982;57(6):769-774.
67. Chung EM. Transcranial Doppler embolus dtection: a primer. *Ultrasound*. 2006;14(4):202-210.
68. Bishop CC, Powell S, Rutt D, Browse NL. Transcranial Doppler measurement of middle cerebral artery blood flow velocity: a validation study. *Stroke*. 1986;17(5): 913-915.
69. Grocott HP, Amory DW, Lowry E, Croughwell ND, Newman MF. Transcranial Doppler blood flow velocity versus 133Xe clearance cerebral blood flow during mild hypothermic cardiopulmonary bypass. *J Clin Monit Comput*. 1998;14(1): 35-39.
70. Trivedi UH, Patel RL, Turtle MR, Venn GE, Chambers DJ. Relative changes in cerebral blood flow during cardiac operations using xenon-133 clearance versus transcranial Doppler sonography. *Ann Thorac Surg*. 1997;63(1):167-174.
71. Groom RC, Quinn RD, Lennon P, et al. Detection and elimination of microemboli related to cardiopulmonary bypass. *Circ Cardiovasc Qual Outcomes*. 2009;2(3):191-198.
72. Rodriguez RA, Cornel G, Semelhago L, Splinter WM, Weerasena NA. Cerebral effects in superior vena caval cannula obstruction: the role of brain monitoring. *Ann Thorac Surg*. 1997;64(6):1820-1822.
73. Siegel LC, St Goar FG, Stevens JH. Monitoring considerations for port-access cardiac surgery. *Circulation*. 1997; 96(2):562-568.
74. Grocott HP, Smith MS, Glower DD, Clements FM. Endovascular aortic balloon clamp malposition during minimally invasive cardiac surgery: detection by transcranial Doppler monitoring. *Anesthesiology*. 1998;88(5): 1396-1399.
75. O'Hare B, Bissonnette B, Bohn D, Cox P, Williams W. Persistent low cerebral blood flow velocity following profound hypothermic circulatory arrest in infants. *Can J Anaesth*. 1995;42(11):964-971.
76. Astudillo R, van der Linden J, Ekroth R, et al. Absent diastolic cerebral blood flow velocity after circulatory arrest but not after low flow in infants. *Ann Thorac Surg*. 1993;56(3): 515-519.

77. Zimmerman AA, Burrows FA, Jonas RA, Hickey PR. The limits of detectable cerebral perfusion by transcranial Doppler sonography in neonates undergoing deep hypothermic low-flow cardiopulmonary bypass. *J Thorac Cardiovasc Surg*. 1997;114(4):594-600.
78. Neri E, Sassi C, Barabesi L, et al. Cerebral autoregulation after hypothermic circulatory arrest in operations on the aortic arch. *Ann Thorac Surg*. 2004;77(1):72-79.
79. Tanoue Y, Tominaga R, Ochiai Y, et al. Comparative study of retrograde and selective cerebral perfusion with transcranial Doppler. *Ann Thorac Surg*. 1999;67(3):672-675.
80. Ganzel BL, Edmonds HL Jr, Pank JR, Goldsmith LJ. Neurophysiologic monitoring to assure delivery of retrograde cerebral perfusion. *J Thorac Cardiovasc Surg*. 1997; 113(4):748-755.
81. Saver JL, Feldman E. Basic transcranial Doppler examination: technique and anatomy. In: Babakian VL, Wechsler LR, eds. *Transcranial Doppler Ultrasonography*. St Louis: Mosby; 1993.
82. Doblar DD, Plyushcheva NV, Jordan W, McDowell H. Predicting the effect of carotid artery occlusion during carotid endarterectomy: comparing transcranial doppler measurements and cerebral angiography. *Stroke*. 1998; 29(10):2038-2042.
83. Adams R, McKie V, Nichols F, et al. The use of transcranial ultrasonography to predict stroke in sickle cell disease. *N Engl J Med*. 1992;326(9):605-610.
84. Grosset DG, Georgiadis D, Kelman AW, Lees KR. Quantification of ultrasound emboli signals in patients with cardiac and carotid disease. *Stroke*. 1993;24(12):1922-1924.
85. Georgiadis D, Mallinson A, Grosset DG, Lees KR. Coagulation activity and emboli counts in patients with prosthetic cardiac valves. *Stroke*. 1994;25(6):1211-1214.
86. Georgiadis D, Grosset DG, Quin RO, Nichol JA, Bone I, Lees KR. Detection of intracranial emboli in patients with carotid disease. *Eur J Vasc Surg*. 1994;8(3):309-314.
87. Grosset DG, Cowburn P, Georgiadis D, Dargie HJ, Faichney A, Lee KR. Ultrasound detection of cerebral emboli in patients with prosthetic heart valves. *J Heart Valve Dis*. 1994;3(2):128-132.
88. Grosset DG, Georgiadis D, Abdullah I, Bone I, Lees KR. Doppler emboli signals vary according to stroke subtype. *Stroke*. 1994;25(2):382-384.
89. Tong DC, Bolger A, Albers GW. Incidence of transcranial Doppler-detected cerebral microemboli in patients referred for echocardiography. *Stroke*. 1994;25(11):2138-2141.
90. Streifler JY, Katz M. Cardiogenic cerebral emboli: diagnosis and treatment. *Curr Opin Neurol*. 1995;8(1):45-54.
91. Muller HR, Lyrer P, Boccalini P. Doppler monitoring of middle cerebral artery emboli from carotid stenoses. *J Neuroimaging*. 1995;5(2):71-7 5.
92. Aasen J, Kerty E, Russell D, Bakke SJ, Nyberg-Hansen R. Amaurosis fugax: clinical, Doppler and angiographic findings. *Acta Neurol Scand*. 1988;77(6):450-455.
93. Dittrich R, Ritter MA, Kaps M, et al. The use of embolic signal detection in multicenter trials to evaluate antiplatelet efficacy: signal analysis and quality control mechanisms in the CARESS (Clopidogrel and Aspirin for Reduction of Emboli in Symptomatic carotid Stenosis) trial. *Stroke*. 2006;37(4):1065-1069.
94. Spencer MP, Thomas GI, Nicholls SC, Sauvage LR. Detection of middle cerebral artery emboli during carotid endarterectomy using transcranial Doppler ultrasonography. *Stroke*. 1990;21(3):415-423.
95. Arrowsmith JE, Stygall J, Timberlake N, et al. The intra-aortic balloon pump is a source of cerebral microemboli. Perfusion. 1997;12(1):33.
96. von Knobelsdorff G, Brauer P, Tonner PH, et al. Transmyocardial laser revascularization induces cerebral microembolization. Anesthesiology. 1997;87(1):58-62.
97. Dagirmanjian A, Davis DA, Rothfus WE, Goldberg AL, Deeb ZL. Detection of clinically silent intracranial emboli ipsilateral to internal carotid occlusions during cerebral angiography. Am J Roentgenol. 2000;174(2):367-369.
98. Edmonds CR, Barbut D, Hager D, Sharrock NE. Intraoperative cerebral arterial embolization during total hip arthroplasty. Anesthesiology. 2000;93(2):315-318.
99. Rodriguez RA, Sinclair B, Weatherdon D, Letts M. Patent foramen ovale and brain microembolization during scoliosis surgery in adolescents. Spine. 2001;26(15):1719-1721.
100. Nabavi DG, Stockmann J, Schmid C, et al. Doppler microembolic load predicts risk of thromboembolic complications in Novacor patients. *J Thorac Cardiovasc Surg*. 2003; 126(1):160-167.
101. Ferrari J, Baumgartner H, Tentschert S, et al. Cerebral microembolism during transcatheter closure of patent foramen ovale. *J Neurol*. 2004;251(7):825-829.
102. Ehrlich R, Mutzmacher L, Averbuch L, Dotan G, Hirsh R. Do complaints of amaurosis fugax and blurred vision after transcatheter device closure of atrial septal defect indicate microemboli to retinal vessels? *J Interv Cardiol*. 2005; 18(1):21-25.
103. van der Linden J, Casimir-Ahn H. When do cerebral emboli appear during open heart operations? A transcranial Doppler study. *Ann Thorac Surg*. 1991;51(2):237-241.
104. Barbut D, Hinton RB, Szatrowski TP, et al. Cerebral emboli detected during bypass surgery are associated with clamp removal. *Stroke*. 1994;25(12):2398-2402.
105. Hartman GS, Yao FS, Bruefach M 3rd, et al. Severity of aortic atheromatous disease diagnosed by transesophageal echocardiography predicts stroke and other outcomes associated with coronary artery surgery: a prospective study. *Anesth Analg*. 1996;83(4):701-708.
106. O'Brien JJ, Butterworth J, Hammon JW, Morris KJ, Phipps JM, Stump DA. Cerebral emboli during cardiac surgery in children. *Anesthesiology*. 1997;87(5):1063-1069.
107. Taylor RL, Borger MA, Weisel RD, Fedorko L, Feindel CM. Cerebral microemboli during cardiopulmonary bypass: increased emboli during perfusionist interventions. *Ann Thorac Surg*. 1999;68(1):89-93.
108. Borger MA, Feindel CM. Cerebral emboli during cardiopulmonary bypass: effect of perfusionist interventions and aortic cannulas. *J Extra Corpor Technol*. 2002;34(1): 29-33.
109. Cassie AB, Riddell AG, Yates PO. Hazard of antifoam emboli from a bubble oxygenator. *Thorax*. 1960;15:22-29.
110. Helmsworth JA, Gall EA, Perrin EV, et al. Occurrence of emboli during perfusion with an oxygenator pump. *Surgery*. 1963;53:177-185.
111. Deverall PB, Padayachee TS, Parsons S, Theobold R, Battistessa SA. Ultrasound detection of micro-emboli in

the middle cerebral artery during cardiopulmonary bypass surgery. *Eur J Cardiothorac Surg*. 1988;2(4):256-260.
112. Padayachee TS, Parsons S, Theobold R, Linley J, Gosling RG, Deverall PB. The detection of microemboli in the middle cerebral artery during cardiopulmonary bypass: a transcranial Doppler ultrasound investigation using membrane and bubble oxygenators. *Ann Thorac Surg*. 1987;44(3): 298-302.
113. Novitzky D, Boswell BB. Total myocardial revascularization without cardiopulmonary bypass utilizing computer-processed monitoring to assess cerebral perfusion. *Heart Surg Forum*. 2000;3(3):198-202.
114. Watters MP, Cohen AM, Monk CR, Angelini GD, Ryder IG. Reduced cerebral embolic signals in beating heart coronary surgery detected by transcranial Doppler ultrasound. *Br J Anaesth*. 2000;84(5):629-631.
115. Skjelland M, Bergsland J, Lundblad R, et al. Cerebral microembolization during off-pump coronary artery bypass surgery with the Symmetry aortic connector device. *J Thorac Cardiovasc Surg*. 2005;130(6):1581-1585.
116. Murkin JM. Con: Blood gases should not be corrected for temperature during hypothermic cardiopulmonary bypass: alpha-stat mode. *J Cardiothorac Anesth*. 1988;2(5): 705-707.
117. Murkin JM. Alpha-stat acid-base regulation during cardiopulmonary bypass. *J Thorac Cardiovasc Surg*. 1997;113(3): 619-620.
118. Pugsley W, Klinger L, Paschalis C, Treasure T, Harrison M, Newman S. The impact of microemboli during cardiopulmonary bypass on neuropsychological functioning. *Stroke*. 1994;25(7):1393-1399.
119. BhaskerRao B, VanHimbergen D, Edmonds HL Jr, et al. Evidence for improved cerebral function after minimally invasive bypass surgery. *J Card Surg*. 1998;13(1):27-31.
120. Braekken SK, Reinvang I, Russell D, Brucher R, Svennevig JL. Association between intraoperative cerebral microembolic signals and postoperative neuropsychological deficit: comparison between patients with cardiac valve replacement and patients with coronary artery bypass grafting. *J Neurol Neurosurg Psychiatry*. 1998;65(4):573-576.
121.Malheiros SM, Brucki SM, Gabbai AA, et al. Neurological outcome in coronary artery surgery with and without cardiopulmonary bypass. *Acta Neurol Scand*. 1995;92(3):256-260.
122. Jacobs A, Neveling M, Horst M, et al. Alterations of neuropsychological function and cerebral glucose metabolism after cardiac surgery are not related only to intraoperative microembolic events. *Stroke*. 1998;29(3):660-667.
123. Katz ES, Tunick PA, Rusinek H, Ribakove G, Spencer FC, Kronzon I. Protruding aortic atheromas predict stroke in elderly patients undergoing cardiopulmonary bypass: experience with intraoperative transesophageal echocardiography. *J Am Coll Cardiol*. 1992;20(1):70-77.
124. Mackensen GB, Ti LK, Phillips-Bute BG, Mathew JP, Newman MF, Grocott HP. Cerebral embolization during cardiac surgery: impact of aortic atheroma burden. *Br J Anaesth*. 2003;91(5):656-661.
125. Pugsley WB, Klinger L, Paschalis C, Newman SN, Harrison M, Treasure T. Does arterial line filtration affect the bypass related cerebral impairment observed in patients undergoing coronary artery surgery? *Clin Sci*. 1988;75(Suppl 19):30-31.
126. Calafiore AM, Bar-El Y, Vitolla G, et al. Early clinical experience with a new sutureless anastomotic device for proximal anastomosis of the saphenous vein to the aorta. *J Thorac Cardiovasc Surg*. 2001;121(5):854-858.
127. Mullges W, Franke D, Reents W, Babin-Ebell J. Brain microembolic counts during extracorporeal circulation depend on aortic cannula position. *Ultrasound Med Biol*. 2001;27(7):933-936.
128. Borger MA, Taylor RL, Weisel RD, et al. Decreased cerebral emboli during distal aortic arch cannulation: a randomized clinical trial. *J Thorac Cardiovasc Surg*. 1999;118(4): 740-745.
129. Caton R. The electric currents of the brain. *BMJ*. 1875; 2:278.
130. Swartz BE, Goldensohn ES. Timeline of the history of EEG and associated fields. *Electroencephalogr Clin Neurophysiol*. 1998;106(2):173-176.
131. Berger H. Uber das Elektroenkelogram des Menchen. *Arch f Psychiat*. 1929;87:527-570.
132. Jenkinson JL. The monitoring of central nervous system funciton in anesthesia and intensive care. *Curr Anaesth Crit Care*. 1990;1(2):115-121.
133. Rampil IJ. A primer for EEG signal processing in anesthesia. *Anesthesiology*. 1998;89(4):980-1002.
134. McCormick DA. Neurotransmitter actions in the thalamus and cerebral cortex and their role in neuromodulation of thalamocortical activity. *Prog Neurobiol*. 1992;39(4): 337-388.
135. American Electroencephalographic Society guidelines for standard electrode position nomenclature. *J Clin Neurophysiol*. 1991;8(2):200-202.
136. Klem GH, Luders HO, Jasper HH, Elger C. The ten-twenty electrode system of the International Federation. The International Federation of Clinical Neurophysiology. *Electroencephalogr Clin Neurophysiol Suppl*. 1999; 52:3-6.
137. Cooley JW, Tukey JW. An algorithm for the machine calculation of complex Fourier series. *Math Comput*. 1965; 19:297-301.
138. Maynard DE, Jenkinson JL. The cerebral function analysing monitor. Initial clinical experience, application and further development. *Anesthesia*. 1984;39(7):678-690.
139. Prichep LS, Gugino LD, John ER, et al. The Patient State Index as an indicator of the level of hypnosis under general anesthesia. *Br J Anaesth*. 2004;92(3):393-399.
140. Sachdev NS, Carter CC, Swank RL, Blachly PH. Relationship between post-cardiotomy delirium, clinical neurological changes, and EEG abnormalities. *J Thorac Cardiovasc Surg*. 1967;54(4):557-563.
141. Sotaniemi KA. Clinical and prognostic correlates of EEG in open-heart surgery patients. *J Neurol Neurosurg Psychiatr*. 1980;43(10):941-947.
142. Sotaniemi KA, Sulg IA, Hokkanen TE. Quantitative EEG as a measure of cerebral dysfunction before and after open-heart surgery. *Electroencephalogr Clin Neurophysiol*. 1980;50(1-2):81-95.
143. Sotaniemi K. Five-year neurological and EEG outcome after open-heart surgery. *J Neurol Neurosurg Psychiatr*. 1985;48(6):569-575.
144. Levy WJ. Quantitative analysis of EEG changes during hypothermia. *Anesthesiology*. 1984;60(4):291-297.

145. Frank M, Maynard DE, Tsanaclis LM, Major E, Coutinho PE. Changes in cerebral electrical activity measured by the Cerebral Function Analysing Monitor following bolus injections of thiopentone. *Br J Anaesth*. 1984;56(10):1075-81.
146. Sebel PS, Bovill JG, Wauquier A, Rog P. Effects of high-dose fentanyl anesthesia on the electroencephalogram. *Anesthesiology*. 1981;55(3):203-211.
147. John ER, Prichep LS, Kox W, et al. Invariant reversible QEEG effects of anesthetics. *Conscious Cogn*. 2001;10(2):165-183.
148. Gugino LD, Chabot RJ, Prichep LS, John ER, Formanek V, Aglio LS. Quantitative EEG changes associated with loss and return of consciousness in healthy adult volunteers anaesthetized with propofol or sevoflurane. *Br J Anaesth*. 2001;87(3):421-428.
149. Woodcock TE, Murkin JM, Farrar JK, Tweed WA, Guiraudon GM, McKenzie FN. Pharmacologic EEG suppression during cardiopulmonary bypass: cerebral hemodynamic and metabolic effects of thiopental or isoflurane during hypothermia and normothermia. *Anesthesiology*. 1987;67(2):218-224.
150. Bonhomme V, Plourde G, Meuret P, Fiset P, Backman SB. Auditory steady-state response and bispectral index for assessing level of consciousness during propofol sedation and hypnosis. *Anesth Analg*. 2000;91(6):1398-1403.
151. Drover DR, Lemmens HJ, Pierce ET, et al. Patient State Index: titration of delivery and recovery from propofol, alfentanil, and nitrous oxide anesthesia. *Anesthesiology*. 2002;97(1):82-89.
152. Adam N, Sebel PS. BIS monitoring: awareness and catastrophic events. *Semin Cardiothorac Vasc Anesth*. 2004;8(1):9-12.
153. Ekman A, Lindholm ML, Lennmarken C, Sandin R. Reduction in the incidence of awareness using BIS monitoring. *Acta Anaesthesiol Scand*. 2004;48(1):20-26.
154. Vakkuri A, Yli-Hankala A, Talja P, et al. Time-frequency balanced spectral entropy as a measure of anesthetic drug effect in central nervous system during sevoflurane, propofol, and thiopental anesthesia. *Acta Anaesthesiol Scand*. 2004;48(2):145-153.
155. Guaracino F. Cerebral monitoring during cardiovascular surgery. *Curr Opin Anesthesiol*. 2008;21:50-54.
156. Edmonds HL Jr. Multi-modality neurophysiologic monitoring for cardiac surgery. *Heart Surg Forum*. 2002;5(3): 225-228.
157. Schwartz RB, Jones KM, LeClercq GT, et al. The value of cerebral angiography in predicting cerebral ischemia during carotid endarterectomy. *Am J Roentgenol*. 1992;159(5): 1057-1061.
158. Hanowell LH, Soriano S, Bennett HL. EEG power changes are more sensitive than spectral edge frequency variation for detection of cerebral ischemia during carotid artery surgery: a prospective assessment of processed EEG monitoring. *J Cardiothorac Vasc Anesth*. 1992;6(3):292-294.
159. Hans SS, Jareunpoon O. Prospective evaluation of electroencephalography, carotid artery stump pressure, and neurologic changes during 314 consecutive carotid endarterectomies performed in awake patients. *J Vasc Surg*. 2007; 45(3):511-515.
160. Theye RA, Patrick RT, Kirklin JW. The electro-encephalogram in patients undergoing open intracardiac operations with the aid of extracorporeal circulation. *J Thorac Surg*. 1957;34(6):709-717.
161. Branthwaite MA. Factors affecting cerebral activity during open-heart surgery. *Anesthesia*. 1973;28(6):619-625.
162. Branthwaite MA. Detection of neurological damage during open-heart surgery. *Thorax*. 1973;28(4):464-472.
163. Branthwaite MA. Prevention of neurological damage during open-heart surgery. *Thorax*. 1975;30(3):258-261.
164. Kritikou PE, Branthwaite MA. Significance of changes in cerebral electrical activity at onset of cardiopulmonary bypass. *Thorax*. 1977;32(5):534-538.
165. Arom KV, Cohen DE, Strobl FT. Effect of intraoperative intervention on neurological outcome based on electroencephalographic monitoring during cardiopulmonary bypass. *Ann Thorac Surg*. 1989;48(4):476-483.
166. Bashein G, Nessly ML, Bledsoe SW, et al. Electroencephalography during surgery with cardiopulmonary bypass and hypothermia. *Anesthesiology*. 1992;76(6): 878-891.
167. Edmonds HL Jr, Griffiths LK, van der Laken J, Slater AD, Shields CB. Quantitative electroencephalographic monitoring during myocardial revascularization predicts postoperative disorientation and improves outcome. *J Thorac Cardiovasc Surg*. 1992;103(3):555-563.
168. Hauser E, Seidl R, Rohrbach D, Hartl I, Marx M, Wimmer M. Quantitative EEG before and after open heart surgery in children. A significant decrease in the beta and alpha 2 bands postoperatively. *Electroencephalogr Clin Neurophysiol*. 1993;87(5):284-290.
169. Chabot RJ, Gugino LD, Aglio LS, Maddi R, Cote W. QEEG and neuropsychological profiles of patients after undergoing cardiopulmonary bypass surgical procedures. *Clin Electroencephalogr*. 1997;28(2):98-105.
170. Gugino LD, Chabot RJ, Aglio LS, Maddi R, Gosnell J, Aranki S. QEEG and neuropsychological profiles of patients prior to undergoing cardiopulmonary bypass surgical procedures. *Clin Electroencephalogr*. 1997;28(2): 87-97.
171. Banoub M, Tetzlaff JE, Schubert A. Pharmacologic and physiologic influences affecting sensory evoked potentials: implications for perioperative monitoring. *Anesthesiology*. 2003;99(3):716-737.
172. Gugino LD, Chabot RJ, Aglio LS, Aranki S, Dekkers R, Maddi R. QEEG changes during cardiopulmonary bypass: relationship to postoperative neuropsychological function. *Clin Electroencephalogr*. 1999;30(2):53-63.
173. Arroyo S, Lesser RP, Gillinov AM, et al. EEG and prognosis of neurologic recovery of dogs under profound hypothermic circulatory arrest. *Electroencephalogr Clin Neurophysiol*. 1993;87(4):242-249.
174. Edmonds HL Jr, Rodriguez RA, Audenaert SM, Austin EH 3rd, Pollock SB Jr, Ganzel BL. The role of neuromonitoring in cardiovascular surgery. *J Cardiothorac Vasc Anesth*. 1996;10(1):15-23.
175. Stecker MM, Cheung AT, Pochettino A, et al. Deep hypothermic circulatory arrest: II Changes in electroencephalogram and evoked potentials during rewarming. *Ann Thorac Surg*. 2001;71(1):22-28.
176. Newberg LA, Michenfelder JD. Cerebral protection by isoflurane during hypoxemia or ischemia. *Anesthesiology*. 1983;59(1):29-35.

177. Newberg LA, Milde JH, Michenfelder JD. The cerebral metabolic effects of isoflurane at and above concentrations that suppress cortical electrical activity. *Anesthesiology.* 1983;59(1):23-28.
178. Michenfelder JD. A valid demonstration of barbiturate-induced brain protection in man-at last. *Anesthesiology.* 1986;64(2):140-142.
179. Nussmeier NA, Arlund C, Slogoff S. Neuropsychiatric complications after cardiopulmonary bypass: cerebral protection by a barbiturate. *Anesthesiology.* 1986;64(2):165-170.
180. Pascoe EA, Hudson RJ, Anderson BA, et al. High-dose thiopentone for open-chamber cardiac surgery: a retrospective review. *Can J Anaesth.* 1996;43(6):575-579.
181. Newman MF, Murkin JM, Roach G, et al. Cerebral physiologic effects of burst suppression doses of propofol during nonpulsatile cardiopulmonary bypass CNS Subgroup of McSPI. *Anesth Analg.* 1995;81(3):452-457.
182. Newman MF, Croughwell ND, White WD, Sanderson I, Spillane W, Reves JG. Pharmacologic electroencephalographic suppression during cardiopulmonary bypass: a comparison of thiopental and isoflurane. *Anesth Analg.* 1998;86(2):246-251.
183. Roach GW, Newman MF, Murkin JM, et al. Ineffectiveness of burst suppression therapy in mitigating perioperative cerebrovascular dysfunction. Multicenter Study of Perioperative Ischemia (McSPI) Research Group. *Anesthesiology.* 1999;90(5):1255-1264.
184. Mourisse J, Booij L. Bispectral index detects period of cerebral hypoperfusion during cardiopulmonary bypass. *J Cardiothorac Vasc Anesth.* 2003;17(1):76-78.
185. Villacorta J, Kerbaul F, Collart F, et al. Perioperative cerebral ischemia in cardiac surgery and BIS. *Anaesth Intensive Care.* 2005;33(4):514-517.
186. Puri GD, Murthy SS. Bispectral index monitoring in patients undergoing cardiac surgery under cardiopulmonary bypass. *Eur J Anaesthesiol.* 2003;20(6):451-456.
187. Kumar A, Bhattacharya A, Makhija N. Evoked potential monitoring in anesthesia and analgesia. *Anesthesia.* 2000; 55(3):225-241.
188. American Electroencephalographic Society. Guideline eleven: guidelines for intraoperative monitoring of sensory evoked potentials. *J Clin Neurophysiol.* 1994;11(1):77-87.
189. American Electroencephalographic Society. Guideline nine: guidelines on evoked potentials. *J Clin Neurophysiol.* 1994;11(1):40-73.
190. American Electroencephalographic Society. Guideline one: minimum technical requirements for performing clinical electroencephalography. *J Clin Neurophysiol.* 1994;11(1): 2-5.
191. Denys EH. AAEM minimonograph #14: The influence of temperature in clinical neurophysiology. *Muscle Nerve.* 1991;14(9):795-811.
192. Markand ON, Warren C, Mallik GS, King RD, Brown JW, Mahomed Y. Effects of hypothermia on short latency somatosensory evoked potentials in humans. *Electroencephalogr Clin Neurophysiol.* 1990;77(6):416-424.
193. Markand ON, Warren C, Mallik GS, Williams CJ. Temperature-dependent hysteresis in somatosensory and auditory evoked potentials. *Electroencephalogr Clin Neurophysiol.* 1990;77(6):425-435.
194. Stecker MM, Cheung AT, Pochettino A, et al. Deep hypothermic circulatory arrest: I Effects of cooling on electroencephalogram and evoked potentials. *Ann Thorac Surg.* 2001;71(1):14-21.
195. Cantor RS. The lateral pressure profile in membranes: a physical mechanism of general anesthesia. *Biochemistry.* 1997;36(9):2339-2344.
196. Rosenberg PH, Heavner JE. Temperature-dependent nerve-blocking action of lidocaine and halothane. *Acta Anaesthesiol Scand.* 1980;24(4):314-320.
197. Zhou JX, Liu J. The effect of temperature on solubility of volatile anesthetics in human tissues. *Anesth Analg.* 2001;93(1):234-238.
198. Stecker MM, Kent G, Escherich A, Patterson T, Cheung AT. Anesthesia and temperature effects on somatosensory evoked potentials produced by train stimuli. *Int J Neurosci.* 2002;112(3):349-369.
199. Stecker MM, Cheung AT, Patterson T, et al. Detection of stroke during cardiac operations with somatosensory evoked responses. *J Thorac Cardiovasc Surg.* 1996;112(4):962-972.
200. Cheung AT, Savino JS, Weiss SJ, et al. Detection of acute embolic stroke during mitral valve replacement using somatosensory evoked potential monitoring. *Anesthesiology.* 1995;83(1):208-210.
201. Guerit JM, Verhelst R, Rubay J, et al. The use of somatosensory evoked potentials to determine the optimal degree of hypothermia during circulatory arrest. *J Card Surg.* 1994;9(5):596-603.
202. Cheung AT, Bavaria JE, Pochettino A, Weiss SJ, Barclay DK, Stecker MM. Oxygen delivery during retrograde cerebral perfusion in humans. *Anesth Analg.* 1999;88(1):8-15.
203. Hickey C, Gugino LD, Aglio LS, Mark JB, Son SL, Maddi R. Intraoperative somatosensory evoked potential monitoring predicts peripheral nerve injury during cardiac surgery. *Anesthesiology.* 1993;78(1):29-35.
204. Jellish WS, Martucci J, Blakeman B, Hudson E. Somatosensory evoked potential monitoring of the brachial plexus to predict nerve injury during internal mammary artery harvest: intraoperative comparisons of the Rultract and Pittman sternal retractors. *J Cardiothorac Vasc Anesth.* 1994;8(4):398-403.
205. Jellish WS, Blakeman B, Warf P, Slogoff S. Somatosensory evoked potential monitoring used to compare the effect of three asymmetric sternal retractors on brachial plexus function. *Anesth Analg.* 1999;88(2):292-297.
206. Seal D, Balaton J, Coupland SG, et al. Somatosensory evoked potential monitoring during cardiac surgery: an examination of brachial plexus dysfunction. *J Cardiothorac Vasc Anesth.* 1997;11(2):187-191.
207. Porkkala T, Kaukinen S, Hakkinen V, Jantti V. Effects of hypothermia and sternal retractors on median nerve somatosensory evoked potentials. *Acta Anaesthesiol Scand.* 1997;41(7):843-848.
208. Rodriguez RA. Human auditory evoked potentials in the assessment of brain function during major cardiovascular surgery. *Semin Cardiothorac Vasc Anesth.* 2004;8(2):85-99.
209. Thornton C. Evoked potentials in anesthesia. *Eur J Anaesthesiol.* 1991;8(2):89-107.
210. Thornton C, Jones JG. Evaluating depth of anesthesia: review of methods. *Int Anesthesiol Clin.* 1993;31(4): 67-88.

211. Rodriguez RA, Audenaert SM, Austin EH 3rd, Edmonds HL Jr. Auditory evoked responses in children during hypothermic cardiopulmonary bypass: report of cases. *J Clin Neurophysiol.* 1995;12(2):168-176.
212. Soltani M, Knight RT. Neural origins of the P300. *Crit Rev Neurobiol.* 2000;14(3–4):199-224.
213. Baudena P, Halgren E, Heit G, Clarke JM. Intracerebral potentials to rare target and distractor auditory and visual stimuli. III. Frontal cortex. *Electroencephalogr Clin Neurophysiol.* 1995;94(4):251-264.
214. Halgren E, Baudena P, Clarke JM, et al. Intracerebral potentials to rare target and distractor auditory and visual stimuli. I. Superior temporal plane and parietal lobe. *Electroencephalogr Clin Neurophysiol.* 1995;94(3):191-220.
215. Halgren E, Baudena P, Clarke JM, et al. Intracerebral potentials to rare target and distractor auditory and visual stimuli. II. Medial, lateral and posterior temporal lobe. *Electroencephalogr Clin Neurophysiol.* 1995;94(4): 229-250.
216. Guerit JM, Verougstraete D, de Tourtchaninoff M, Debatisse D, Witdoeckt C. ERPs obtained with the auditory oddball paradigm in coma and altered states of consciousness: clinical relationships, prognostic value, and origin of components. *Clin Neurophysiol.* 1999;110(7):1260-1259.
217. Mazzini L, Zaccala M, Gareri F, Giordano A, Angelino E. Long-latency auditory-evoked potentials in severe traumatic brain injury. *Arch Phys Med Rehabil.* 2001;82(1): 57-65.
218. Cheour M, Korpilahti P, Martynova O, Lang AH. Mismatch negativity and late discriminative negativity in investigating speech perception and learning in children and infants. *Audiol Neurootol.* 2001;6(1):2-11.
219. Korpilahti P, Krause CM, Holopainen I, Lang AH. Early and late mismatch negativity elicited by words and speech-like stimuli in children. *Brain Lang.* 2001;76(3):332-339.
220. Jemel B, Oades RD, Oknina L, Achenbach C, Ropcke B. Frontal and temporal lobe sources for a marker of controlled auditory attention: the negative difference (Nd) event-related potential. *Brain Topogr.* 2003;15(4): 249-262.
221. Alho K. Cerebral generators of mismatch negativity (MMN) and its magnetic counterpart (MMNm) elicited by sound changes. *Ear Hear.* 1995;16(1):38-51.
222. Naatanen R, Alho K. Mismatch negativity–a unique measure of sensory processing in audition. *Int J Neurosci.* 1995; 80(1–4):317-337.
223. Kraus N, McGee T. The middle latency response generating system. *Electroencephalogr Clin Neurophysiol Suppl.* 1995;44:93-101.
224. Rodriguez RA, Cornel G, Austin EH 3rd, Auden SM, Weerasena NA. Brain function monitoring during bidirectional Glenn procedures. *J Thorac Cardiovasc Surg.* 2000; 119(3):617-619.
225. Rodriguez RA, Edmonds HL Jr, Auden SM, Austin EH 3rd. Auditory brainstem evoked responses and temperature monitoring during pediatric cardiopulmonary bypass. *Can J Anaesth.* 1999;46(9):832-839.
226. Kress JP, Pohlman AS, O'Connor MF, Hall JB. Daily interruption of sedative infusions in critically ill patients undergoing mechanical ventilation. *N Engl J Med.* 2000; 342(20):1471-1477.
227. Yppärilä H, Karhu J, Westerén-Punnonen S, Musialowicz T, Partanen J. Evidence of auditory processing during postoperative propofol sedation. *Clin Neurophysiol.* 2002; 113(8):1357-1364.
228. Schwender D, Kaiser A, Klasing S, Peter K, Poppel E. Midlatency auditory evoked potentials and explicit and implicit memory in patients undergoing cardiac surgery. *Anesthesiology.* 1994;80(3):493-501.
229. Kilo J, Czerny M, Gorlitzer M, et al. Cardiopulmonary bypass affects cognitive brain function after coronary artery bypass grafting. *Ann Thorac Surg.* 2001;72(6):1926-1932.
230. Grimm M, Zimpfer D, Czerny M, et al. Neurocognitive deficit following mitral valve surgery. *Eur J Cardiothorac Surg.* 2003;23(3):265-271.
231. Zimpfer D, Kilo J, Czerny M, et al. Neurocognitive deficit following aortic valve replacement with biological/mechanical prosthesis. *Eur J Cardiothorac Surg.* 2003;23(4): 544-551.
232. Korpelainen JT, Kauhanen ML, Tolonen U, et al. Auditory P300 event related potential in minor ischemic stroke. *Acta Neurol Scand.* 2000;101(3):202-208.
233. Austin EH 3rd, Edmonds HL Jr, Auden SM, et al. Benefit of neurophysiologic monitoring for pediatric cardiac surgery. *J Thorac Cardiovasc Surg.* 1997;114(5):707-715.
234. Malmivuo J, Plonsey R. Bioelectromagnetism – Principles and Applications of Bioelectric and Biomagnetic Fields. New York: Oxford University Press; 1995.

Near-Infrared Spectroscopy Monitoring in Cardiac Surgery: Theory, Practice, and Utility[1]

11

John M. Murkin, Miguel F. Arango, Alain Deschamps, and André Y. Denault

Patients undergoing cardiac surgical procedures are at increased risk of central nervous system (CNS) complications from a variety of causes. The increase in age and associated incidence of comorbidities give rise to significant cerebrovascular disease in upwards of 50% of adult cardiac surgical patients, rendering them more susceptible to cerebral ischemic events.[1,2] In specific circumstances, for example, selective cerebral perfusion (SCP), or even more generally, during cardiac surgery, relative cerebral hypoperfusion can engender cerebral ischemia and negatively impact outcome. As such, the ability to monitor and optimize cerebral perfusion in real time represents an important development.

In this chapter, we provide an overview of the basic principles of near-infrared spectroscopic (NIRS) cerebral oximetry, a description of the limitations of current clinical NIRS cerebral monitoring devices, a review of clinical outcome studies, and a discussion of the clinical scenarios in which such monitoring may be beneficial. Furthermore, a clinical algorithm designed to assist in the diagnosis and treatment of lowered cerebral saturation developing in the perioperative period is provided.

J.M. Murkin (✉)
Director, Cardiac Anesthesiology Research,
Department of Anesthesiology and Perioperative Medicine,
University of Western Ontario, London, ON, Canada
e-mail: John.Murkin@lhsc.on.ca

11.1 Near-Infrared Spectroscopy

In a landmark paper in December 1977, Jobsis described how the relatively high degree of transparency of myocardial and brain tissue in the near-infrared (NIR) range allows for real-time, noninvasive near-infrared spectroscopic (NIRS) monitoring of tissue oxygenation.[3] Initially based on the absorption properties of tissue cytochrome c oxidase, he soon began to report on the absorption properties of hemoglobin. By 1982, Ferrari and colleagues were studying noninvasive near-infrared spectroscopy in rat brain, and in 1985, they presented findings from among the first human cerebral oximetry studies using near-infrared spectroscopy.[4]

As these early investigators had reported, NIRS light can be used to measure regional cerebral tissue oxygen saturation (rSO_2). This is based on the fact that biological material, including skull, is relatively transparent in the near-infrared range as can be readily demonstrated by transillumination of an anatomy laboratory skull by a laser pointer or other such device. Techniques employing principles of optical spectrophotometry can exploit this fact to measure absorption characteristics of deeper tissues. Knowledge of the photon pathlength, the presence of nonheme chromophores, and variable light absorption by overlying extracerebral tissue represent some of the challenges posed in utilizing noninvasive transcranial NIRS to measure cerebral tissue oxygen saturation. The challenges posed by these fundamental aspects of cerebral NIRS are discussed below.[1]

[1]Adapted from Murkin JM, Arango M. Near-infrared spectroscopy as an index of brain and tissue oxygenation. Br J Anaesth 2009; 103 (suppl 1) i3–i13.

R.S. Bonser et al. (eds.), *Brain Protection in Cardiac Surgery*,
DOI: 10.1007/978-1-84996-293-3_11, © Springer-Verlag London Limited 2011

11.2 Beer–Lambert and the Measure of Tissue Oxygen Saturation

The ability to measure cerebral tissue oxygen saturation, as well as tissue hemoglobin content and potentially other substances, is rooted in the concept that the concentration of a substance in a solution can be determined by measuring the difference in intensity between a transmitted and subsequently received light, as delivered at specific wavelengths. This is what is described by the Beer–Lambert law (see below), wherein a change in light intensity is equivalent to the quantity (depth of penetration) of the substance and the amount of light that is absorbed by a known quantity of that substance. The depth of penetration is defined as the mean pathlength of the photons through the tissue, and the amount of light absorbed by the substance is determined by its absorption coefficient, a factor which varies with the incident-light wavelength.

Light transmission through tissue depends on a combination of reflectance, scattering, and absorption effects. Reflectance is a function of the surface characteristics and the angle of the light beam to the tissue surface and decreases with increasing wavelength thus favoring transmission of near-infrared (NIR) light, conventionally defined as light comprised of wavelengths from 650 to 1,100 nm. Scattering is, in part, a function of the tissue composition and the number of various tissue interfaces. Absorption occurs at specific wavelengths, determined by the molecular properties of the materials in the light path. Absorption of light by such chromophores – *molecules where the energy difference between molecular orbits falls within the wavelength of the incident NIR light, causing photon absorption by exciting an electron from its ground state to an excited state* – can be detected and quantified by spectral analysis. Over a pathlength of a few millimeters, all photons at wavelengths above 1,300 nm are absorbed by water (H_2O) with a secondary absorptive peak between 950 and 1,050 nm. At wavelengths below 700 nm, more intense absorption bands of hemoglobin and increased light scattering prevent effective transmission. However, NIR light penetrates tissue several centimeters within the 700–1,300 nm range.[5]

The primary light absorbing molecules within the NIR range in biological tissue are metal complex chromophores: hemoglobin, bilirubin, and cytochrome. Figure 11.1 shows the absorption spectra of oxyhemoglobin (HbO_2), demonstrating a broad peak between 700 and 1,150, whereas deoxyhemoglobin ranges from 650 to 1,000 nm, and a broad peak at 820–840 nm represents absorption by cytochrome oxidase aa3 (Caa3).[3]

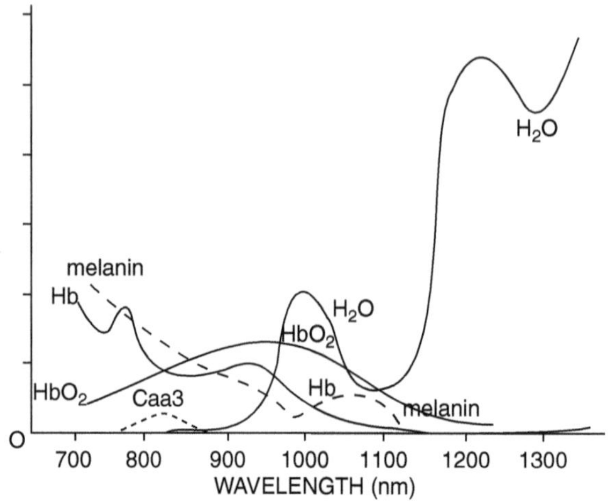

Fig. 11.1 Absorption spectra for oxygenated hemoglobin (HbO_2), deoxygenated hemoglobin (Hb), cytochrome oxidase aa3 (Caa3), melanin and water (H_2O) over wavelengths in near-infrared range. Note the relatively low peak for Caa3. Commercial cerebral near-infrared spectroscopy devices currently utilize wavelengths in 700–850 nm range to maximize separation between Hb and HbO_2. Presence of melanin as found in human hair can significantly attenuate Hb, HbO_2, and Caa3 signals (Murkin JM. Arango M. Near-infrared spectroscopy as an index of brain and tissue oxygenation. Br J Anaesth 2009; 103 (suppl 1) i3–i13

Commercial devices employ wavelengths of NIR light selected to be sensitive to these biologically important chromophores. These generally utilize wavelengths between 700 and 850 nm where there is minimal overlap with H_2O and the absorption spectra of Hb and HbO_2 are maximally separated. The isobestic point, or wavelength at which hemoglobin species (Hb/HbO_2) have the same molar absorptivity is 810 nm. The absorption spectra at this wavelength can be utilized to measure total hemoglobin concentration.

The Beer-Lambert law describes the absorption of NIR light in tissue and relates the pathlength of NIR light to the concentration and absorption spectra of various tissue chromophores. It is conventionally written as:

$$\Delta A = L \bullet \mu$$

where ΔA is the amount of light attenuation,
L is the differential photon pathlength through tissue,
μ is absorption coefficient of the chromophore and can be expressed as $[X] \bullet \varepsilon$,

where [X] is the tissue concentration of the chromophore, and ε is the extinction co-efficient of the chromophore thus, thus $[X] = \Delta A / L \bullet \varepsilon$,
thus, in theory, permitting measurement of tissue oxygen saturation (SO_2)

11.2.1 Multiwavelength NIRS and Absolute Versus Relative Oxygen Saturation

Absolute chromophore concentration [X] is inversely proportional to the optical pathlength, since Δ(delta)A is measured directly and ε(epsilon) has been determined for various tissue chromophores. However, due to reflection and refraction in the various tissue layers involved, photon pathlength cannot be measured directly and unless pathlength can be determined, only relative change in chromophore concentration can be assessed. In practice, successive approximation from tissue modeling and computer simulation can be used to estimate photon tissue pathlength and an analysis algorithm can be calibrated to provide a measure of relative change of chromophore concentration.

A different approach is employed in order to measure absolute tissue chromophore concentrations. This is based on radiative transport theory and uses multiple wavelengths and frequency-domain NIRS (fdNIRS) or time-domain NIRS (tdNIRS) analyses to determine tissue absorption coefficients (μ[mu]). Theoretically, these approaches, fdNIRS or tdNIRS, avoid the need for actual photon pathlength determination.[6,7] Fundamental to such techniques is that tissue absorption coefficients can be measured directly using multiwavelength NIRS, and, since $(mu) = [X] \bullet \varepsilon(epsilon)$ Tissue chromophore concentration can thus be measured absolutely, since there is no requirement for determination of optical pathlength. With time-domain or frequency domain spectroscopy, detected light is time or intensity modulated and thus is phaseshifted in comparison to the source intensity. In tdNIRS, light attenuation is thus measured as a function of time relative to a pulsed light source, whereas in fdNIRS, light attenuation is measured as a function of a light source which is intensity modulated.[8]

In these analyses, the ratio of the phase angle difference between several wavelengths (nominally three wavelengths, λ(lambda)$_1$, λ(lambda)$_2$, λ(lambda)$_3$) is equivalent to the sum of the ratio of the extinction coefficient difference of hemoglobin chromophore between those wavelengths and the product of tissue oxygen saturation (SO_2) and the ratio of the difference between extinction coefficients for oxy- and deoxyhemoglobin between wavelengths one and three, and the extinction coefficients for deoxyhemoglobin between wavelengths two and three according to:

$$\theta(\lambda_1-\lambda_3)/\theta(\lambda_2-\lambda_3) = \varepsilon^{Hb}(\lambda_1-\lambda_3)/\varepsilon^{Hb}(\lambda_2-\lambda_3) + SO_2(\varepsilon^{HbO2}-\varepsilon^{Hb})(\lambda_1-\lambda_3) / \varepsilon^{Hb}(\lambda_2-\lambda_3)$$

such that $SO_2 = \{[\theta(\lambda_1 - \lambda_3)/\theta(\lambda_2 - \lambda_3)] - \varepsilon^{Hb}(\lambda_1-\lambda_3)/\varepsilon^{Hb}(\lambda_2-\lambda_3)\}/(\varepsilon^{HbO2}-\varepsilon^{Hb})(\lambda_1-\lambda_3)/\varepsilon^{Hb}(\lambda_2-\lambda_3)$

where $\theta(\lambda_1 - \lambda_3)$ is the phase angle difference between wavelengths one and three,

$\theta(\lambda_2 - \lambda_3)$ is the phase angle difference between wavelengths two and three,

$\varepsilon^{Hb}(\lambda_1 - \lambda_3)$ is the extinction coefficient difference for deoxygenated hemoglobin (ε^{Hb}) between wavelengths one and three,

$\varepsilon^{Hb}(\lambda_2 - \lambda_3)$ is the extinction coefficient difference for deoxygenated hemoglobin between wavelengths two and three, and

$(\varepsilon^{HbO2} - \varepsilon^{Hb})(\lambda]_1 - \lambda_3)$ is the extinction coefficient difference between oxygenated hemoglobin (ε^{HbO2}) and deoxygenated hemoglobin between wavelengths one and three.

11.3 Temporal Resolution

With tdNIRS techniques, those photons detected as arriving at a receiver later relative to those detected sooner following a pulsed optical signal have a longer tissue pathlength. This longer pathlength may be assumed to correspond to greater depth of tissue penetration and thus reflective of cerebral tissue. An important assumption in this analysis is the homogeneity of interrogated tissue – a condition that is not necessarily consistent with biological reality.

Using an in vitro model of human skull and brain, fdNIRS has been shown to yield reasonable fidelity, but hemoglobin concentration less than 6 gm/dL yields error of approximately 15%, and increasing skull thickness produces error as high as 32%.[8] Accordingly, some correction for extracerebral tissue must still be made even with such "absolute" measurements.

11.3.1 Extracerebral Tissue

In order for noninvasive NIRS interrogation of cerebral tissue, photons must penetrate several tissue layers

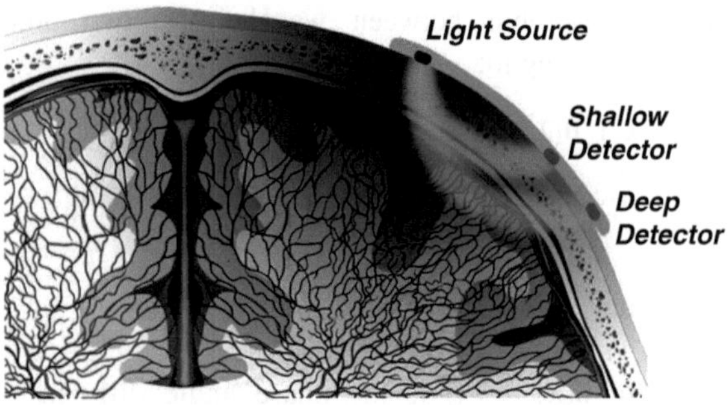

Fig. 11.2 A computer simulation of the characteristic ellipsoidal optical pathways traversed by transcranial near-infrared light. The technique of spatial resolution enables correction for extracerebral tissue by use of differentially spaced receiving optodes (i.e., shallow detector and deep detector) as illustrated (Reprinted with permission, Somanetics Corp, Troy MI)

including scalp, skull, and dura, which may contain various concentrations of blood and tissue-derived chromophores which potentially confounds the signal derived from cortical brain tissue. As shown in Fig. 11.2, various models employing both computer simulation and experimental tissue preparations have demonstrated an elliptical photon distribution centered around the transmitter, whose mean depth is proportional to the separation of the optodes by a factor of approximately 1/3.[9] Increasing transmitter/receptor distance increases depth of penetration, but within the safe power limits to prevent direct thermal tissue damage, and since signal intensity decreases exponentially with increasing distance, 5 cm separation appears to be the functional maximal spacing providing a mean depth of NIRS penetration approximating 1.7 cm giving an increasing weighting to cerebral versus extracerebral tissue.[9] There is still significant attenuation from extracerebral tissue even with increased transmitter/receiver separation, so further techniques can be utilized.

11.4 Spatial Resolution

By utilizing two differentially spaced receiving optodes – one spaced more closely and the other spaced farther from the transmitter – a degree of spatial resolution can be achieved since mean depth of photon penetration approximates 1/3 the transmitter/receiver separation. As such, it is primarily superficial tissue that is detected by the closer receiver (e.g., 3 cm separation) while deeper cortical tissue is detected by the farther optode (e.g., 4 cm separation). Calculation of the difference between the two signals by incorporation of a subtraction algorithm thus provides a measure of deeper cortical tissue saturation. Differential spacing of receiving optodes thus provides a degree of spatial resolution to distinguish signals from cerebral versus extracerebral tissue.[10]

11.5 Cerebral Arterial/Venous Blood Partitioning

It is important to recognize that all cerebral NIRS devices measure mean tissue oxygen saturation and, as such, reflect hemoglobin saturation in venous, capillary, and arterial blood comprising the sampling volume. For cerebral cortex, it can be demonstrated that, on average, tissue hemoglobin is distributed in a proportion of 70% venous and 30% arterial-based correlations between position emission tomography (PET) and NIRS.[10] Clinical studies, however, have demonstrated that there may be considerable biologic variation in individual cerebral arterial/venous ratios between patients. This further emphasizes that use of a fixed ratio in the device analysis algorithm may produce significant divergence from actual in vivo tissue oxygen saturation thus confounding even "absolute" measures of cerebral oxygenation, for example, fdNIRS and tdNIRS.[11]

Therefore, in patients undergoing coronary artery bypass (CAB) surgery, use of cerebral NIRS as a trend monitor with interventions designed to preserve a patient's cerebral saturation values close to their individual baseline values (e.g., equating each patient's unique baseline saturation value to 100%, and treating deviations from that 100% baseline), has been shown to produce a significantly lower incidence of adverse clinical events.[12] Employing a trend monitoring approach thus minimizes the impact of confounds introduced by biologic variation in individual cerebral arterial/venous ratios and outer layer tissue composition, since these can result in inaccurate therapy if it is assumed that a device is measuring "absolute" in vivo cerebral oxygenation rather than recognizing that an offset may be present.

11.6 NIRS Devices

Commercially available NIRS devices employ either direct laser light or sequentially pulsed light emitting diodes (LED) to emit NIR light transcutaneously and detect returning photons either by photodiodes or fiberoptic transmission to a photomultiplier and can be used to determine the oxygen saturation status of cerebral tissue. While several new devices are currently in development or undergoing evaluation before the Food and Drug Administration (FDA), there are currently two FDA-approved cerebral oximeters: INVOS 5100 (Somanetics Corporation, Troy, MI) and Foresight (CAS Medical Systems, Branford, CT). There appears to be some difference in approach between these devices.

INVOS is a multichannel continuous wave spatially resolved spectrometer which has been designed to measure change in rSO_2. Using a proprietary subtraction algorithm, this device uses light emitting diodes (LED) at 730 and 810 nm and differentially spaced receiving optodes located 3 and 4 cm distal to the transmitter to assess bi-frontal cortical oxygenation. It has been determined by modeling that at a 4-cm source–detector spacing and with no signal subtraction, the overlying tissue and skull contribute, on average, about 45% of the signal while 55% is cerebral in origin. Subtracting the data from the 3-cm spacing (as the INVOS does) reduces this extracerebral contribution to less than 15%. Accordingly, the noninvasive Somanetics INVOS Cerebral Oximeter provides a predominately cerebral measurement where, on average, 85% of the signal is derived exclusively from the brain.[13]

Foresight is a dual-channel continuous wave NIRS device utilizing discrete wavelengths at 690, 780, 805, and 850 nm and reported as measuring absolute brain tissue oxygen saturation.[15] To date, there have been no direct comparisons between these two technologies. A third device, NIRO-300 (Hamamatsu Photonics KH, Hamamatsu City, Japan), which in North America is currently for investigational use only, employs spatially resolved spectroscopy to measure light attenuation as a function of source-detector separation which is theoretically not influenced by photon path length and can also potentially provide a measure of absolute tissue oxygen saturation.[10] As noted above, however, all these devices make an assumption regarding the relative venous/arterial composition of cerebral tissue and saturation values thus derived are "absolute" in theory only, subject as they are to interindividual variations in regional cerebral venous/arterial distribution and the presence of various nonheme tissue chromophores.

There is now evidence that in adult cardiac surgical patients resting baseline rSO_2 is a strong predictor of perioperative morbidity and 30 day and 1-year mortality. In particular, in high risk patients rSO_2 <50% has been shown to be a stronger predictor than EUROscore or high sensitivity biomarkers for early and later postoperative mortality.[14]

11.7 NIRS Limitations and Confounds

In a study of 103 cardiac surgical and neurosurgical patients, cerebral rSO_2 from NIRO-100 was compared with INVOS 4100 after consideration of computed tomographic assessment of skull thickness (t-skull), cerebrospinal fluid area (a-CSFL), and hemoglobin concentration.[16] It was reported that INVOS rSO_2 values were potentially influenced by hemoglobin concentration, t-skull, and a-CSFV. However, as there was no assessment of superficial tissue attenuation of NIR light, the authors did indicate that there was a potential confound in this evaluation since INVOS does employ a subtraction algorithm as compensation for extracerebral tissue.[16] The potential for artifact and signal attenuation when extracerebral tissue is thickened or edematous does have clinical implications as discussed above. Extracranial or subdural hemorrhage can artifactually influence measured cerebral saturation values since hemoglobin represents the primary chromophore at the wavelengths utilized. Based, in part, on positron emission tomography (PET) studies, the analysis algorithms of most clinical NIRS devices assume a fixed venous/arterial distribution of cortical tissue (approximately 70/30%).[17] Consequently, resting cerebral rSO_2 may vary between individuals, in part, as a consequence of interindividual variations in cerebral A/V ratio. It is also important to recognize that changes in rSO_2 may largely reflect alterations in cerebral venous rather than arterial blood.

11.7.1 NIRS Device Sensitivity

In an in vivo animal study comparing sensitivity between INVOS 5100 and NIRO-300 (Hamamatsu

Photonics KH, Hamamatsu City, Japan), a swine model involving induced events including circulatory arrest, altered blood flow rate, core cooling, and rewarming during CPB was employed.[18] In this comparison, the authors concluded that NIRO-300 measured a higher tissue oxygen index (TOI) than INVO 5100 rSO_2 during low concentrations of oxygenated hemoglobin and lower values during high concentrations of oxygenated hemoglobin which may indicate a difference in sensitivity between these devices. This sensitivity difference was confirmed later in a human study using the INVOS 5100 and NIRO 200 in 31 children with congenital heart disease, where NIRS readings were compared to jugular bulb (SjO_2) and superior vena cava (SvO_2) blood oxygen saturations.[18] In this study, INVOS rSO_2 showed significant correlation with SjO_2 ($r=0.83$) and excellent correlation with $SvO_2$2 ($r = 0.93$) as compared with NIRO TOI correlations with SjO_2 ($r = 0.56$) and SvO_2 ($r = 0.74$).[19] There are currently no interdevice correlation data available for Foresight NIRS.

11.7.2 Melanin and Other Tissue Chromophores

Optimal placement of transmitting and receiving optodes is high on the frontal eminences, approximately 2–3 cm above the orbital ridge, in order to avoid frontal sinuses and hair follicles. Melanin pigmentation, particularly as found in hair,[20] can significantly attenuate light transmission and impede NIRS measurements (see Fig. 11.1). Since cutaneous melanin is confined to the epidermal layer at a depth of 50–100 μ(mu)m, it does not produce significant attenuation of NIRS signal. Conjugated bilirubin, however, has an absorption peak at 730 nm, and is deposited throughout all tissue layers. As such, concern has been raised about the ability of NIRS to assess cerebral oxygenation in the presence of jaundice.[21] In a study of 48 patients undergoing orthotopic liver transplantation, total plasma bilirubin was shown to be related to cerebral rSO_2 effectively producing a variable offset. During reperfusion of the grafted liver, however, an average increase in rSO_2 of 7% ($P<0.05$) was detected and plasma bilirubin concentration did not appear to influence the ability to detect this increase. It was concluded that while bilirubin concentration may dampen cerebral NIRS, even at high bilirubin values, changes in cerebral perfusion may still be discerned.[21] This further supports the approach that rather than relying primarily upon a specific threshold value, clinicians should establish a baseline value in each patient individually and observe for perturbations from that baseline – particularly given the demonstrated potential for interference/offset of rSO_2 from various nonheme tissue chromophores.

11.7.3 Nonmetabolizing Tissue

In nonmetabolizing tissue, oxygen saturation values may be high or low. Even in dead or nonmetabolizing brain tissue, oxygen saturation may be near normal because of blood sequestered in cerebral capillaries and venous capacitance vessels.[22] In a study in 18 adult human cadavers, Scharwtz et al. examined cerebral rSO_2 and found values in one third of the specimens that exceeded the lowest values that they had previously recorded in normal subjects.[23] This raised concern regarding the validity of the rSO_2 measurement. However, in a study of cerebral venous oxygen saturation obtained during 214 autopsies, Maeda et al. found O_2 saturation values to range from 0.3 to 95.1% apparently as a consequence of total hemoglobin content, cause of death, and cadaver storage conditions.[24] Accordingly, the pathophysiology of nonmetabolizing yet nonperfused tissue is such that rSO_2 or other measures of cerebral oxygen saturation may appear discordantly high, but rather than being indicative of error in the device, may rather reflect in vivo oxygenation.[24] In clinical practice, it is thus the context-sensitive change in 'cerebral rSO_2 (e.g., during cooling or rewarming), that is of fundamental importance.

11.8 Overview of NIRS Clinical Studies

Previous studies have indicated a positive predictive value between low intraoperative rSO_2 and adverse CNS outcomes. Data is also accruing that preoperative rSO_2 is a strong predictor of postoperative morbidity and mortality.[25] The use of cerebral oximetry has identified a number of otherwise unrecognized causes of cerebral hypoperfusion both during conventional CPB[26] and during beating heart surgery.[27] Various causes of cerebral hypoperfusion including inadvertent positioning of the head turned to extreme left side, cannula-obstructed venous outflow from the brain, hypocapnia, low perfusion pressure, and inadequate hemoglobin concentration have all been detected and successfully treated by applied rSO_2 oximetry.[28,29] During beating heart procedures, compromised cerebral perfusion can occur relatively frequently with an incidence nearly twice that which occurs during CPB, as demonstrated using jugular oximetry in a randomized clinical study of 187 patients.[30] In a series of 550 beating heart patients, combined electroencephalographic (EEG) and cerebral oximetry rSO_2 monitoring identified episodes of cerebral ischemia in 15% of patients, who were treated with a combination of pharmacologically improved cardiac output, increased perfusion pressure, and cardiac repositioning.[27] Postoperative length of stay has also been reported as decreased in CAB patients in whom cerebral NIRS had been utilized, in comparison to a group without such monitoring.[31]

The use of rSO_2 has also demonstrated correlations between CAB patients having low rSO_2 values and cognitive dysfunction,[32] prolonged hospital stay,[33] and most recently, perioperative cerebrovascular accident (CVA).[34] Dunham et al. showed that rSO_2 values correlated with cerebral perfusion pressure (CPP), Glasgow Outcome Score, and mortality in patients with traumatic brain injuries,[35] and several other groups have demonstrated the ability of rSO_2 to provide an early warning of potentially catastrophic cerebral ischemia.[36–38]

In a recent large nonrandomized series of 1,034 cardiac surgical patients reported by Goldman and colleagues, a significant reduction in perioperative stroke rate, from 2.01 to 0.97%, was observed in patients in whom INVOS rSO_2 cerebral oximetry was used to optimize and maintain intraoperative cerebral oxygenation in comparison to an untreated comparator group of 1,245 similar patients operated on in the immediately preceding 18 month interval.[34]

In a recent prospective, randomized blinded study by Murkin et al. in 200 patients undergoing coronary artery grafting, it was demonstrated that treatment of declining INVOS rSO_2 values prevented prolonged desaturations. This was an important demonstration in that utilization of an intervention protocol was effective in restoring 84% of cerebral desaturations. Patients in the treatment group had a shorter intensive care unit (ICU) length of stay and a significantly reduced incidence of major organ morbidity or mortality.[12,39] As outlined in detail below, the intervention protocol undertaken to return rSO_2 to baseline did not add undue risk to the patient, including no increase in allogeneic blood transfusions, and resulted in a rapid improvement in rSO_2 in most instances.[12] Directionally consistent with previous studies, there were also numerically fewer clinical CVA in monitored patients.[35]

Studies assessing the utility of Foresight as a clinical monitor are also beginning to appear.[40]

11.9 NIRS in the Setting of Cerebral Ischemia

The proper management of brain oxygenation is without doubt one of the principal end points of all anesthesia procedures, but paradoxically the brain is still the least monitored organ during clinical anesthesia.[41] There are some surgical procedures where iatrogenic brain ischemia is induced (e.g., carotid endarterectomy [CEA], temporal clipping in brain aneurysm surgery, selective cerebral perfusion [SCP] for aortic arch procedures, etc.). We shall discuss some of the data pertaining to these situations and the role of cerebral NIRS in detecting and potentially ameliorating cerebral ischemia.

11.9.1 Carotid Endarterectomy

Carotid endarterectomy is a widely accepted and established procedure in symptomatic patients with high-grade carotid stenosis to reduce subsequent ischemic stroke.[42,43] In patients with poor collateral flow, temporary cross clamping of the internal carotid artery (ICA) can produce brain ischemia; yet, this is integral to CEA. Unfortunately, the incidence of perioperative stroke during CEA can be as high as 5%[44,45]; a setting in which NIRS monitoring of intraoperative brain oxygen saturation may be beneficial.[46]

Despite the existence of various cerebral monitoring techniques for patients under general anesthesia, the traditional assessment of cerebral ischemia is still relatively cumbersome; intraoperative monitoring methods such as transcranial Doppler (TCD), EEG, and somatosensory evoked potentials (SSEP) provide only an indirect evidence of the ischemic insult while having other logistic limitations and technical disadvantages.[47–51] The adequacy of collateral flow through the Circle of Willis can be estimated by measurement of distal ICA stump pressure after external and common carotid clamping. As SP can be affected by numerous factors including blood pressure, $PaCO_2$, type of anesthetic agent, etc.,[52,53] and has the disadvantage of being a single static measurement unavailable during the actual surgical endarterectomy, it is not as widely employed.

Multiple recent studies have shown cerebral NIRS to be a potentially important and valuable tool for the detection of cerebral ischemia during CEA.[53–59] As described above, cerebral NIRS is a simple and easy-to-use noninvasive monitor, suited to the operating room environment, which can provide a continuous measure of brain oxygenation.

In 1998, Kirkpatrick et al. published an important study describing standard brain ischemia monitoring (three lead cerebral function monitor [CFM], and TCD) and NIRS in 103 patients.[60] Using a regression model correlating percentage change in the middle cerebral artery (MCA) flow and change in the NIRS saturation, the authors demonstrated a positive, statistically significant correlation ($r=0.68$, $p<0.001$) between change in flow and change in NIRS saturation. Using CMF for diagnosis of severe ischemia, the authors concluded that usage of cerebral NIRS was a valuable monitor for detection of brain ischemia in the operation room. In 2000, Samra et al. reported on a study of 99 awake patients undergoing CEA using regional anesthesia and evaluated cerebral NIRS as a method to detect intraoperative brain ischemia.[61] These authors performed a logistic regression analysis to evaluate the specificity and sensitivity of various cutoff points of the NIRS value relative to the onset of cerebral ischemia, where ischemia was detected clinically as an inability to respond appropriately to verbal commands, unconsciousness, slurring of speech, or the development of motor weakness. They demonstrated that cerebral NIRS had a sensitivity of 80% with a specificity of 82% using as a cutoff point a 20% relative decrease in SrO_2, with a false-positive and false-negative rate of 66.7% and 2.6%, respectively. Similar results were found by Hirofumi et al. in a smaller study of 19 patients showing that a reduction of 15.6–18.2% in the NIRS cerebral oxygen saturation was associated with ipsilateral EEG changes and was predictive of poor neurological outcome.[56] The authors also reported that brain ischemia with possible neurologic compromise could occur when a cerebral oxygen saturation less than 54–56% was reached during carotid cross-clamping.

In 2004, Mille et al. reported their study analyzing INVOS cerebral NIRS data from 594 carotid endarterectomies performed under general anesthesia during which all patients were tested after extubation for development of a new neurological deficit.[62] Patients who had a neurological deficit with complete recovery within 24 h were classified as having sustained a transient ischemic attack, while those with neurological deficit persisting for more than 24 h were classified as having sustained a stroke. The main objective was to determine the reliability of NIRS in predicting postoperative complications. Sensitivity, specificity, and predictive values were computed to appraise the ability of determining a cutoff point of NIRS saturation to predict the need for shunting or risk of neurological complications. Utilizing a 20% reduction, as previously described by Samra et al.[61] was found to have a very high specificity (98%) but a low sensitivity – 30%, with a positive and negative predictive value of 37% and 98%, respectively. A cutoff point of 11.7% was identified as optimal, having a sensitivity of 75% and a specificity of 77% with a positive predictive value of 37% and negative value of 98%.

Most recently, Rigamonti et al. in 2005 published their results analyzing 50 patients having CEA under cervical plexus block during which an independent neurologist evaluated clinical and EEG signs of ischemia while NIRS was continuously recorded.[63] Ten percent of the patients experienced clinical and EEG brain ischemia requiring shunt placement and showed a reduction in NIRS saturation of $17\pm4\%$. The NIRS reduction in patients with no clinical or EEG ischemia averaged only $8\pm6\%$ ($p=0.01$). However, in this study, they were unable to identify an rSO_2 threshold that can be used alone to predict the need of shunt placement because of a low sensitivity and specificity.

Rebound increases in cerebral blood flow (CBF) after surgical repair of the carotid stenosis have been associated with postoperative neurological complication after CEA and may be related to impaired autoregulation as a consequence of chronic brain ischemia. As such, rapid restoration of regional perfusion can generate a hyperperfusion syndrome characterized by headache, brain edema, seizures, and in severe cases, intracerebral hemorrhage.[64] Ogasawara et al. found a significant linear correlation ($r^2=0.247$ $p=0.0002$) between NIRS values immediately after declamping and CBF.[65] Using a cutoff point of 5%, the sensitivity and specificity of cerebral NIRS for detection of patients at risks of developing hyperperfusion syndrome were 100% and 86.4%, respectively. Cerebral

NIRS demonstrated a positive predictive value of 50% and a negative predictive value of 100% using a cutoff point of 5%, such that if there is an increase of 5% from the NIRS baseline value, the sensitivity and specificity for finding a hyperperfusion syndrome is 100 and 86.2%, respectively. Increasing the cutoff point to 10% achieved 100% sensitivity and specificity.

11.9.2 Retrograde and Selective Anterograde Cerebral Perfusion

During complex aortic arch repair, surgical access may require interruption of systemic perfusion for relatively protracted periods. While moderate (25–30 °C) and deep (<25 °C) hypothermia remain a mainstay for cerebral and systemic protection, there is relatively little ability to monitor cerebral well-bring during such times since EEG becomes progressively attenuated below 25 °C. Accordingly, cerebral NIRS has been advocated to understand some of the cerebral responses to deep hypothermia and as a means of monitoring and detecting onset of cerebral ischemia during deep hypothermic circulatory arrest (DHCA).[66,67] While some groups monitor jugular venous oxygen saturation (SjO_2) using retrograde cannulation of the internal jugular vein as an index of cerebral metabolic suppression during cooling, correlation has not been demonstrated between SjO_2 and cerebral NIRS during DHCA,[68] likely indicative of the fact that NIRS is a highly regional measure of cerebral cortical oxygen tissue saturation, whereas SjO_2 is a measure of cerebral mixed venous oxygen saturation and thus reflective of global changes in venous oxygenation and, as such, potentially less sensitive to regional perfusion inhomogeneities.

In addition to DHCA, some centers utilize retrograde cerebral perfusion (RCP) via the superior vena cava or, increasingly, selective anterograde cerebral perfusion (SACP) via the innominate or subclavian artery. There have been a variety of case reports of the ability of cerebral NIRS to detect onset of cerebral ischemia during aortic arch surgeries and there is growing interest in the role of cerebral NIRS as a measure of adequacy of perfusion in this setting.[69–73] There is increasing recognition that RCP does not provide sufficient nutritive flow to sustain cerebral integrity for an extended interval,[74] as has been reflected in lower rSO_2 values seen during NIRS monitoring in RCP versus SACP.[75,76]

In a review of the role of NIRS monitoring during SACP, a study was undertaken in 46 consecutive patients in whom SACP was established by separate concomitant perfusion of the innominate and the left carotid arteries or by perfusion of the right subclavian artery (with or without left carotid artery perfusion) and during which bilateral regional cerebral tissue oxygen saturation index was monitored by INVOS 4100 NIRS and which used stroke as the primary clinical end point, along with indices of diagnostic performance of the NIRS device.[77] In this series, six patients died in the hospital, and six patients (13%) in whom regional cerebral tissue oxygen saturation values were significantly lower during SACP experienced a perioperative stroke. Regional cerebral tissue oxygen saturation decreasing to between 76% and 86% of baseline during selective antegrade cerebral perfusion had a sensitivity of up to 83% and a specificity of up to 94% in identifying individuals with stroke. It was concluded that using NIRS monitoring of regional cerebral tissue oxygen saturation during SACP allows detection of clinically important cerebral desaturations and can help predict perioperative neurologic sequelae supporting its use as a noninvasive trend monitor of cerebral oxygenation.[77]

In adult patients, cerebral malperfusion can occur either as a consequence of ascending aortic dissection with occlusion of carotid lumen,[38] kinking, or obstruction of perfusion cannula during selective cerebral perfusion for circulatory arrest procedures, or due to migration of aortic endoclamp cannula during minimal access cardiac surgery with potential compromise of cerebral perfusion.[78,79] There are increasing reports that bilateral rSO_2 monitoring can detect contralateral desaturation during unilateral selective cerebral perfusion. This can result from an incomplete circle of Willis which in some series has a prevalence of up to 50% and has been estimated to be a factor in cerebral malperfusion in approximately 15% of patients.[80,81] In a more recent case report, cerebral rSO_2 monitoring was utilized during selective cerebral perfusion in the absence of systemic CPB during repair of traumatic aortic arch rupture and detected both episodes of cerebral malperfusion and, most critically, acute thrombosis of carotid artery graft leading to thrombectomy and restoration of flow.[82]

11.10 Cerebral NIRS and Systemic Outcomes

In previous studies, cerebral deoxygenation has been associated with various adverse systemic outcomes. In a randomized, prospective study of 200 patients undergoing coronary artery bypass (CAB) surgery, it has recently been shown that by using the brain as an index organ, interventions to improve cerebral oxygenation enhanced overall outcomes in cardiac surgical patients.[12] It was hypothesized that by detection and correction of factors giving rise to cerebral desaturations, the interventions taken would also result in improved perfusion to other organ systems thus enhancing overall clinical outcomes. In this study, significantly more patients in the control group demonstrated prolonged cerebral desaturation ($p=0.014$) and longer duration of ICU stay ($p = 0.029$) versus monitored intervention patients. There was no difference in overall incidence of adverse complications, but significantly more control patients had major organ morbidity or mortality (MOMM: death, ventilation > 48 h, stroke, myocardial infarction, return for reexploration) versus intervention group patients ($p=0.048$). Patients experiencing MOMM had lower baseline and mean rSO_2, greater cerebral desaturations, and longer lengths of stay in ICU and postoperative hospitalization, than patients without such complications. As has been demonstrated in previous studies, there was a weak but significant ($r^2=0.29$) inverse correlation between intraoperative rSO_2 and duration of postoperative hospitalization in patients requiring ≥ 10 days postoperative length of stay. The overall conclusion was that monitoring cerebral rSO_2 in CAB patients avoids profound cerebral desaturation and is associated with significantly lower incidences of major organ dysfunction.[12]

11.11 Clinical Strategies for Low rSO_2

In order to develop a practical way to use cerebral NIRS on a routine clinical basis, an algorithm has been developed (Fig. 11.3) that we are currently using perioperatively.[83] This algorithm is based on optimizing those factors that can affect cerebral oxygen

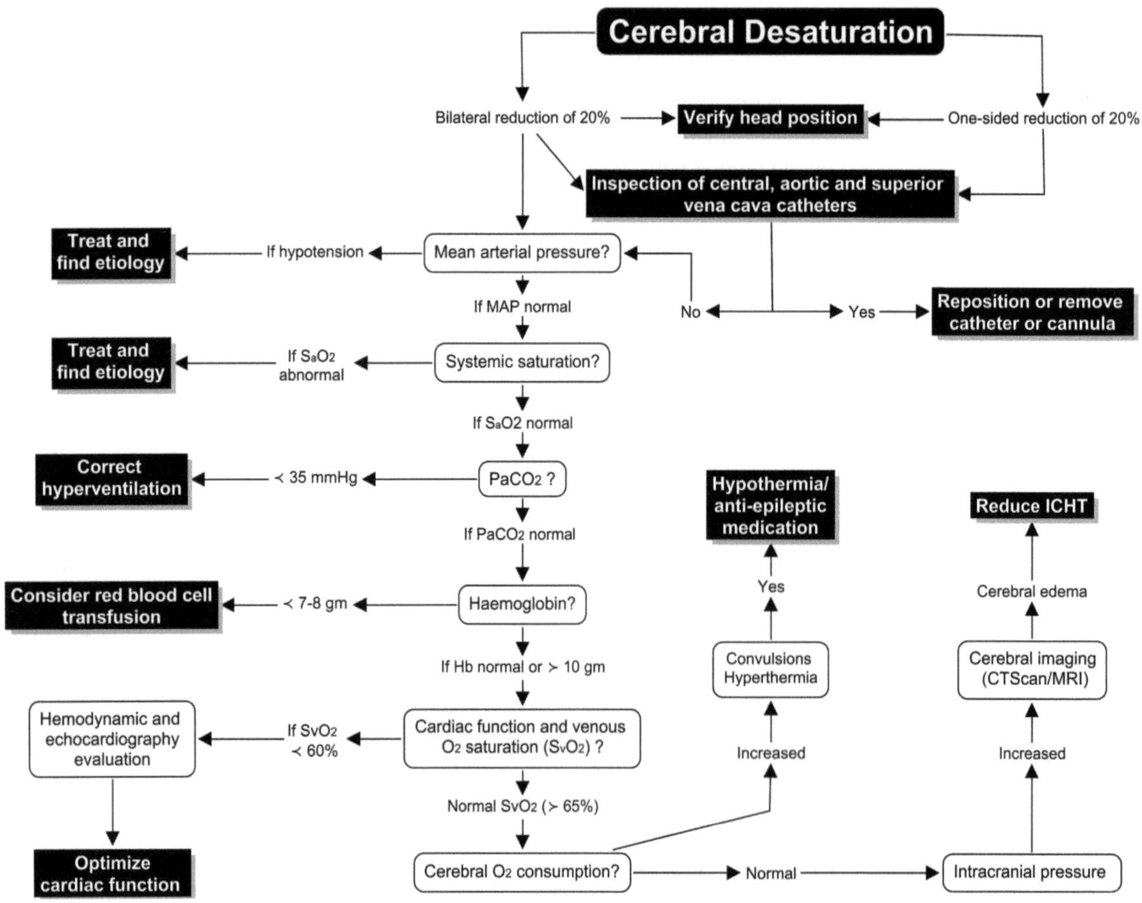

Fig. 11.3 Proposed algorithm in the use of brain oximetry. *CT* computed tomography, *ICHT* intracranial hypertension, *MAP* mean arterial pressure, *MRI* magnetic resonance imaging (From Denault et al.[83] Reprinted by permission of SAGE Publications, Inc.)

supply/demand such as perfusion pressure, cardiac output, arterial oxygen content, partial pressure of carbon dioxide ($PaCO_2$), cerebral metabolic rate, etc. Other factors, such as blood pH, body temperature, the presence of abnormal hemoglobin, or changes in the level of 2–3 DPG can modify hemoglobin affinity for oxygen, influencing the amount of oxygen released to the tissues, and thus can also affect NIRS. Furthermore, brain oxygen consumption or the cerebral metabolic rate of oxygen ($CMRO_2$) is influenced by factors such as the activation status, brain temperature, anesthetic agents, and pulsatile or laminar perfusion. Finally, some studies have also reported a relationship between rSO_2 and cardiac function.[84–86] Therefore, the algorithm is based on these considerations. Several examples illustrating the use of NIRS in the operating room environment are also presented. This approach, based on our experience, goes through several comprehensive and logical steps to help correct decreases in cerebral saturation values with the intention of improving patient outcome. Ideally, baseline values should be obtained when the patient is awake, resting comfortably with O_2 supplementation. We define abnormal rSO_2 as a 20% bilateral or unilateral reduction from baseline values or an absolute decrease below 50%.[31]

11.11.1 Rule Out Mechanical Obstruction

11.11.1.1 Arterial Malperfusion

When the value of rSO_2 decreases, the first and most important step is to rule out a mechanical obstruction to cerebral blood flow. For instance, in minimally invasive cardiac surgery, the endoclamping aortic cannula inserted through a femoral access could migrate in a position in the aortic arch where cerebral blood flow could be acutely compromised.[79] Also, with use of a j-tip arterial cannula in the ascending aorta, malrotation of the cannula can cause perfusion directly into the innominate artery giving rise to unilateral cerebral hyperemia manifest as "harlequin facies" with an abrupt fall in contralateral rSO_2 and invariably associated with extensive cerebral injury unless detected.[87] This occurs with a relatively greater frequency during congenital surgery and is one of the reasons why NIRS is increasingly employed during pediatric cardiac surgery.[88] In such situations, if the carotid arteries are partially occluded or malperfused, the decreases in rSO_2 will be sudden and rapid, and once diagnosed, repositioning the aortic cannula can be easily effected with relief of malperfusion. As noted above, during SACP, cannula malposition can be detected with relief of cerebral hypoperfusion.[78]

11.11.1.2 Superior Vena Cava Obstruction

Since cerebral perfusion pressure (CPP) reflects the difference between inflow mean arterial pressure (MAP) and outflow (jugular venous) pressures, unrecognized cerebral venous obstruction via dislocation of the heart or venous cannula malposition can compromise cerebral perfusion. This has been well documented[89,90] and it has been observed during cardiac transplantation[83], but may occur more frequently than clinicians may appreciate even during nonpump beating heart procedures.[32] It is also possible that the position of the head could impede venous return. As noted by Edmonds et al., repositioning the patient's head when rSO_2 decreases ensures that it had not been inadvertently rotated and also rules out facial plethora.[31]

11.11.2 Increase Mean Arterial Pressure

The incidence of occult or overt cerebrovascular disease in the cardiac surgical population has been estimated at over 50%,[1,2] thus increasing the potential for hypoperfusion due to impaired autoregulation and requirement for elevated CPP. One of the most common interventions in the treatment of brain desaturation is to maintain CPP as reported by Murkin et al.[12] With decreased rSO_2, the goal is to maintain mean arterial pressure (MAP) within 15% of the patient's awake resting baseline MAP using vasopressors as required during CPB. However, if this intervention does not correct the abnormality, rapidly move to the next step.

11.11.3 Verify Systemic Oxygenation

Because it does not necessitate pulsatile flow, NIRS can also be used to confirm the presence or absence of peripheral desaturation in a variety of clinical settings.

This can be particularly useful in patients with cardiovascular disease or in shock. The signals obtained from noninvasive peripheral pulse oximeter are often absent in these critically ill patients because of the peripheral vasoconstriction. During CPB, pulse oximetry is nonfunctional and cerebral oximetry has been used to detect sudden vaporizer failure, prior to any decrease in mixed venous oxygenation.[91] Studies have also demonstrated the particular benefit of hyperoxia in preserving cells in ischemic cerebral penumbral tissue.[92] Hyperoxia has not been shown to increase oxygen-free radical generation,[93] during rewarming after hypothermic circulatory arrest, and has been associated with less histological evidence of brain injury.[94] Accordingly, we will increase FiO_2 during CPB if previous measures have not restored rSO_2. Unexpected brain and peripheral desaturation can also lead to specific diagnoses such as the detection of a nonsuspected cause of hypoxia such as an undiagnosed patient foramen ovale with associated right-to-left shunting as previously reported.[83]

11.11.4 Normalize $PaCO_2$

One of the most powerful determinants of cerebral blood flow is $PaCO_2$ with the effects of hypocapnia and hypercapnia on brain circulation being well known to clinicians. Yao, for instance, has observed that during hyperventilation, brain oximetry signals will reduce and during hypoventilation, they will increase.[95] Kolb et al. described a protocol to determine acute cerebrovascular and ventilatory response to hypoxia.[96] They measured flow velocity in the middle cerebral artery and rSO_2. Hypoxia was associated with a reduction in rSO_2, whereas during hypercapnia, both the rSO_2 and velocity of the MCA increased. In our experience, one of the most common causes of decreased rSO_2 is inadvertent hyperventilation after induction of anesthesia and during rewarming on CPB. Such unexpected brain desaturation can occur particularly during rewarming on CPB when the $PaCO_2$ may often be below 35 mmHg. Normalization of $PaCO_2$ was the third most common intervention in the recent large prospective trial.[12]

11.11.5 Optimize Hemoglobin

Hemoglobin is a key element in oxygen transport, and reduction in hemoglobin can be associated with reduction in rSO_2 values. Torella et al. have proposed that NIRS could be used as a monitor of blood loss.[97] They monitored 10 blood donors during and 10 min after blood collection of 470 mL. A good correlation between blood losses and NIRS parameters was observed. The significant reduction in hemoglobin due to acute hemodilution observed during initiation of cardiopulmonary bypass (CPB), combined with reduction in MAP due to decreased viscosity is often reflected in decreased rSO_2 with onset of CPB. Whether refractory low rSO_2 values should be used as an indication for transfusion is currently contentious, but may be beneficial when other interventions listed (Fig. 11.3) have proven ineffective.

11.11.6 Evaluate Cardiac Function

During CPB, increasing pump flow is the most common and efficacious technique used in the correction of brain desaturations.[12] In non-CPB settings, some studies have reported a direct relationship between rSO_2 and cardiac function.[84–86] As cardiac performance is reduced, increased brain oxygen extraction would be encountered and lower brain oximetry values would be observed. In that regard, Madsen observed that rSO_2 values are lower in patients with normotensive acute heart failure and improved with the treatment of heart failure.[84] In addition, cerebral oxygen saturation has been shown to correlate with the presence of left ventricular dysfunction in patients with valvular disease during exercise testing.[85] Lower cerebral saturation values were observed in patients who did not increase their cardiac output. To further explore the relationship between cardiac function and brain oximetry, Paquet et al. analyzed 99 patients using NIRS, pulmonary artery catheter, and transesophageal echocardiography.[86] Correlations were observed between mean rSO_2 values, hemodynamic and echocardiographic values. A model to predict baseline mean rSO_2 was developed. The key variables identified in the model were the presence of normal left ventricular systolic function which tended to raise the mean rSO_2 value, and LV dilatation, mitral valve replacement, female gender, central venous pressure, and the use of beta-blockers all of which contributed to lower rSO_2 values.

11.11.7 Decrease $CMRO_2$

If reductions in rSO_2 values are observed despite the above measures, then a relative increase in $CMRO_2$ or other processes may be operative. Cerebral hyperthermia may occur after rewarming during CPB and would be associated with reduction in rSO_2 values through an increase in $CMRO_2$. In this instance, measurements of tympanic or nasopharyngeal temperature can be obtained to detect hyperthermia and brain cooling should be initiated.[98] For refractory cerebral desaturations during CPB reduction of $CMRO_2$ through deepening of anesthesia (e.g., incremental bolus of propofol or thiopental) may be used.[12] Similarly, in the postoperative interval, the presence of unexpected low rSO_2 may be due to cortical seizures which have been reported to occur with a frequency of 3.5% in one study of adult patients[2] and has been reported to occur with increasing frequency after longer duration DHCA.[99]

11.11.8 Other Therapeutic Alternatives

In the presence of persistent low rSO_2, particularly if unilateral, an intracranial process should be ruled out. Early postoperative neurological assessment with cerebral imaging might be considered. Finally, there is some evidence that laminar flow during CPB decreases CBF to a greater extent than pulsatile perfusion.[100, 101] In the setting of low rSO_2 during CPB, pulsatile perfusion may be introduced. Improvements have been noted in rSO_2 in certain patients treated with pulsatile perfusion during CPB.[12]

11.12 Other Applications for NIRS

Brain oximetry electrodes normally used on the forehead can also be placed on peripheral sites. Harel et al. from the Montreal Heart Institute have validated the use of NIRS as a monitor of peripheral perfusion and compared it to strain gauge and radionuclide plethysmography.[102] An excellent correlation was observed between these modalities. Therefore, NIRS could be used as a monitor for vascular peripheral perfusion. For example, they were able to detect an unexpected arterial embolic event in the contralateral extremity during a femoro-femoral bypass (Fig. 11.4).[102] The combined use of peripheral and central NIRS parameters has been reported in pediatric patients as a useful way to discriminate a reduction in rSO_2 results from a ce ntral or a peripheral process.[88]

Finally NIRS has not been limited to cardiac surgery. It has been used and studied either as a neurologic or a tissue perfusion monitor in numerous conditions and procedures such as vascular surgery,[103] laparoscopic surgery,[104] liver transplantation,[105] fluid optimization,[106] and hemorrhagic[107] and septic[108] shock management.

Results from these studies provide an insight into the promising potential of NIRS to improve outcomes in the clinical setting. Overall, we believe that in the absence of feedback from a specific indicator of end-organ compromise as provided by cerebral oximetry (i.e., cerebral desaturations), the ability of the clinician to detect and optimize otherwise silent but potentially adverse perturbations in a variety of clinical settings remains limited.

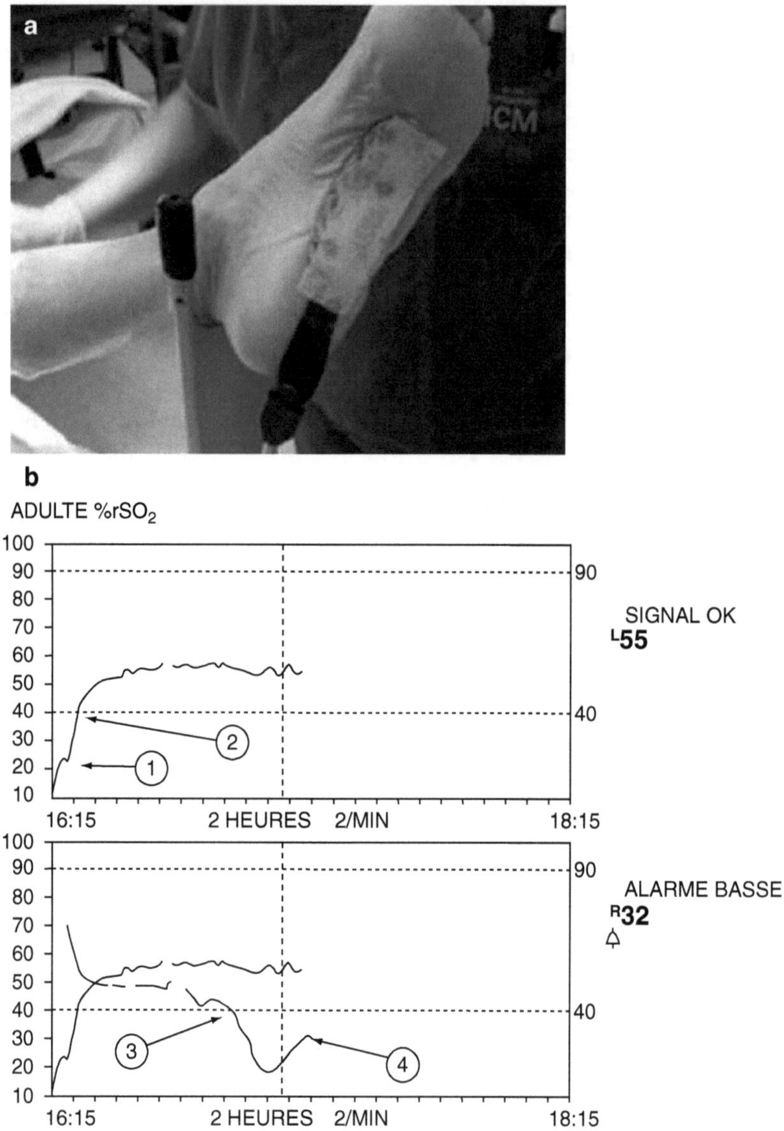

Fig. 11.4 (**a**) NIRS monitoring of the lower extremities during surgery. (**b**) Output of the NIRS device in a patient with occluded left femoral graft. Initially reduction of the signal was observed on the left (*arrow 1*). Following femoro-femoral bypass, restoration of flow was associated with an increase of the signal (*arrow 2*). However, an unexpected reduction of the right side occurred (*arrow 3*). This was secondary to a thrombus in the distal femoral artery that was confirmed and removed using a Fogarty catheter. Restoration of flow was noted (*arrow 4*) (With Permission of Harel et al.[102]

References

1. Uehara T, Tabuchi M, Kozawa S, Mori E. MR angiographic evaluation of carotid and intracranial arteries in Japanese patients scheduled for coronary artery bypass grafting. *Cerebrovasc Dis*. 2001;11(4):341-345.
2. Yoon BW, Bae HJ, Kang DW, et al. Intracranial cerebral artery disease as a risk factor for central nervous system complications of coronary artery bypass graft surgery. *Stroke*. 2001;32:94-99.
3. Josbis FF. Noninvasive, infrared monitoring of cerebral and myocardial oxygen sufficiency and circulatory parameters. *Science*. 1977;198:1264-1267.
4. Ferrari M, Giannini I, Sideri G, Zanette E. Continuous non invasive monitoring of human brain by near infrared spectroscopy. *Adv Exp Med Biol*. 1985;191:873-882.
5. McCormick PW, Stewart M, Goetting MG, et al. Noninvasive cerebral optical spectroscopy for monitoring cerebral oxygen delivery and hemodynamics. *Crit Care Med*. 1991;19:89-97.
6. Matcher SJ, Cope M, Delpy DT. Use of the water absorption spectrum to quantify tissue chromophore concentration changes in near-infrared spectroscopy. *Phys Med Biol*. 1994 Jan;39(1):177-196.
7. Lakowicz JR, Berndt K. Frequency-domain measurements of photon migration in tissues. *Chem Phys Lett*. 1990; 166:246-252.
8. Kurth CD, Thayer WS. A multiwavelength frequency-domain near-infrared cerebral oximeter. *Phys Med Biol*. 1990;44:727-740.
9. Germon TJ, Evans PD, Barnett NJ, Wall P, Manara AR, Nelson RJ. Cerebral near infrared spectroscopy: emitter-detector separation must be increased. *Br J Anaesth*. 1999;82(6):831-837.

10. Ohmae E, Ouchi Y, Oda M, et al. Cerebral hemodynamics evaluation by near-infrared time-resolved spectroscopy: correlation with simultaneous positron emission tomography measurements. *Neuroimage*. 2006 Feb 1;29(3): 697-705.
11. Watzman HM, Kurth CD, Montenegro LM, Rome J, Steven JM, Nicolson SC. Arterial and venous contributions to near-infrared cerebral oximetry. *Anesthesiology*. 2000 Oct;93(4): 947-953.
12. Adams MJM, SJ NRJ, Iglesias I, et al. Monitoring brain oxygen saturation during coronary bypass surgery: a randomized, prospective study. *Anesth Analg*. 2007;104: 51-58.
13. http://www.somanetics.com/invos_principles.htm
14. Heringlake M, Garbers C, Kabler JH, Anderson I, Heinze H, Schon J, Berger KU, Dibbelt L, Sievers HH, Hanke T. Perioperative cerebral oxygen saturation and clinical outcomes in cardiac surgery. Anesthesiology (in press) 2011
15. http://www.casmed.com/foresight.html
16. Yoshitani K, Kawaguchi M, Miura N, et al. Effects of hemoglobin concentration, skull thickness, and the area of the cerebrospinal fluid layer on near-infrared spectroscopy measurements. *Anesthesiology*. 2007;106:458-462.
17. Ito H, Kanno I, Fukuda H. Human cerebral circulation: positron emission tomography studies. *Ann Nucl Med*. 2005 Apr;19(2):65-74.
18. Gagnon RE, Macnab AJ, Gagnon FA, Blackstock D, LeBlanc JG. Comparison of two spatially resolved NIRS oxygenation indices. *J Clin Monit Comput*. 2002;17:385-391.
19. Nagdyman N, Ewert P, Peters B, Miera O, Fleck T, Berger F. Comparison of different near-infrared spectroscopic cerebral oxygenation indices with central venous and jugular venous oxygenation saturation in children. *Paediatr Anaesth*. 2008;18:460-466.
20. Pringle J, Roberts C, Kohl M, Lekeux P. Near infrared spectroscopy in large animals: optical pathlength and influence of hair covering and epidermal pigmentation. *Vet J*. 1999;158(1):48-52.
21. Madsen PL, Skak C, Rasmussen A, Secher NH. Interference of cerebral near-infrared oximetry in patients with icterus. *Anesth Analg*. 2000 Feb;90(2):489-493.
22. Dunham C, Sosnowski C, Porter J. Correlation of noninvasive cerebral oximetry with cerebral perfusion in the severe head injured patients: a pilot study. *J Trauma*. 2002;52:40-46.
23. Schwartz G, Litscher G, Kleinert R. Cerebral oximetry in dead subjects. *J Neurosurg Anesthesiol*. 1996;8:189-193.
24. Maeda H, Fukita K, Oritani S. Evaluation of post-mortem oximetry with references to the causes of death. *Forensic Sci Int*. 1997;87:201-210.
25. Newman MF, Lowry E, Croughwell ND, et al. Near infrared spectroscopy (INVOS 3100A) and cognitive outcome after cardiac surgery. *Anesth Analg*. 1997;84:S111.
26. Murkin JM. Neurologic monitoring during cardiac surgery. *Sem Cardiothorac Vasc Anesth*. 2002;6:35-38.
27. Novistky D, Boswell BB. Total myocardial revascularization without cardiopulmonary bypass utilizing computer-processed monitoring to assess cerebral perfusion. *Heart Surg Forum*. 2000;3:198-202.
28. Edmonds HL Jr. Multi-modality neurophysiologic monitoring for cardiac surgery. *Heart Surg Forum*. 2002;5: 225-228.
29. Edmonds HL, Ganzel BL, Austin EH. Cerebral oximetry for cardiac and vascular surgery. *Sem Cardiothorac Vasc Anesth*. 2004;8:147-166.
30. Diephuis JC, Moons KG, Nierich AN, Bruens M, van Dijk D, Kalkman CJ. Jugular bulb desaturation during coronary artery surgery: a comparison of off-pump and on-pump procedures. *Br J Anaesth*. 2005;94:715-720.
31. Alexander HC, Kronenefeld MA, Dance GR. Reduced postoperative length of stay may result from using cerebral oximetry monitoring to guide treatment. *Ann Thorac Surg*. 2002;73:373–C (abstract).
32. Yao FF, Tseng CA, Ho CA, Levin SK, Illner P. Cerebral oxygen desaturations is associated with early postoperative neuropsychological dysfunction in patients undergoing cardiac surgery. *J Cardiothorac Vasc Anesth*. 2004;18:552-558.
33. Yao FSF, Levin SK, Wu D, Illner P, Yu J, Huang SW, Tseng CC. Maintaining cerebral oxygen saturation during cardiac surgery shortened ICU and hospital stays. *Anesth Analg*. 2001;92:SCA 86.
34. Goldman S, Sutter F, Ferdinand F, Trace C. Optimizing intraoperative cerebral oxygen delivery using noninvasive cerebral oximetry decreases the incidence of stroke for cardiac surgical patients. *Heart Surg Forum*. 2004;7(5):E376-381.
35. Dunham CM, Ransom KJ, Flowers LL, Siegal JD, Kohli CM. Cerebral hypoxia in severely brain-injured patients is associated with admission Glasgow Coma Score, computed tomographic severity, cerebral perfusion pressure, and survival. *J Trauma*. 2004;56:482-491.
36. Papadimos TJ, Marco AP. Cerebral oximetry and an unanticipated circulatory arrest (letter). *Anaesthesia*. 2004;59: 309-310.
37. Fukada J, Morishita K, Kawaharada N, et al. Isolated cerebral perfusion for interoperative cerebral malperfusion in type A aortic dissection. *Ann Thor Surg*. 2003;75:266-268.
38. Janelle GM, Mnookin S, Gravenstein N, Martin TD, Urdaneta F. Unilateral cerebral oxygen desaturations during emergent repair of DeBakey type 1 aortic dissection: potential aversion of a major catastrophe. *Anesthesiology*. 2002;96:1263-1265.
39. Murkin JM, Bainbridge D, Novick R. In response. Do the data really support the conclusion? (letter). *Anesth Analg*. 2007;105:536-538.
40. Fischer GW, Reich D, Plestis KA, Griepp RB. Results using absolute cerebral oximetry monitoring suggest the need for tailored patient management during cardiac surgery. *Heart Surg Forum*. 2006 (abstract)
41. Cullen DJ, Kirby RR. Beachchair position may decrease cerebral perfusion. Catastrophic outcomes have occurred. *APSF Newslett*. 2007;22(2):25-26.
42. North American Symptomatic Carotid Endarterectomy Trial Collaborators. Beneficial effect of carotid endarterectomy in symptomatic patients with high-grade carotid stenosis. *N Engl J Med*. 1991;325:445-453.
43. The European Carotid Surgery Trialists Collaborative Group. Risk of stroke in the distribution of an asymptomatic carotid artery. *Lancet*. 1995;345:209-212.
44. Barnett HJ, Taylor DW, Eliasziw M, et al. Benefit of carotid endarterectomy in patients with symptomatic moderate or severe stenosis. North American Symptomatic Carotid Endarterectomy Trial Collaborators. *N Engl J Med*. 1998; 339:1415-1425.

45. Rothwell PM, Eliasziw M, Gutnikov SA, et al. Analysis of pooled data from the randomised controlled trials of endarterectomy for symptomatic carotid stenosis. *Lancet*. 2003; 361:107-116.
46. Naylor AR, Bell PR, Ruckley CV. Monitoring and cerebral protection during carotid endarterectomy. *Br J Surg*. 1992; 79:735-741.
47. Beese U, Langer H, Lang W, Dinkel M. Comparison of near-infrared spectroscopy and somatosensory evoked potentials for the detection of cerebral ischemia during carotid endarterectomy. *Stroke*. 1998;29:2032-2037.
48. Cho H, Nemoto EM, Yonas H, Balzer J, Sclabassi RJ. Cerebral monitoring by means of oximetry and somatosensory evoked potentials during carotid endarterectomy. *J Neurosurg*. 1998;89:533-538.
49. de Letter JA, Sie HT, Thomas BM, et al. Near-infrared reflected spectroscopy and electroencephalography during carotid endarterectomy – in search of a new shunt criterion. *Neurol Res*. 1998;20(Suppl 1):S23-27.
50. Williams IM, Picton A, Farrell A, Mead GE, Mortimer AJ, McCollum CN. Light-reflective cerebral oximetry and jugular bulb venous oxygen saturation during carotid endarterectomy. *Br J Surg*. 1994;81:1291-1295.
51. Howell SJ. Carotid endarterectomy. *Br J Anaesth*. 2007;99:119-131.
52. Moritz S, Kasprzak P, Arlt M, Taeger K, Metz C. Accuracy of cerebral monitoring in detecting cerebral ischemia during carotid endarterectomy: a comparison of transcranial Doppler sonography, near-infrared spectroscopy, stump pressure, and somatosensory evoked potentials. *Anesthesiology*. 2007;107:563-569.
53. Calderon-Arnulphi M, Alaraj A, Amin-Hanjani S, et al. Detection of cerebral ischemia in neurovascular surgery using quantitative frequency-domain near-infrared spectroscopy. *J Neurosurg*. 2007;106:283-290.
54. Carlin RE, McGraw DJ, Calimlim JR, Mascia MF. The use of near-infrared cerebral oximetry in awake carotid endarterectomy. *J Clin Anesth*. 1998;10:109-113.
55. Casati A, Spreafico E, Putzu M, Fanelli G. New technology for noninvasive brain monitoring: continuous cerebral oximetry. *Minerva Anestesiol*. 2006;72:605-625.
56. Hirofumi O, Otone E, Hiroshi I, et al. The effectiveness of regional cerebral oxygen saturation monitoring using near-infrared spectroscopy in carotid endarterectomy. *J Clin Neurosci*. 2003;10:79-83.
57. Vets P, ten Broecke P, Adriaensen H, Van Schil P, De Hert S. Cerebral oximetry in patients undergoing carotid endarterectomy: preliminary results. *Acta Anaesthesiol Belg*. 2004;55:215-220.
58. Yamamoto K, Komiyama T, Miyata T, et al. Contralateral stenosis as a risk factor for carotid endarterectomy measured by near infrared spectroscopy. *Int Angiol*. 2004;23: 388-393.
59. Yamamoto K, Miyata T, Nagawa H. Good correlation between cerebral oxygenation measured using near infrared spectroscopy and stump pressure during carotid clamping. *Int Angiol*. 2007;26:262-265.
60. Kirkpatrick PJ, Lam J, Al-Rawi P, Smielewski P, Czosnyka M. Defining thresholds for critical ischemia by using near-infrared spectroscopy in the adult brain. *J Neurosurg*. 1998;89:389-394.
61. Samra SK, Dy EA, Welch K, Dorje P, Zelenock GB, Stanley JC. Evaluation of a cerebral oximeter as a monitor of cerebral ischemia during carotid endarterectomy. *Anesthesiology*. 2000;93:964-970.
62. Mille T, Tachimiri ME, Klersy C, et al. Near infrared spectroscopy monitoring during carotid endarterectomy: which threshold value is critical? *Eur J Vasc Endovasc Surg*. 2004;27:646-650.
63. Rigamonti A, Scandroglio M, Minicucci F, Magrin S, Carozzo A, Casati A. A clinical evaluation of near-infrared cerebral oximetry in the awake patient to monitor cerebral perfusion during carotid endarterectomy. *J Clin Anesth*. 2005;17:426-430.
64. Ogasawara K, Sakai N, Kuroiwa T, et al. Intracranial hemorrhage associated with cerebral hyperperfusion syndrome following carotid endarterectomy and carotid artery stenting: retrospective review of 4494 patients. *J Neurosurg*. 2007;107:1130-1136.
65. Ogasawara K, Konno H, Yukawa H, Endo H, Inoue T, Ogawa A. Transcranial regional cerebral oxygen saturation monitoring during carotid endarterectomy as a predictor of postoperative hyperperfusion. *Neurosurgery*. 2003;53:309-14. discussion 314–315.
66. Kurth CD, Steven JM, Nicolson SC. Cerebral oxygenation during pediatric cardiac surgery using deep hypothermic circulatory arrest. *Anesthesiology*. 1995 Jan;82(1):74-82.
67. Kurth CD, Steven JM, Nicolson SC, Chance B, Delivoria-Papadopoulos M. Kinetics of cerebral deoxygenation during deep hypothermic circulatory arrest in neonates. *Anesthesiology*. 1992 Oct;77(4):656-661.
68. Leyvi G, Bello R, Wasnick JD, Plestis K. Assessment of cerebral oxygen balance during deep hypothermic circulatory arrest by continuous jugular bulb venous saturation and near-infrared spectroscopy. *J Cardiothorac Vasc Anesth*. 2006 Dec;20(6):826-833.
69. Ogino H, Ueda Y, Sugita T, et al. Monitoring of regional cerebral oxygenation by near-infrared spectroscopy during continuous retrograde cerebral perfusion for aortic arch surgery. *Eur J Cardiothorac Surg*. 1998 Oct;14(4):415-418.
70. Orihashi K, Sueda T, Okada K, Imai K. Near-infrared spectroscopy for monitoring cerebral ischemia during selective cerebral perfusion. *Eur J Cardiothorac Surg*. 2004 Nov;26(5):907-911.
71. Ogino H, Ueda Y, Sugita T, Morioka K, Sakakibara Y, Matsubayashi K. Nomoto T Monitoring of regional cerebral oxygenation by near-infrared spectroscopy during continuous retrograde cerebral perfusion for aortic arch surgery. *Eur J Cardiothorac Surg*. 1998 Oct;14(4):415-418.
72. Hofer A, Haizinger B, Geiselseder G, Mair R, Rehak P, Gombotz H. Monitoring of selective antegrade cerebral perfusion using near infrared spectroscopy in neonatal aortic arch surgery. *Eur J Anaesthesiol*. 2005 Apr;22(4):293-298.
73. Higami T, Kozawa S, Asada T, et al. A comparison of changes of cerebrovascular oxygen saturation in retrograde and selective cerebral perfusion during aortic arch surgery. *Nippon Kyobu Geka Gakkai Zasshi*. 1995 Dec;43(12):1919-1923.
74. Matalanis G, Hata M, Buxton BF. A retrospective comparative study of deep hypothermic circulatory arrest, retrograde, and antegrade cerebral perfusion in aortic arch surgery. *Ann Thorac Cardiovasc Surg*. 2003 June;9(3):174-179.
75. Higami T, Kozawa S, Asada T, et al. Retrograde cerebral perfusion versus selective cerebral perfusion as evaluated by

cerebral oxygen saturation during aortic arch reconstruction. *Ann Thorac Surg*. 1999 Apr;67(4):1091-1096.

76. Okita Y, Minatoya K, Tagusari O, Ando M, Nagatsuka K, Kitamura S. Prospective comparative study of brain protection in total aortic arch replacement: deep hypothermic circulatory arrest with retrograde cerebral perfusion or selective antegrade cerebral perfusion. *Ann Thorac Surg*. 2001 July;72(1):72-79.
77. Olsson C, Thelin S. Regional cerebral saturation monitoring with near-infrared spectroscopy during selective antegrade cerebral perfusion: diagnostic performance and relationship to postoperative stroke. *J Thorac Cardiovasc Surg*. 2006 Feb;131(2):371-379.
78. Sakaguchi G, Komiya T, Tamura N, et al. Cerebral malperfusion in acute type A dissection: direct innominate artery cannulation. *J Thorac Cardiovasc Surg*. 2005;129:1190-1191.
79. Schneider F, Falk V, Walther T, Mohr FW. Control of endoaortic clamp position during port-access mitral valve operations using transcranial Doppler echography. *Ann Thorac Surg*. 1998;65:1481.
80. Hoksbergen AW, Legemate DA, Csiba L, et al. Absent collateral function of the circle of Willis as risk factor for ischemic stroke. *Cerebrovasc Dis*. 2003;16:191-198.
81. Merkkola P, Tulla H, Ronkainen A, et al. Incomplete circle of Willis and right axillary artery perfusion. *Ann Thorac Surg*. 2006;82:74-79.
82. Santo KC, Bonser RS, et al. Near-infrared spectroscopy. An important monitroing tool druing hybrid aortic arch replacement. *Anesth Analg*. 2008;107(3):793-796.
83. Denault A, Deschamps A, Murkin JM. A proposed algorithm for the intraoperative use of cerebral near-infrared spectroscopy. *Semin Cardiothorac Vasc Anesth*. 2007;11:274-281.
84. Madsen PL, Nielsen HB, Christiansen P. Well-being and cerebral oxygen saturation during acute heart failure in humans. *Clin Physiol*. 2000;20:158-164.
85. Koike A, Itoh H, Oohara R, et al. Cerebral oxygenation during exercise in cardiac patients. *Chest*. 2004;125:182-190.
86. Paquet C, Deschamps A, Denault AY, et al. Baseline regional cerebral oxygen saturation correlates with left ventricular systolic and diastolic function. *J Cardiothorac Vasc Anesth*. 2008;22(4):840-846. Ref Type: In Press.
87. Gottlieb EA, Fraser CD Jr, Andropoulos DB, Diaz LK. Bilateral monitoring of cerebral oxygen saturation results in recognition of aortic cannula malposition during pediatric congenital heart surgery. *Paediatr Anaesth*. 2006;16: 787-789.
88. Rossi M, Tirotta CF, Lagueruela RG, Madril D. Diminished Blalock-Taussig shunt flow detected by cerebral oximetry. *Paediatr Anaesth*. 2007;17:72-74.
89. Paton B, Pearcy WC, Swan H. The importance of the electroencephalogram during open cardiac surgery with particular reference to superior vena caval obstruction. *Surg Gynecol Obstet*. 1960;111:197-202.
90. Avraamides EJ, Murkin JM. The effect of surgical dislocation of the heart on cerebral blood flow in the presence of a single, two-stage venous cannula during cardiopulmonary bypass. *Can J Anaesth*. 1996;43:A36.
91. Caruso LJ, Gravenstein N, Janelle GM, Gabrielli A. Detection of oxygen delivery failure during cardiopulmonary bypass: an even earlier warning technique. *J Cardiothorac Vasc Anesth*. 2002;16:789.
92. Longhi L, Valeriani V, Rossi S, et al. Effects of hyperoxia on brain tissue oxygen tension in cerebral focal lesions. *Acta Neurochir Suppl*. 2002;81:315-317.
93. Singhal AB, Dijkhuizen RM, Rosen BR, Lo EH. Normobaric hyperoxia reduces MRI diffusion abnormalities and infarct size in experimental stroke. *Neurology*. 2002;58:945-952.
94. Agardh CD, Zhang H, Smith ML, Siesjo BK. Free radical production and ischemic brain damage: influence of postischemic oxygen tension. *Int J Dev Neurosci*. 1991;9:127-138.
95. Yao FSF, Tseng CC, Yu JHN. Relationship between ETCO2 and cerebral oxygen tension. *Anesthesiology*. 2000; A-320.
96. Kolb JC, Ainslie PN, Ide K, Poulin MJ. Protocol to measure acute cerebrovascular and ventilatory responses to isocapnic hypoxia in humans. *Respir Physiol Neurobiol*. 2004;141:191-199.
97. Torella F, McCollum CN. Regional haemoglobin oxygen saturation during surgical haemorrhage. *Minerva Med*. 2004;95:461-467.
98. Shann KG, Likosky DS, Murkin JM, et al. An evidence-based review of the practice of cardiopulmonary bypass in adults: a focus on neurologic injury, glycemic control, hemodilution, and the inflammatory response. *J Thorac Cardiovasc Surg*. 2006;132:283-290.
99. Gaynor JW, Nicolson SC, Jarvik GP, et al. Increasing duration of deep hypothermic circulatory arrest is associated with an increased incidence of postoperative electroencephalographic seizures. *J Thorac Cardiovasc Surg*. 2005 Nov;130(5):1278-1286.
100. Dernevik L, Arvidsson S, William-Olsson G. Cerebral perfusion in dogs during pulsatile and non pulsatile extracorporeal circulation. *J Cardiovasc Surg (Torino)*. 1985; 26:32-5.
101. Murkin JM, Farrar K. The influence of pulsatile vs nonpulsatile cardiopulmonary bypass on cerebral blood flow and cerebral metabolism. *Anesthesiology*. 1989;71:A41.
102. Harel F, Denault A, Ngo Q, et al. Near-infrared spectroscopy to monitor peripheral blood flow perfusion. *J Clin Monit Comput*. 2008;22(1):37-43.
103. Fearn SJ, Hutchinson S, Riding G, et al. Carotid endarterectomy improves cognitive function in patients with exhausted cerebrovascular reserve. *Eur J Vasc Endovasc Surg*. 2003;26:529-536.
104. de Waal EE, de Vries JW, Kruitwagen CL, Kalkman CJ. The effects of low-pressure carbon dioxide pneumoperitoneum on cerebral oxygenation and cerebral blood volume in children. *Anesth Analg*. 2002;94:500-505.
105. Plachky J, Hofer S, Volkmann M, et al. Regional cerebral oxygen saturation is a sensitive marker of cerebral hypoperfusion during orthotopic liver transplantation. *Anesth Analg*. 2004;99:344-349. table.
106. Bundgaard-Nielsen M, Ruhnau B, Secher NH, Kehlet H. Flow-related techniques for preoperative goal-directed fluid optimization. *Br J Anaesth*. 2007;98:38-44.
107. Taylor JH, Mulier KE, Myers DE, Beilman GJ. Use of near-infrared spectroscopy in early determination of irreversible hemorrhagic shock. *J Trauma*. 2005;58:1119-1125.
108. Skarda DE, Mulier KE, Myers DE, et al. Dynamic near-infrared spectroscopy measurements in patients with severe sepsis. *Shock*. 2007;27:348-353.

12 The Design and Methodology of Clinical Studies of Neuroprotection in Cardiac Surgery

Reza Motallebzadeh and Marjan Jahangiri

12.1 Introduction

Despite years of intensive investigation and research, cerebral injury following cardiac surgery remains a major cause of postoperative morbidity and has been associated with as much as a 10% increase in hospital mortality, increased length of stay, and expensive rehabilitation.[1] The clinical manifestations of neurological impairment include almost all the possible deficits and modalities of dysfunction depending on the nature and localization (single or multiple) of the injury,[2] with the spectrum of deficits ranging from subtle changes in cognitive function to overt stroke.[3] The cognitive deficits after cardiac surgery are similar to those occurring with aging: attention, concentration, memory, and speed of response are the most affected areas.[4]

Stroke is the most important measure of central nervous system dysfunction after cardiac surgery. However, as the incidence of stroke is relatively low, affecting between 1% and 5% of patients,[5–7] any randomized study intended to investigate the impact of an intervention with respect to the incidence of stroke after cardiac surgery would require a very large number of patients. This is one of the main reasons for research to be focused on neurocognitive dysfunction, which is a more prevalent postoperative complication than stroke. In fact, it has been said that cardiac surgery provides a convenient model in which to study neuroprotective agents as a large number of patients are susceptible to neurological deficits at a predictable time.[8]

The aims of neuroprotective strategies are to prevent the occurrence of cerebral injury, for example, by use of pharmacologic agents[9] and limiting cerebral emboli,[10] and to increase the ischemic tolerance of the brain, for example, by control of body temperature[11,12] and preventing hyperglycemia.[13,14] In operations on the aortic arch, neuroprotective strategies take on an even more important role as a period of circulatory arrest, and thus interruption of cerebral blood flow is required to replace the aorta in a dry field.[15] Besides inducing deep hypothermia,[16] additional maneuvers such as antegrade perfusion of the cerebral circulation via the inominate arteries[17] or retrograde cerebral perfusion via the superior vena cava[18] are used to extend the "safety-period" of circulatory arrest.

Previous prospective randomized studies which have compared the efficacy of neuroprotective strategies in cardiac surgery have focused on neurocognitive outcomes, for example, degree of hypothermia and rewarming rate,[19–21] use of arterial filters,[10] acid-base management: pH-stat versus α (alpha)-stat,[22] control of hyperglycemia during cardiopulmonary bypass (CPB),[23] avoiding CPB in coronary bypass surgery,[24–29] antegrade versus retrograde cerebral perfusion in aortic arch surgery,[30,31] and use of pharmacologic neuroprotective agents.[9,32,33]

What is common to all these studies is that a measure of neurocognitive function has been derived. Therefore, we shall focus on the merits of using different methods that assess neurocognitive function.

R. Motallebzadeh (✉)
Specialist Registrar and Wellcome Trust Clinical Research Fellow, Department of Surgery, Addenbrooke's Hospital, Cambridge, Cambridgeshire, UK
e-mail: rmz1001@yahoo.co.uk

R.S. Bonser et al. (eds.), *Brain Protection in Cardiac Surgery*,
DOI: 10.1007/978-1-84996-293-3_12,

12.2 Neurocognitive Testing

12.2.1 Background

Since the 1960s, neurocognitive testing has become an established method of identifying cerebral dysfunction after cardiac surgery. A battery of tests used to measure varying aspects of cognitive function is usually administered before surgery and at various time points afterwards. Despite the extensive use of neurocognitive testing in the field of cardiac surgery, there is uncertainty regarding the precise interpretation of the findings in any given study. In particular, the definition of what constitutes a neuropsychological deficit has been the subject of much discussion. One major advance in addressing the methodological issues was the publication of a consensus statement in 1995 which has laid down a set of guidelines for the use of neurocognitive tests in cardiac research studies.[34] However, it should be noted that most conventional cognitive tests are designed for the identification of brain dysfunction, rather than the assessment of change in function over time. Although these tests are suitable for the investigation of brain-behavior relationships, they possess psychometric properties, as discussed below, which impair their applicability for the serial assessments of neurocognitive function that are required in studies of neuroprotection in cardiac surgery.

Neurocognitive testing has been utilized in two distinct ways in cardiac surgery. It has been used (1) in clinical group studies to determine the size, nature, and severity of neurocognitive dysfunction and (2) in interventional studies to investigate the benefits of neuroprotective strategies.[10] Although related, these represent different aims and as a result, different methods of analysis of neurocognitive data have been employed – group mean and incidence analysis. As most investigators have noted, the two types of analysis do not always give rise to the same conclusions.

12.2.2 Group Mean Analysis

The issue of group mean versus incidence analysis is discussed at length in the second Consensus Statement.[35] Group mean analysis involves looking at changes for the group as a whole or mean differences in change scores for the target and comparison groups. One advantage of this analysis is that it allows the use of parametric statistics. Group mean analyses have repeatedly found a pattern of significant deterioration immediately after surgery and either no significant change or improved performance a few months later.[36,37]

One significant limitation of group mean analysis is that it does not take into account "practice effects." Neurocognitive assessment almost always requires the repeated use of the same tests on at least two occasions (preoperatively and postoperatively). It is an established fact that repeat testing on neurocognitive tests leads to changes in performance independent of any changes in underlying function or capacity. The most problematic of these changes is the practice effect, leading to an apparent recovery in function in the absence of any true improvement.[38,39] In other words, patients can exhibit a practice effect due to learning and show a slight improvement in test score. In any given group of patients assessed over a period of time, some patients will sustain cerebral injury and thus show a decline in neurocognitive function, but others will actually improve due to practice effects. As a result, there will be a small change in the overall mean and a large increase in the standard deviation, which in turn decreases the detectability of group differences using parametric statistics. The overall conclusion is that there has been no overall change in cognitive function. Hence, group analysis is not a sensitive method for detecting neurocognitive dysfunction as it fails to identify those patients with deficits. Practice effects can be minimized by the use of alternative forms of tests (parallel tests), and tests which have an objective measure of performance such as time to completion, rather than subjective measures such as scoring nuances of recalled material.[34] It should, however, be noted that practice effects are still observed in studies where alternate forms of the same test have been used.[39] Also, using long follow-up intervals or including an age- and education-matched control/comparison group that undergoes the same assessments at the same time points will minimize the practice effect.[34,38,40] The spouses of patients undergoing surgery can be used as a matched control group to eliminate the confounding effects of practice and anxiety/distress.[41] Without a control/comparison group it is not possible to distinguish the effects of brain dysfunction from practice.

12.2.3 Incidence Analysis

Incidence analysis has been endorsed as the preferred method of defining cognitive impairment.[35] Incidence analysis looks at the number of individuals in a group who show evidence of substantial deterioration after surgery. Each patient is used as his or her own control. Although such numbers superficially provide a convenient summation of the incidence of postoperative neurocognitive impairment, it must be recognized that they are calculated by imposing an arbitrary statistical decision on individual test measures. As such, overall incidence data will vary according to which statistical criteria are used to define neurocognitive dysfunction, the sensitivity of the tests, the type and number of tests used, and the range of cognitive domains they assess.[42] Any approach that essentially dichotomizes patients as "impaired" or "unimpaired" promotes a one-dimensional view of brain dysfunction, and leads to a reduction in the statistical power to detect cognitive dysfunction.[43]

Many studies have used the following definitions to classify patients as "significantly declined": decline of one standard deviation (SD) or more on some number of tests, or decline of 20% or more on some number of tests compared to the preoperative test results.[44–46] At present, there is no agreement as to what degree of change constitutes neuropsychological dysfunction. In one study of patients undergoing coronary artery bypass graft (CABG) surgery, the incidence of postoperative neurocognitive dysfunction was compared using four commonly used criteria of impairment. The incidence of postoperative neurocognitive decline ranged from 15% to 66% before hospital discharge and from 3% to 19% at 6 months follow-up.[45] This highlights the arbitrariness of the definitions used to define neurocognitive dysfunction. There are a number of other limitations to using incidence analysis. First, chance fluctuations in test scores are not adequately dealt with. For a reliable (that is, statistically significant) change to occur, the change has to exceed the margin of measurement error, which is not necessarily the case with a change of one SD or more.[47] The definition of what constitutes neurocognitive impairment can thus be too sensitive as a one SD decline would be expected to occur by chance alone with a likelihood of about 14% (α (alpha) $= 0.14$).[48] For instance, an individual assessed on a test that has poor reliability can be classified as having significant cognitive decline purely as a result of changes in sources of measurement error (e.g., fatigue, anxiety). In fact, the risk of detecting a deficit by chance is increased after repeated testing and when a large test battery is used.[49,50] Second, the SD that is used is calculated from the preoperative assessment and in fact reflects the variability of performance between subjects in a population. It is therefore the "wrong" SD that is being used. In a test-retest study, the distribution of change scores between baseline and retest is of interest and not the variability of scores at baseline alone. Only if the SD of change (the difference between test and retest) is used, can one tell if retest performance has been affected. In any case, the SDs from the preoperative assessment will differ between studies. This makes it very difficult to compare the reported incidences of postoperative neurocognitive dysfunction. Third, the SD method of analysis does not correct for the effects of learning and so the "true" changes in cognitive scores become obscured.

12.2.4 Regression to the Mean

In addition, it has been suggested that "regression to the mean" (RTM) explains much of the neurocognitive deficits that have been reported with the use of incidence analysis.[51] Regression to the mean is the statistical phenomenon, whereby extreme baseline scores tend to become less extreme after repeated examinations, even though true change has not occurred.[52,53] The effect of RTM is present whenever there is an intrasubject variation on a repeated test and is thus an inevitable feature of cognitive testing. With respect to cognitive testing, RTM suggests that high scoring individuals will do worse on repeat testing, and that lower scoring people will do better. The magnitude of RTM is exacerbated when the tests used to define cognitive status have poor reliability, as greater amounts of measurement error result in greater RTM. To overcome the influence of RTM on neurocognitive scores, multiple data points are required.[54] This would involve multiple preoperative cognitive assessments that could be averaged to obtain a patient's "real" baseline score. Similar multiple assessments would be required in the postoperative period to again establish a reliable level of neurocognitive function. However, the difficulties of performing a large number of tests, in addition to the increased chance of practice effects, preclude the use of this methodology. An alternative method would be the use of group mean analysis.[54] Group mean analysis allows the use of parametric statistical methods that are free from the influence of RTM. However, as mentioned earlier, group mean analysis fails to take into account the individuals who have deteriorated or improved cognitive function.

An alternative method to the SD definition of neurocognitive decline is the use of z change scores, which are derived by dividing the difference between the retest and baseline score with the SD of all the scores.[9] These scores can be left as raw numbers and can be used to give a mean for each test or a battery of tests. This method has the advantage of increased sensitivity as it is a continuous measure without absolute cut-offs.

Another alternative to the SD definition involves use of the reliable change index (RCI). RCI looks at the dispersion of change scores that occurs in the absence of real change, by using the 90% confidence interval as the criterion for defining reliable change. Originally proposed by Jacobson and Truax, the RCI is calculated by dividing the individual's test-retest difference score by the standard error of that difference score.[55] Subsequently, Naugle and associates introduced a modified RCI.[56] The modified RCI corrects for practice effects based on a control group's mean change scores across two test sessions. Patients whose assessment scores fall outside of the RCI are defined as impaired or improved, depending on the direction of index. Advantages of the RCI method is that it accounts for test reliability at both baseline and follow-up assessments, thus allowing for RTM, and it corrects for practice effects. There are some limitations of this method though, as RCI methodology is only as good as the control group on which the actual RCIs are derived. In addition, because the 90% CI is used, the chance of a Type I error on a single test is 5%. When several tests are used, Type I errors increase in proportion to the number of assessments in the test battery.[57]

In a recent prospective randomized study of neurocognitive function after on-pump versus off-pump CABG, we have used a composite neurocognitive score as the primary outcome measure.[24] Patients were given a battery of neurocognitive tests to perform before and after surgery. Each battery of tests yielded 21 different outcome variables, and was combined to a single measure, a composite score, by using principal component analysis. It has been argued however that using composite scores is counterintuitive in that each test reflects a particular function or specific brain area, and that useful information will be lost.[40] Nevertheless, comparing cognitive domains instead of overall cognitive function will result in multiple comparisons that cannot be adequately corrected for. Hence, the use of composite scores has been recommended for analysis of postoperative cognitive function.[58] Comparison of postoperative scores was carried out adjusting for the preoperative scores by using analysis of covariance (ANCOVA). ANCOVA takes RTM into account and is a powerful method of analyzing test-retest data.[59] This is similar to analyzing the difference between before and after, but is a better method. For example, it allows for the possibility that people with higher initial values may be more likely to experience greater declines.

Whatever method is used to classify a patient as cognitively impaired, one important point needs to be recognised. While a specific definition of neurocognitive impairment is required when the study objective is to determine the incidence of postoperative neurocognitive dysfunction, it is not necessary when one wants to test a specific hypothesis such as the effects of an intervention, for example, off-pump surgery, or a putative neuroprotective agent. Incidence figures superficially provide a convenient summation of the extent of acquired impairment, but it must be understood that they are calculated by imposing an arbitrary statistical intervention on individual test measures. As such, overall incidence data will vary according to which statistical criteria are used, the sensitivity of the tests, the number of tests used, and the range of cognitive domains they assess.[34,45] Any approach that essentially dichotomizes patients as "impaired" or "unimpaired" promotes a one-dimensional view of brain dysfunction, and is a costly way of data handling that reduces statistical power.[40] It is far better to use continuous measures and look at change and its relative difference between groups, which greatly enhances the power of the analysis.[60]

Neurocognitive testing can provide a reliable, sensitive, and objective means to evaluate the function of the brain to determine the presence of injury. Many conventional neuropsychometric tests are inappropriate for the serial assessment of cognitive function, as they may have poor psychometric properties. As suggested in a review by Collie and colleagues, a number of modifications are required in order for these tests to be applied in longitudinal and repeated-measures studies.[61] They suggested that the test battery should have multiple and equivalent forms, not have floor and ceiling effects when administered to normal and impaired individuals, and provide a range of possible scores, so that minor changes in cognition are reflected as changes in test score. In addition, the test battery should be brief enough so that the effects of fatigue and boredom do not adversely affect assessment.

12.3 Biochemical Markers of Cerebral Injury

Neuropsychometric tests have been the mainstay of assessing cognitive function after cardiac surgery, but have major drawbacks. They are time-consuming, taking as much as an hour to perform, and there must be a preoperative baseline assessment so that change can be determined. Their use is therefore limited to elective, stable patients who can cooperate with the testing process before and after surgery. Certain groups of patients such as the critically ill, and those whose language skills are deficient are excluded. Furthermore, practice effects, mood state, and medication obscure the results of neurocognitive testing. As a result, research has focused on finding biochemical markers that can reflect the degree of brain injury sustained during cardiac surgery.

During the past 2 decades, a variety of substances have been suggested as possible biochemical markers of cerebral injury such as adenylate kinase, creatinine phosphokinase isoenzyme BB, lactate, myelin basic protein, S100β (beta), neuron-specific enolase, and glial fibrillary acidic protein.[62,63] Most of these substances are not ideal markers. For example, adenylate kinase and lactate have to be sampled directly from cerebrospinal fluid, and creatinine phosphokinase isoenzyme BB lacks brain specificity. An ideal biochemical marker of cerebral injury would have the following properties: it would be specific for the central nervous system, be rapidly and significantly released into blood after injury, and its serum concentration would correlate to the degree of injury. In this regard, most research has focused on neuron-specific enolase (NSE) and S100β (beta).

NSE has a molecular weight of 78 kDa and is mainly located in the cytoplasm of endocrine tissues and axonal processes.[64] Small cell lung cancer and tumors of neuroendocrine origin may also produce NSE.[65] Unfortunately, it is also present in platelets and erythrocytes, which can lead to errors in interpretation because a small amount of hemolysis or platelet damage can substantially increase plasma levels.[66] Hence, its usefulness as a biochemical marker of cerebral injury is questionable.

S100 protein is an acidic calcium binding protein with a molecular weight of 21 kDa.[67] The S100 family comprises 17 monomers, each of which exhibits a unique pattern of tissue-specific expression. The term "S100" refers to a mixture of dimeric proteins consisting of two subunits of M_r 10,500 termed A and B. Two of the monomers, S100A1 and S100B, are found in high concentrations in the nervous system of vertebrates. In the biologically active form, A1 and B form dimeric proteins called S100A1–A1, S100A1B, and S100BB.[68] S100BB is present in high concentration in glial and Schwann cells, and S100A1B is present mostly in glial cells, but can also be found in melanocytes, adipocytes, chondrocytes, and epidermal Langerhans cells. S100BB dominates 30–100-fold, and collectively these two dimers (S100A1B and S100BB) are known as S100β (beta).[67,69] S100β (beta) protein is metabolized in the kidney and excreted in urine, and has a biological half-life of less than 1 h.[70]

Serum elevations of S100β (beta) and/or NSE have been reported in patients with a variety of cerebral lesions, including head injury, multiple sclerosis, status epilepticus, and brain tumors.[71–74] S100β (beta) is normally detected at low concentrations in the serum. It is postulated that damaged brain cells release S100β (beta) into cerebrospinal fluid, but cerebral S100β (beta) will appear in serum only if there is a concomitant increase in the permeability of the blood-brain barrier.[75]

After an acute stroke, serum levels of both S100β (beta) and NSE are elevated. Unlike NSE, S100β (beta) levels appear to be related both to the volume of brain damage and clinical outcome of acute stroke.[76,77] Furthermore, one study has shown that patients with neuropsychological impairment after an acute stroke have a higher, albeit nonsignificant, serum S100β (beta) concentration than patients without neurocognitive impairment.[78] Because of the relationship to the volume of injured brain, many studies have investigated the use of postoperative S100β (beta) levels to estimate the amount of brain injury in patients undergoing cardiac surgery.

Blomquist and colleagues studied the pattern of S100β (beta) protein release during and after CABG.[79] Maximum levels were found at the end of bypass, which stabilized for a few hours, and was then followed by a continuous decline. Serum S100β (beta) has been correlated with age, duration of cardiopulmonary bypass, duration of aortic-cross clamping, duration of deep hypothermic circulatory arrest, preoperative renal impairment, and pre-operative cerebral complications.[80]

The relationship of S100β (beta) to neurocognitive dysfunction after cardiac surgery is controversial in that there are extracerebral sources of S100β (beta) that can significantly contribute to serum levels. Jönsson and colleagues discovered a significant amount of S100β both in blood from the surgical field and in shed mediastinal blood from patients undergoing cardiac surgery.[70] They also found that elevations of serum S100β (beta) were significantly decreased after washing shed blood with a cell-saver, before transfusing it back to the patient. Hence, it was suggested that blood from the surgical wound, containing very high concentrations of S100β (beta) derived from lipolysis of mediastinal fat, is reintroduced into the circulation via cardiotomy suckers. In turn, this could account for the high serum S100β (beta) levels seen at the end of cardiopulmonary bypass.

As a result of these findings, Vaage and Anderson suggest that the extracerebral sources of S100β (beta) make the interpretation of early S100β (beta) blood concentration difficult, and a valid conclusion concerning neurological injury can be drawn only if cardiotomy suction is avoided.[81] They imply that many of the conclusions of early studies that did not consider the extracerebral sources of S100β (beta) will have to be revised. To overcome this problem, they have proposed either sampling serum S100β (beta) at 24–48 h after surgery or analyzing CSF for S100β (beta).

12.4 Neuroimaging

Until recently, neuroimaging had added little to the understanding of neurological dysfunction after CABG. Computed tomography (CT) scans can demonstrate if a patient has suffered a cerebral infarct, either as a result of hypoperfusion (watershed infarct) or cerebral emboli. Because of its superiority to other imaging methods, magnetic resonance imaging (MRI) has been increasingly employed in studies before and after cardiac surgery. Using conventional MRI, some investigators have found new focal brain lesions (e.g., cerebral infarcts, deep white matter lesions) after CABG in up to one third of patients without overt neurological complications.[82,83] Correlation of the presence of new lesions on MRI scans with cognitive dysfunction is variable in the few studies that have assessed cognition.[84,85] At the 1 year neuropsychological assessment in Kohn's study of 27 patients undergoing CABG, the number of new infarcts on MRI did correlate with the number of tests showing a one SD decline.[84] However, many patients undergoing CABG have old ischemic changes on baseline MRI scans that may obscure small new lesions, and this may account for the lack of correlation between MRI lesions and neurocognitive impairment found in other studies.

Advances in MRI techniques, such as diffusion-weighted imaging, can detect ischemic changes within minutes after onset and are therefore superior to conventional imaging.[86] The correlation between the presence of new lesions on diffusion-weighted imaging with postoperative neurocognitive decline is again variable.[87]

In essence, MRI is very sensitive in detecting new ischemic lesions, but the inconsistent correlation between these lesions and cognitive dysfunction, as measured by neuropsychometric tests, limits its usefulness. Recently however, one study from Oxford has used functional MRI, instead of neurocognitive tests, to measure cerebral injury after on-pump and off-pump CABG.[88,89] This modality could be more sensitive than neuropsychometric testing in future studies of neuroprotective agents.[90]

12.5 Conclusion

Central nervous system complications of cardiac surgery are due to a variety of patho-physiologic changes. Causative factors include cerebral embolization, cerebral hypoperfusion, cerebral hypoxia, blood-brain barrier dysfunction, hyperthermia, and genetic susceptibility to cerebral injury, for example, the presence of the apolipoprotein E ε-4 ($E_{epsilon}$-4) allele.[91] Because there are a myriad of factors that can affect neurocognitive function after cardiac surgery, in some studies of neuroprotection it has not been possible to standardize all of these. For instance, there are intraoperative characteristics that are unique to on-pump surgery, for example, nonpulsatile perfusion and systemic hypothermia, that cannot be replicated in an equivalent group undergoing off-pump CABG, where patients are maintained at near-normothermia and arterial blood flow is pulsatile. Nonpulsatile flow during cardiopulmonary bypass may induce cerebral edema and cortical cerebral oxygen desaturation.[92,93] There are also patient characteristics such as the degree of aortic atheromatous disease that cannot be matched. Evidence has accumulated that the single largest risk factor for neurological complications in cardiac surgery is the presence of aortic atheromatous disease.[94–96] As a result, one cannot attribute the potential neurocognitive benefits of off-pump surgery just on the absence of cardiopulmonary bypass.

Previous studies which have examined the effect of neuroprotective agents/strategies have been limited by the use of different definitions of neurocognitive decline, inappropriate statistical handling of neurocognitive data, and assessment of neurocognitive function at different time points, thus making comparisons of studies difficult. The design of future studies must take into account the different mechanisms that contribute to cerebral injury, and include patients who are at higher risk of neurocognitive injury, for example, advanced age and previous cerebrovascular disease, so that the potential benefit of the neuroprotective agent/strategy is likely to be shown.

References

1. Roach GW, Kanchuger M, Mangano CM, et al. Adverse cerebral outcomes after coronary bypass surgery. *Multicenter Study of Perioperative Ischemia Research Group and the Ischemia Research and Education Foundation Investigators N Engl J Med.* 1996;335(25):1857.
2. Opie JC. Cardiac surgery and acute neurological injury. In: Willner A, ed. *Cerebral Damage Before and After Cardiac Surgery.* Dordrecht: Kluwer; 1993. 15.
3. Harrison MJ. Neurologic complications of coronary artery bypass grafting: diffuse or focal ischemia? *Ann Thorac Surg.* 1995;59(5):1356.
4. Deslauriers R, Saunders JK, McIntyre MC. Magnetic resonance studies of the effects of cardiovascular surgery on brain metabolism and function. *J Cardiothorac Vasc Anesth.* 1996;10(1):127.
5. Dacey LJ, Likosky DS, Leavitt BJ, et al. Perioperative stroke and long-term survival after coronary bypass graft surgery. *Ann Thorac Surg.* 2005;79(2):532.
6. Hogue CW Jr, Murphy SF, Schechtman KB, Davila-Roman VG. Risk factors for early or delayed stroke after cardiac surgery. *Circulation.* 1999;100(6):642.
7. McKhann GM, Grega MA, Borowicz LM Jr, et al. Encephalopathy and stroke after coronary artery bypass grafting: incidence, consequences, and prediction. *Arch Neurol.* 2002;59(9):1422.
8. Arrowsmith JE, Grocott HP, Reves JG, Newman MF. Central nervous system complications of cardiac surgery. *Br J Anaesth.* 2000;84(3):378.
9. Arrowsmith JE, Harrison MJ, Newman SP, Stygall J, Timberlake N, Pugsley WB. Neuroprotection of the brain during cardiopulmonary bypass: a randomized trial of remacemide during coronary artery bypass in 171 patients. *Stroke.* 1998;29(11):2357.
10. Pugsley W, Klinger L, Paschalis C, Treasure T, Harrison M, Newman S. The impact of microemboli during cardiopulmonary bypass on neuropsychological functioning. *Stroke.* 1994;25(7):1393.
11. Busto R, Dietrich WD, Globus MY, Ginsberg MD. The importance of brain temperature in cerebral ischemic injury. *Stroke.* 1989;20(8):1113.
12. Busto R, Globus MY, Dietrich WD, Martinez E, Valdes I, Ginsberg MD. Effect of mild hypothermia on ischemia-induced release of neurotransmitters and free fatty acids in rat brain. *Stroke.* 1989;20(7):904.
13. Li PA, Shuaib A, Miyashita H, He QP, Siesjo BK, Warner DS. Hyperglycemia enhances extracellular glutamate accumulation in rats subjected to forebrain ischemia. *Stroke.* 2000;31(1):183.
14. Pulsinelli WA, Waldman S, Rawlinson D, Plum F. Moderate hyperglycemia augments ischemic brain damage: a neuropathologic study in the rat. *Neurology.* 1982;32(11):1239.
15. Griepp RB, Stinson EB, Hollingsworth JF, Buehler D. Prosthetic replacement of the aortic arch. *J Thorac Cardiovasc Surg.* 1975;70(6):1051.
16. Borst HG, Schaudig A, Rudolph W. Arteriovenous fistula of the aortic arch: repair during deep hypothermia and circulatory arrest. *J Thorac Cardiovasc Surg.* 1964;48:443.
17. Frist WH, Baldwin JC, Starnes VA, et al. A reconsideration of cerebral perfusion in aortic arch replacement. *Ann Thorac Surg.* 1986;42(3):273.
18. Ueda Y, Miki S, Kusuhara K, Okita Y, Tahata T, Yamanaka K. Surgical treatment of aneurysm or dissection involving the ascending aorta and aortic arch, utilizing circulatory arrest and retrograde cerebral perfusion. *J Cardiovasc Surg (Torino).* 1990;31(5):553.
19. Regragui I, Birdi I, Izzat MB, et al. The effects of cardiopulmonary bypass temperature on neuropsychologic outcome after coronary artery operations: a prospective randomized trial. *J Thorac Cardiovasc Surg.* 1996;112(4):1036.
20. Grigore AM, Mathew J, Grocott HP, et al. Prospective randomized trial of normothermic versus hypothermic cardiopulmonary bypass on cognitive function after coronary artery bypass graft surgery. *Anesthesiology.* 2001;95(5):1110.
21. Grigore AM, Grocott HP, Mathew JP, et al. The rewarming rate and increased peak temperature alter neurocognitive outcome after cardiac surgery. *Anesth Analg.* 2002;94(1):4.
22. Murkin JM, Martzke JS, Buchan AM, Bentley C, Wong CJ. A randomized study of the influence of perfusion technique

and pH management strategy in 316 patients undergoing coronary artery bypass surgery. II. Neurologic and cognitive outcomes. *J Thorac Cardiovasc Surg*. 1995;110(2):349.
23. Butterworth J, Wagenknecht LE, Legault C. Attempted control of hyperglycemia during cardiopulmonary bypass fails to improve neurologic or neurobehavioral outcomes in patients without diabetes mellitus undergoing coronary artery bypass grafting. *J Thorac Cardiovasc Surg*. 2005; 130(5):1319.
24. Motallebzadeh R, Bland JM, Markus HS, Kaski JC, Jahangiri M. Neurocognitive function and cerebral emboli: randomized study of on-pump versus off-pump coronary artery bypass surgery. *Ann Thorac Surg*. 2007;83(2):475.
25. Lee JD, Lee SJ, Tsushima WT, et al. Benefits of off-pump bypass on neurologic and clinical morbidity: a prospective randomized trial. *Ann Thorac Surg*. 2003;76(1):18.
26. Diegeler A, Hirsch R, Schneider F, et al. Neuromonitoring and neurocognitive outcome in off-pump versus conventional coronary bypass operation. *Ann Thorac Surg*. 2000;69(4):1162.
27. Taggart DP, Browne SM, Halligan PW, Wade DT. Is cardiopulmonary bypass still the cause of cognitive dysfunction after cardiac operations? *J Thorac Cardiovasc Surg*. 1999;118(3):414.
28. Van Dijk D, Jansen EW, Hijman R, et al. Cognitive outcome after off-pump and on-pump coronary artery bypass graft surgery: a randomized trial. *JAMA*. 2002;287(11):1405.
29. Zamvar V, Williams D, Hall J, et al. Assessment of neurocognitive impairment after off-pump and on-pump techniques for coronary artery bypass graft surgery: prospective randomised controlled trial. *BMJ*. 2002;325(7375):1268.
30. Svensson LG, Nadolny EM, Penney DL, et al. Prospective randomized neurocognitive and S-100 study of hypothermic circulatory arrest, retrograde brain perfusion, and antegrade brain perfusion for aortic arch operations. *Ann Thorac Surg*. 2001;71(6):1905.
31. Svensson LG, Husain A, Penney DL, et al. A prospective randomized study of neurocognitive function and s-100 protein after antegrade or retrograde brain perfusion with hypothermic arrest for aortic surgery. *J Thorac Cardiovasc Surg*. 2000;119(1):163.
32. Nussmeier NA, Arlund C, Slogoff S. Neuropsychiatric complications after cardiopulmonary bypass: cerebral protection by a barbiturate. *Anesthesiology*. 1986;64(2):165.
33. Legault C, Furberg CD, Wagenknecht LE, et al. Nimodipine neuroprotection in cardiac valve replacement: report of an early terminated trial. *Stroke*. 1996;27(4):593.
34. Murkin JM, Newman SP, Stump DA, Blumenthal JA. Statement of consensus on assessment of neurobehavioral outcomes after cardiac surgery. *Ann Thorac Surg*. 1995; 59(5):1289.
35. Murkin JM, Stump DA, Blumenthal JA, McKhann G. Defining dysfunction: group means versus incidence analysis – a statement of consensus. *Ann Thorac Surg*. 1997; 64(3):904.
36. Benedict RH. Cognitive function after open-heart surgery: are postoperative neuropsychological deficits caused by cardiopulmonary bypass? *Neuropsychol Rev*. 1994;4(3):223.
37. Townes BD, Bashein G, Hornbein TF, et al. Neurobehavioral outcomes in cardiac operations. A prospective controlled study. *J Thorac Cardiovasc Surg*. 1989;98(5 Pt 1):774.
38. Newman SP. Analysis and interpretation of neuropsychologic tests in cardiac surgery. *Ann Thorac Surg*. 1995;59(5): 1351.
39. Benedict RH, Zgaljardic DJ. Practice effects during repeated administrations of memory tests with and without alternate forms. *J Clin Exp Neuropsychol*. 1998;20(3):339.
40. Lezak MD. *Neuropsychological Assessment*. 3rd ed. New York: Oxford University Press; 1995.
41. Bruggemans EF, Van Dijk JG, Huysmans HA. Residual cognitive dysfunctioning at 6 months following coronary artery bypass graft surgery. *Eur J Cardiothorac Surg*. 1995;9(11): 636.
42. Borowicz LM, Goldsborough MA, Selnes OA, McKhann GM. Neuropsychologic change after cardiac surgery: a critical review. *J Cardiothorac Vasc Anesth*. 1996;10(1):105.
43. MacCallum RC, Zhang S, Preacher KJ, Rucker DD. On the practice of dichotomization of quantitative variables. *Psychol Methods*. 2002;7:19.
44. Blumenthal JA, Mahanna EP, Madden DJ, White WD, Croughwell ND, Newman MF. Methodological issues in the assessment of neuropsychologic function after cardiac surgery. *Ann Thorac Surg*. 1995;59(5):1345.
45. Mahanna EP, Blumenthal JA, White WD, et al. Defining neuropsychological dysfunction after coronary artery bypass grafting. *Ann Thorac Surg*. 1996;61(5):1342.
46. Newman S. The incidence and nature of neuropsychological morbidity following cardiac surgery. *Perfusion*. 1989;4:93.
47. Jacobson NS, Follette WC, Revenstorf D, Baucom DH, Hahlweg K, Margolin G. Variability in outcome and clinical significance of behavioral marital therapy: a reanalysis of outcome data. *J Consult Clin Psychol*. 1984;52(4):497.
48. Keith JR, Puente AE, Malcolmson KL, Tartt S, Coleman AE, Marks HF Jr. Assessing postoperative cognitive change after cardiopulmonary bypass surgery. *Neuropsychology*. 2002;16(3):411.
49. Savageau JA, Stanton BA, Jenkins CD, Frater RW. Neuropsychological dysfunction following elective cardiac operation. II. A six-month reassessment. *J Thorac Cardiovasc Surg*. 1982;84(4):595.
50. Moller JT, Cluitmans P, Rasmussen LS, et al. Long-term postoperative cognitive dysfunction in the elderly ISPOCD1 study. ISPOCD investigators. International study of postoperative cognitive dysfunction. *Lancet*. 1998;351(9106): 9857.
51. Browne SM, Halligan PW, Wade DT, Taggart DP. Cognitive performance after cardiac operation: implications of regression toward the mean. *J Thorac Cardiovasc Surg*. 1999; 117(3):481.
52. Bland JM, Altman DG. Some examples of regression towards the mean. *BMJ*. 1994;309(6957):780.
53. Bland JM, Altman DG. Regression towards the mean. *BMJ*. 1994;308(6942):1499.
54. Yudkin PL, Stratton IM. How to deal with regression to the mean in intervention studies. *Lancet*. 1996;347(8996):241.
55. Jacobson NS, Truax P. Clinical significance: a statistical approach to defining meaningful change in psychotherapy research. *J Consult Clin Psychol*. 1991;59(1):12.
56. Naugle RI, Chelune GJ, Cheek R, Luders H, Awad IA. Detection of changes in material-specific memory following temporal lobectomy using the Wechsler memory scale-revised. *Arch Clin Neuropsychol*. 1993;8(5):381.

57. Sawrie SM. Analysis of cognitive change: a commentary on Keith et al. (2002). *Neuropsychology*. 2002;16(3):429.
58. Rasmussen LS, Larsen K, Houx P, Skovgaard LT, Hanning CD, Moller JT. The assessment of postoperative cognitive function. *Acta Anaesthesiol Scand*. 2001;45(3):275.
59. Vickers AJ, Altman DG. Statistics notes: analysing controlled trials with baseline and follow up measurements. *BMJ*. 2001;323(7321):1123.
60. Whitaker D. The use of Z scores in assessing neuropsychological change after cardiac operations. *Ann Thorac Surg*. 2003;75(3):1066. author reply 1066.
61. Collie A, Darby DG, Falleti MG, Silbert BS. Maruff P. Determining the extent of cognitive change after coronary surgery: a review of statistical procedures. *Ann Thorac Surg*. 2002;73(6):2005.
62. Johnsson P. Markers of cerebral ischemia after cardiac surgery. *J Cardiothorac Vasc Anesth*. 1996;10(1):120.
63. Missler U, Wiesmann M, Wittmann G, Magerkurth O, Hagenstrom H. Measurement of glial fibrillary acidic protein in human blood: analytical method and preliminary clinical results. *Clin Chem*. 1999;45(1):138.
64. Marangos PJ, Schmechel D, Parma AM, Clark RL, Goodwin FK. Measurement of neuron-specific (NSE) and non-neuronal (NNE) isoenzymes of enolase in rat, monkey and human nervous tissue. *J Neurochem*. 1979;33(1):319.
65. Pahlman S, Esscher T, Bergh J, Steinholtz L, Nou E, Nilsson K. Neuron-specific enolase as a marker for neuroblastoma and small-cell carcinoma of the lung. *Tumour Biol*. 1984;5(2):119.
66. Pahlman S, Esscher T, Bergvall P, Odelstad L. Purification and characterization of human neuron-specific enolase: radioimmunoassay development. *Tumour Biol*. 1984; 5(2):127.
67. Zimmer DB, Cornwall EH, Landar A, Song W. The S100 protein family: history, function, and expression. *Brain Res Bull*. 1995;37(4):417.
68. Barger SW, Wolchok SR, Van Eldik LJ. Disulfide-linked S100 beta dimers and signal transduction. *Biochim Biophys Acta*. 1992;1160(1):105.
69. Abraha HD, Butterworth RJ, Bath PM, Wassif WS, Garthwaite J, Sherwood RA. Serum S-100 protein, relationship to clinical outcome in acute stroke. *Ann Clin Biochem*. 1997;34(Pt 5):546.
70. Jonsson H, Johnsson P, Alling C, Backstrom M, Bergh C, Blomquist S. S100beta after coronary artery surgery: release pattern, source of contamination, and relation to neuropsychological outcome. *Ann Thorac Surg*. 1999;68(6):2202.
71. Ross SA, Cunningham RT, Johnston CF, Rowlands BJ. Neuron-specific enolase as an aid to outcome prediction in head injury. *Br J Neurosurg*. 1996;10(5):471.
72. Missler U, Wandinger KP, Wiesmann M, Kaps M, Wessel K. Acute exacerbation of multiple sclerosis increases plasma levels of S-100 protein. *Acta Neurol Scand*. 1997;96(3):142.
73. DeGiorgio CM, Gott PS, Rabinowicz AL, Heck CN, Smith TD, Correale JD. Neuron-specific enolase, a marker of acute neuronal injury, is increased in complex partial status epilepticus. *Epilepsia*. 1996;37(7):606.
74. van de Pol M, Twijnstra A, ten Velde GP. Menheere PP. Neuron-specific enolase as a marker of brain metastasis in patients with small-cell lung carcinoma. *J Neurooncol*. 1994;19(2):149.
75. Persson L, Hardemark HG, Gustafsson J, et al. S-100 protein and neuron-specific enolase in cerebrospinal fluid and serum: markers of cell damage in human central nervous system. *Stroke*. 1987;18(5):911.
76. Fassbender K, Schmidt R, Schreiner A, et al. Leakage of brain-originated proteins in peripheral blood: temporal profile and diagnostic value in early ischemic stroke. *J Neurol Sci*. 1997;148(1):101.
77. Missler U, Wiesmann M, Friedrich C, Kaps M. S-100 protein and neuron-specific enolase concentrations in blood as indicators of infarction volume and prognosis in acute ischemic stroke. *Stroke*. 1997;28(10):1956.
78. Wunderlich MT, Ebert AD, Kratz T, Goertler M, Jost S, Herrmann M. Early neurobehavioral outcome after stroke is related to release of neurobiochemical markers of brain damage. *Stroke*. 1999;30(6):1190.
79. Blomquist S, Johnsson P, Luhrs C, et al. The appearance of S-100 protein in serum during and immediately after cardiopulmonary bypass surgery: a possible marker for cerebral injury. *J Cardiothorac Vasc Anesth*. 1997;11(6):699.
80. Ali MS, Harmer M, Vaughan R. Serum S100 protein as a marker of cerebral damage during cardiac surgery. *Br J Anaesth*. 2000;85(2):287.
81. Vaage J, Anderson R. Biochemical markers of neurologic injury in cardiac surgery: the rise and fall of S100beta. *J Thorac Cardiovasc Surg*. 2001;122(5):853.
82. Toner I, Peden CJ, Hamid SK, Newman S, Taylor KM, Smith PL. Magnetic resonance imaging and neuropsychological changes after coronary artery bypass graft surgery: preliminary findings. *J Neurosurg Anesthesiol*. 1994; 6(3):163.
83. Harris DN, Bailey SM, Smith PL, Taylor KM, Oatridge A, Bydder GM. Brain swelling in first hour after coronary artery bypass surgery. *Lancet*. 1993;342(8871):586.
84. Kohn A. Magnetic resonance imaging registration and quantitation of the brain before and after coronary artery bypass graft surgery. *Ann Thorac Surg*. 2002;73(1):S363.
85. Bendszus M, Reents W, Franke D, et al. Brain damage after coronary artery bypass grafting. *Arch Neurol*. 2002; 59(7):1090.
86. Warach S, Gaa J, Siewert B, Wielopolski P, Edelman RR. Acute human stroke studied by whole brain echo planar diffusion-weighted magnetic resonance imaging. *Ann Neurol*. 1995;37(2):231.
87. Knipp SC, Matatko N, Wilhelm H, et al. Evaluation of brain injury after coronary artery bypass grafting. A prospective study using neuropsychological assessment and diffusion-weighted magnetic resonance imaging. *Eur J Cardiothorac Surg*. 2004;25(5):791.
88. Abu-Omar Y, Cifelli A, Matthews PM, Taggart DP. The role of microembolisation in cerebral injury as defined by functional magnetic resonance imaging. *Eur J Cardiothorac Surg*. 2004;26(3):586.
89. Abu-Omar Y, Cader S, Guerrieri Wolf L, Pigott D, Matthews PM, Taggart DP. Short-term changes in cerebral activity in on-pump and off-pump cardiac surgery defined by functional magnetic resonance imaging and their relationship to microembolization. *J Thorac Cardiovasc Surg*. 2006;132(5):1119.
90. Matthews PM, Clare S, Adcock J. Functional magnetic resonance imaging: clinical applications and potential. *J Inherit Metab Dis*. 1999;22(4):337.

91. Tardiff BE, Newman MF, Saunders AM, et al. Preliminary report of a genetic basis for cognitive decline after cardiac operations. The Neurologic Outcome Research Group of the Duke Heart Center. *Ann Thorac Surg*. 1997;64(3):715.
92. Edmonds HL Jr. Advances in neuromonitoring for cardiothoracic and vascular surgery. *J Cardiothorac Vasc Anesth*. 2001;15(2):241.
93. Anderson RE, Li TQ, Hindmarsh T, Settergren G, Vaage J. Increased extracellular brain water after coronary artery bypass grafting is avoided by off-pump surgery. *J Cardiothorac Vasc Anesth*. 1999;13:698.
94. Tunick PA, Rosenzweig BP, Katz ES, Freedberg RS, Perez JL, Kronzon I. High risk for vascular events in patients with protruding aortic atheromas: a prospective study. *J Am Coll Cardiol*. 1994;23(5):1085.
95. Wareing TH, Davila-Roman VG, Barzilai B, Murphy SF, Kouchoukos NT. Management of the severely atherosclerotic ascending aorta during cardiac operations. A strategy for detection and treatment. *J Thorac Cardiovasc Surg*. 1992;3(3):453.
96. Davila-Roman VG, Murphy SF, Nickerson NJ, Kouchoukos NT, Schechtman KB, Barzilai B. Atherosclerosis of the ascending aorta is an independent predictor of long-term neurologic events and mortality. *J Am Coll Cardiol*. 1999;33(5):1308.

Temperature and Brain Protection in Cardiac Surgery

13

George Djaiani, Harish Ramakrishna, and Alina M. Grigore

13.1 The Role of Temperature in Cerebral Physiology and Physiopathology

It is well known and has been clearly demonstrated that temperature plays a significant role in cerebral physiology and physiopathology, particularly in the setting of cardiac surgery with cardiopulmonary bypass (CPB). The human central nervous system (CNS) receives about 15% of the resting cardiac output and consumes about 20% of the oxygen required by the body at rest. The brain, which accounts for 2% of the total body weight, has an oxygen consumption of about 3.5 $mL^{-1} \cdot 100\ g^{-1} \cdot min^{-1}$. This high metabolic rate mandates a high blood flow; therefore, cerebral blood flow (CBF) (Fig. 13.1) is of paramount importance and is normally under metabolic, neural, myogenic, and chemical control.[1]

These issues are critical in cardiac anesthesia and surgery because CPB imposes tremendous demands on cerebral oxygenation and perfusion in the setting of the constant temperature fluctuations and adjustments that cardiac surgery requires. Maintaining steady body temperature preserves the cerebral metabolic rate of oxygen ($CMRO_2$) and is crucial in decreasing the morbidity associated with the use of CPB. Importantly, for every 1°C decrease in body temperature, $CMRO_2$ decreases 7% (Fig. 13.2). The term used to describe this relationship is the metabolic temperature coefficient, Q10, which, by definition, is the ratio of $CMRO_2$ at a given temperature T, divided by the $CMRO_2$ at a temperature 10°C lower (T-10). The value of cerebral Q10 in the physiologic range of 27–37°C is between 2 and 3, reflecting the decrease in rates of basal biochemical actions at this temperature. At temperatures less than 27°C, Q10 increases to approximately 4.5, reflecting

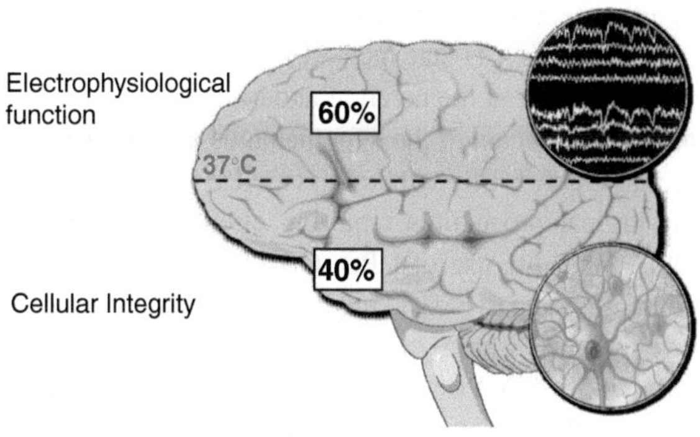

Fig. 13.1 Oxygen requirements of the normal brain

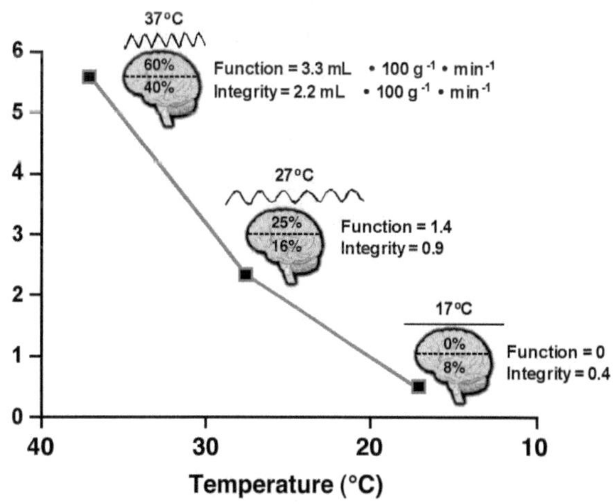

Fig. 13.2 Temperature and cerebral metabolic rate. $CMRO_2$ = cerebral metabolic rate

G. Djaiani (✉)
Department of Anesthesia and Pain Management, Toronto General Hospital, UHN, University of Toronto, Toronto, Ontario, Canada
e-mail: george.djaiani@uhn.on.ca

R.S. Bonser et al. (eds.), *Brain Protection in Cardiac Surgery*,
DOI: 10.1007/978-1-84996-293-3_13, © Springer-Verlag London Limited 2011

the additional effects of the major suppression of neuronal function that occurs between 17°C and 27°C.[2]

Given that moderate hypothermia without major suppression of neuronal function provides better neuroprotection than do isoelectric doses of barbiturates, identifying the mechanisms that control basal $CMRo_2$ is essential.[3] With mild to moderate hypothermia, the coupling of flow to metabolism and vascular responses to $Paco_2$ and Pao_2 are preserved; however, autoregulation may be impaired, even under hypothermic conditions, if the co_2 content of the blood is allowed to rise, which happens when the pH-stat method of blood gas management is used. (See later in this chapter for a discussion of the pH-stat method.) Changes in CBF are most apparent in the cerebral and cerebellar cortex but are not significant in the hypothalamus and brainstem.[4]

Intraoperative hypothermia is used to varying degrees in surgical procedures requiring circulatory arrest or CPB. With the use of CPB, CBF has been shown to decrease by up to 55% at the lowest measured temperature of 26°C, which, in 1 study, correlated with a 56% reduction in $CMRo_2$.[5] At progressively lower temperatures, CBF continues to decrease to the point that the electroencephalogram (EEG) tracing becomes isoelectric, which, in animal studies, has been found to be at approximately 18°C. During profound hypothermia (18–20°C), CBF is disproportionately maintained and is determined more by arterial blood pressure and systemic vascular resistance than by pump flow rates.[6]

When hypothermia is combined with doses of thiopental that produce EEG suppression, the synergistic effects further reduce the $CMRo_2$, leading to an additional decrease in CBF. Although inhaled volatile anesthetic agents, such as isoflurane, also have similar effects on $CMRo_2$, they do not cause the additional drop in CBF.[7]

Hypothermia also attenuates cytokine release during cardiac surgery.[8,9] Moderate hypothermia during CPB protects the myocardium by modifying intramyocardial cytokine balance, with increased synthesis of the anti-inflammatory cytokine interleukin-10 and decreased production of the proinflammatory tumor necrosis factor-α, which provide organ protection.[10] Interleukin-10, a natural monocyte-deactivating cytokine, is a potent inhibitor of tumor necrosis factor-α and cyclooxygenase 2 and has been shown to confer myocardial protection in an animal model of ischemia-reperfusion injury.[11] The mechanism for this effect is postulated to be inhibition of myocardial necrosis and prevention of apoptosis in damaged myocardial cells.[12]

13.2 CNS Injury in the Cardiac Surgical Perioperative Period

13.2.1 Incidence and Risk Factors for the Development of Complications

CNS complications develop in a considerable number of patients after cardiac surgery. These complications range from subtle cognitive changes to clinically evident confusion, delirium, and stroke.[13,14] The prevalence of short-term cognitive dysfunction ranges from 4 to 36% at 6–12 weeks after surgery[15–20] and increases to more than 40% at 5 years after conventional coronary artery bypass graft (CABG) operations.[15,21,22] Independent predictors of early cognitive deficits in low-risk patients undergoing CABG include poor left ventricular function, elevated preoperative creatinine levels, and a higher education level.

Postoperative confusion and delirium occur in 7–16% of patients.[23–26] The predictors of cognitive decline in the long term include older age, lower level of education, and evidence of cognitive decline at discharge.[15]

The rates of clinically apparent frank stroke vary from 1% in low-risk CABG operations to more than 8% in complex valve and aortic repair procedures.[27–32] Independent patient-related predictors of stroke are well known and include age (>70 years), proximal aortic atherosclerosis, previous stroke or transient ischemic attack, diabetes, congestive heart failure, and peripheral vascular disease.[33–38] Intraoperative risk factors include the type of operation, the duration of CPB, hyperglycemia, and low hematocrit levels.[30,32,39] Finally, it is well recognized that the presence of a prior "silent" brain infarction identified by magnetic resonance imaging (MRI) increases the risk of CNS injury after cardiac surgery,[40] and the presence of aortic atheroma is an important risk factor for both silent ischemic brain injury[25] and frank postoperative stroke.[41,42]

13.2.2 Risk Stratification

Various authors have suggested that risk stratification in cardiac surgical patients could be enhanced and streamlined with certain preoperative tests, including brain MRI to test for cerebral vascular disease, aortic MRI to test for atheroma, and psychometric examinations to test for neurocognitive dysfunction.[43–46] However, proposed and validated preoperative risk-stratification models have only modest positive predictive value, particularly when applied to an individual patient. The predictive power of these models can be improved by analyzing the major intraoperative and postoperative factors that influence patients' outcome.

13.2.3 Improving Risk Stratification

The use of neuromonitoring strategies, including performing transcranial Doppler ultrasonography or near-infrared spectroscopy and monitoring jugular bulb (JB) oxygenation, can potentially increase the positive and negative predictive value of the various models. Furthermore, in the future, incorporating data on genetic modulators of stroke and cognitive dysfunction after cardiac surgery may also improve the predictive power of these models.[47,48]

13.2.4 Minimizing the Risk of CNS Injury

In addition to preoperatively eliminating the risk of CNS injury to the extent possible, employing specific intraoperative and postoperative strategies may decrease the risk of a patient developing a CNS injury during or after cardiac surgery. The intraoperative use of ultrasound to examine the ascending aorta and the aortic arch for detection of atheroma may guide surgical technique and minimize aortic manipulation, potentially resulting in better CNS outcomes.[49–51] With respect to temperature management, it has been shown that intraoperative normothermia increases the risk for postoperative cognitive dysfunction[52]; however, the rate of rewarming, rather than intraoperative hypothermia per se, appears to have the greatest effect.[18,53–55]

Close postoperative monitory is essential because between one third and more than one half of postoperative strokes occur after an uneventful recovery from anesthesia[29,38,56–59]; in addition, the neurologic symptoms of the initial insult (i.e., an embolic event during surgery) are not apparent for up to 72 h after surgery because of the slow evolutionary process of ischemic stroke.[60] Postoperative low-output syndrome, heart failure, atrial fibrillation, hyperglycemia, increased thrombin generation,[61] and unrecognized and unaddressed postoperative hyperthermia[32] can all have a significant impact on the rate of neurologic events.

13.3 Perioperative Temperature Management

13.3.1 Temperature Regimens

Temperature is a physiologic variable that can be manipulated to suit the requirements of a particular management strategy. Temperature drift is commonly observed during major surgery, with the amount of drift primarily dependent on the patient's baseline temperature and directly proportional to the duration of surgery unless active measures are taken to maintain normothermia during the operation. Reductions in core temperature force patients' bodies to expend more energy on heat production and to consume more oxygen through postoperative shivering. Frank et al.[62] showed that patients with coronary artery disease who underwent major vascular, thoracic, or abdominal surgery with a mean core temperature of 35.4°C had significantly higher incidences of myocardial ischemia, ventricular tachycardia, myocardial infarction, and cardiac arrest than did patients with a mean core temperature of 36.7°C. Therefore, one of the key components of successful perioperative anesthetic management is maintaining normothermia.

A paradigm shift to fast-tracking cardiac operations by using "warm" CPB has facilitated early extubation and reduced intensive care unit and hospital lengths of stay, thereby reducing costs and improving resource utilization in many cardiac surgical units. Although warm CPB, "tepid" CPB, or both are being used, it is important to note that many cardiac centers in North America and Europe are still using hypothermic CPB (core T = 28°C), even for primary CABG or valve operations. The rationale for this type of practice has been widely debated since the early 1990s. Martin et al.[63] randomly assigned 1,001 patients to warm (≥35°C) or cold (≤28°C) CPB groups and found a threefold increase in the rate of stroke in the warm CPB group (4.5% versus 1.4%).[63] In contrast, the Warm Heart Trials Group (WHTG) study[64] of 1,732 patients randomly assigned to either normothermic (n = 860) or hypothermic (n = 872) CPB techniques found no difference in stroke rates between the two groups (1.6% versus

1.5%, respectively). More recent evidence supports the findings from the WHTG study, suggesting that cold CPB has little advantage over warm CPB in terms of preserving cerebral oxygenation.[65]

The most critical times for ischemic injury are the beginning and end of CPB because these are the times when emboli are most likely to occur. The conflicting results from studies of the use of hypothermic CPB are probably related to the fact that a cerebral ischemic insult (cerebral embolic events) is most likely to occur at the beginning and end of CPB and during cannulation of the aorta, initiation of CPB, and aortic cross-clamping, all of which occur while the patient is normothermic. Furthermore, accelerated rewarming strategies that facilitate separation from CPB may cause cerebral hyperthermia (an overshoot phenomenon), which coincides with another period associated with an increased risk of the development of cerebral ischemia – during aortic declamping and decannulation. All of these events could potentially lead to worse neurologic and neurocognitive outcomes.[53,66] Even though the results of some studies[63,66] suggest that hypothermia during cardiac surgery is beneficial, it is still difficult to distinguish the benefits of hypothermia from the harmful effects of hyperthermia.

13.3.2 The Deleterious Effects of Hyperthermia

13.3.2.1 Background

There is emerging evidence that hyperthermia is an important predictor of adverse neurologic outcomes in patients who have had strokes[67,68] and in patients with cerebral injury.[67,69] Development of early fever is associated with a worse prognosis after stroke.[70] Furthermore, body temperature on admission to the hospital may predict short-term and long-term mortality after acute stroke[71]; low body temperature on admission is considered to be a predictor of good short-term outcome in stroke patients.[72] Kammersgaard et al.[73] showed that a 1°C increase in admission body temperature independently predicted a 30% relative increase in 5-year mortality risk after acute stroke. Thus, treating hyperthermia is a logical therapeutic step toward minimizing neurologic insult; however, it can be difficult to achieve normothermia or hypothermia in critically ill neurologic patients, in whom additional or alternative methods are sometimes required to achieve effective cooling.[68,74,75]

13.3.2.2 Specific Effects of Hyperthermia Related to Cardiac Operations

The potential deleterious effects of hyperthermia after cardiac surgery may include increased free radical production, expansion of the ischemic penumbra, and a mismatch between oxygen supply and demand. Monitoring temperature and aggressively treating cerebral hyperthermia would probably provide an opportunity to minimize the exacerbation of neurologic injury in these patients. A recent evidence-based review supports limiting the arterial inflow temperature to 37°C to prevent cerebral hyperthermia (Class IIa, Level B evidence).[76] Another review agrees that, although hyperthermia is associated with worse neurologic outcomes, there is insufficient evidence that therapeutic hypothermia improves neurologic outcomes.[77]

13.3.3 The Benefits of Hypothermia

Hypothermia has been shown to be neuroprotective in different brain-injury models. Cerebral ischemia is associated with less cytotoxic injury if the brain is rendered hypothermic, even after the initial insult. Hypothermia-induced reduction of $Paco_2$ acts as a direct cerebral vasoconstrictor, reducing CBF and intracranial pressure. These effects are associated with reduced vascular permeability, reduced leukocyte migration within the ischemic brain, and less cerebral edema. Other mechanisms of action, the discovery of which has increased our understanding of the therapeutic effects of hypothermia, include reduced oxygen and glucose utilization, reduced glutamate and free radical formation, membrane stabilization, and reduced release of inflammatory cytokines.[78–83] Furthermore, some evidence suggests that inhibition of apoptosis contributes to the neuroprotective effects of induced hypothermia.[84–86]

The application of hypothermia has improved the functional recovery of patients after cardiac surgery and even after prolonged cardiopulmonary resuscitation from out-of-hospital cardiac arrest.[87,88] Hypothermia may also benefit patients after traumatic brain injury, subarachnoid hemorrhage, and stroke.[69,89–92]

13.3.4 Sites for Temperature Monitoring

Because brain temperature during cardiac surgery with CPB has such a broad and profound effect on the extent and severity of neurologic injury, its adequate monitoring and recording are mandatory for successful outcome, particularly in patients at risk for experiencing neurologic injury.

A wide variety of sites are used for temperature monitoring during cardiac surgery (Fig. 13.3). CPB creates a challenging clinical setting for adequate temperature recording because a significant degree of heat exchange occurs during cooling and rewarming. As a result, thermal changes vary with the specific rates of heat transfer in different tissues.

Because the JB receives 99% of cerebral venous blood flow, JB temperature is considered to be, and has been validated as, the most accurate site for recording brain temperature.[93] Nussmeier and colleagues[94] demonstrated a wide variation between JB temperature and temperature recorded at other sites (Fig. 13.4). Gradients as high as 5°C have been found between JB temperature and bladder and rectal temperatures.[94,95] Thus, if the bladder or rectal temperature is brought to 37°C during the rewarming phase of CPB, the brain temperature could easily reach 40°C or higher and could unnecessarily increase the patient's risk for a poor neurologic outcome.[67,96]

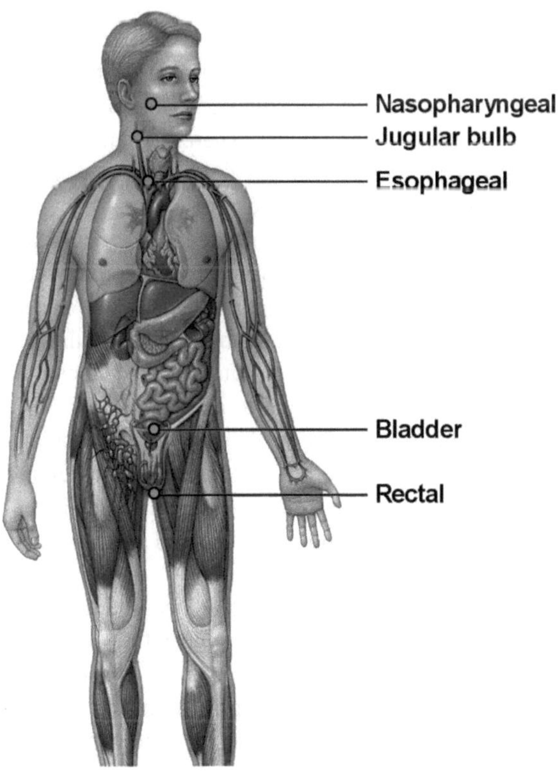

Fig. 13.3 Sites for temperature monitoring

Placing a JB catheter for temperature monitoring can be time consuming and cost inefficient. Nussmeier et al.[94] found that, during CPB, arterial inflow temperatures reliably estimate brain temperatures because equilibration with JB temperatures occurs within the first 5 min after either cooling or rewarming begins (Fig. 13.5).

13.3.5 Methods of Achieving Hypothermia

Cerebral hypothermia can be achieved through either local cooling of the head or global cooling of the whole body. A combination of local brain cooling and normal core temperature maintenance would provide optimally beneficial cerebral hypothermia while minimizing the systemic adverse effects of whole-body cooling.

The presumed mechanisms by which therapeutic hypothermia work include suppression of free radicals, inhibition of destructive enzymatic reactions, reduction of oxygen demand in low-flow regions, and inhibition of the biosynthesis, release, and uptake of excitatory neurotransmitters.[87,97,98] Induced hypothermia of 32–34°C is recommended for most therapeutic purposes and should be maintained for 12–72 h.

Two of the most effective tools for achieving and maintaining hypothermia are conventional cooling blankets and endovascular cooling devices. The conventional cooling blankets (water or air cooling) cool at a rate of 0.9°C per hour. Arctic Sun (Medivance, Inc., Louisville, CO) is a Food and Drug Administration-approved device with gel pads that stick to the skin and can cover up to 40% of the body's surface area. Cold water is circulated through the gel pads.[68] This device cools at a rate of 1.5–2.0°C per hour. Endovascular cooling devices such as Coolgard (Inner Cool Therapeutics, Inc., San Diego, CA) have a 10F catheter that is inserted into a central vein.[99] Cold saline

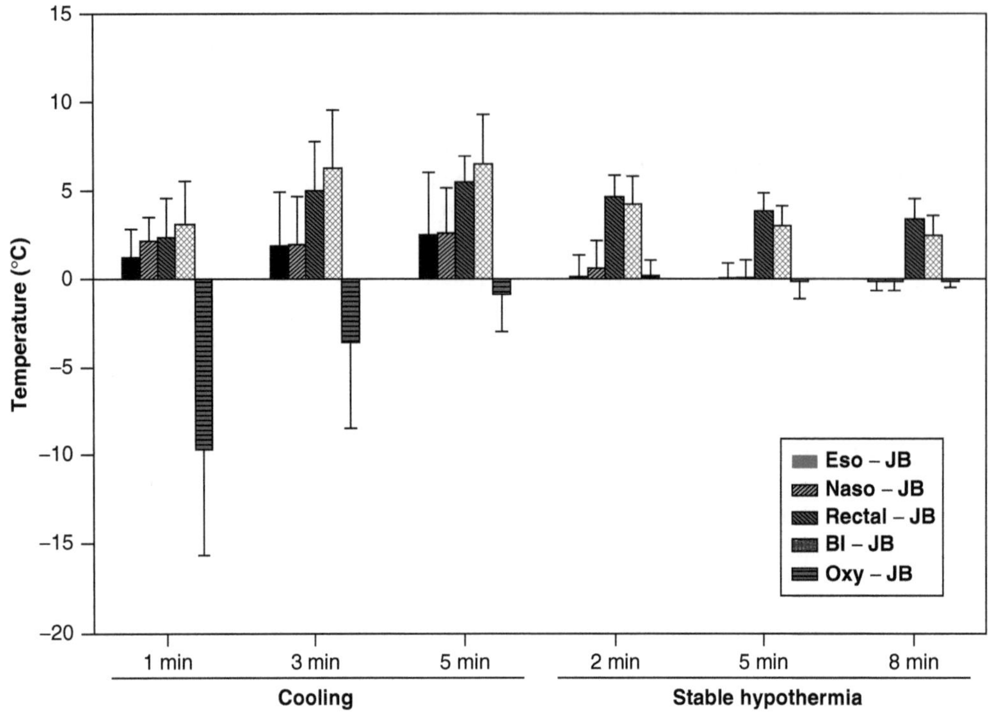

Fig. 13.4 Jugular bulb temperature gradients during cardiopulmonary bypass. JB = jugular bulb; Bl = bladder; Naso = nasopharyngeal; Eso = esophageal, Oxy = oxygenator (Reprinted with permission of the Anesth Analg.[94])

is circulated through this tubing, cooling the patient without coming in contact with the patient's blood. The cooling efficacy of these devices is 4.5°C per hour.

13.3.6 Deep Hypothermic Circulatory Arrest

Deep hypothermic circulatory arrest (DHCA) was one of the earliest applications of induced hypothermia as a neuroprotective measure in cardiac surgery. In 1950, Bigelow et al.[100–102] published the first series of experimental operations using surface cooling and circulatory arrest. A few years later, a number of centers began using surface cooling to 30°C and brief periods of circulatory arrest to repair intracardiac defects such as atrial septal defects. Currently, DHCA is the most common modality used to provide neuroprotection for repairs of the distal ascending aorta, transverse arch, and proximal descending aorta, as well as for other procedures that necessitate complete interruption of CBF (e.g., repairing large brain aneurysms).

Despite a long history of clinical use, the use of DHCA is associated with unpredictable and poorly defined neurologic injury. Therefore, the surgical advantages of a bloodless field must be weighed against the potential drawbacks of prolonged bypass time, coagulopathy, and adverse neurologic outcomes. The actual mechanism by which DHCA protects the brain is not entirely clear, but multiple factors appear to be involved. For one, mild to moderate hypothermia has been shown to reduce glutamate and dopamine release during ischemia and to affect plasma glycine concentrations.[103,104] This pathway affects the activation of NMDA receptors and reduces intracellular calcium accumulation. Before DHCA is instituted, it is important to ensure adequate and homogeneous hypothermia.

Generally, once CPB is initiated, cooling is begun for at least 30 min at perfusate temperatures no lower than 10°C. Cooling to temperatures lower than 18–20°C has been shown to provide better cerebral protection than was once thought[105] because metabolic activity at that range is variable. The most important adjunct for cerebral protection during DHCA is

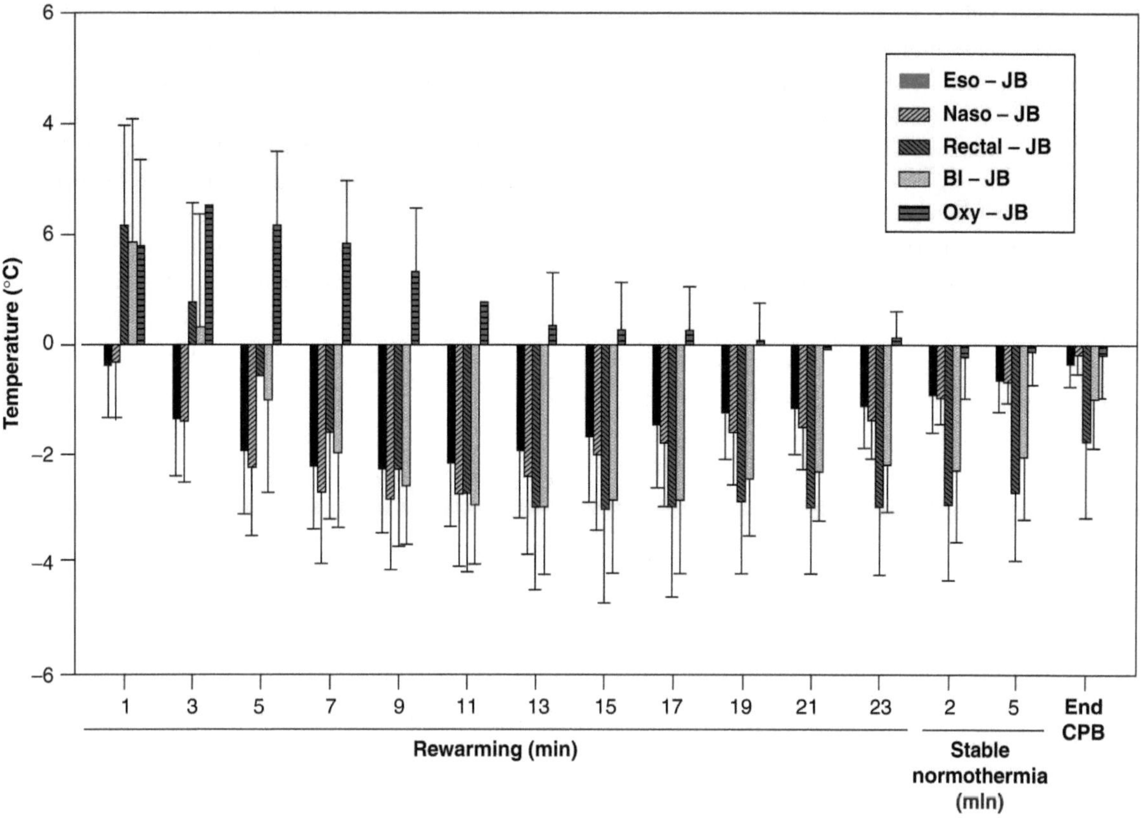

Fig. 13.5 Oxygenator outflow and jugular bulb temperature gradients during rewarming phase of cardiopulmonary bypass. CPB = cardiopulmonary bypass (Reprinted with permission of the Anesth Analg.[94])

surface cooling of the head with ice.[105] In an animal study, Griepp et al.[105] demonstrated that DHCA with head cooling was associated with a significant better postoperative behavioral scores that DHCA with head kept at room temperature. Another important factor is maintenance of CBF during the cooling phase. Some authors suggest inducing truly profound hypothermia before circulatory arrest to achieve maximal metabolic suppression. McCullough et al.[106] have suggested cooling the patient to an esophageal temperature of 10–11°C if a DHCA time of 30 min or greater is expected. Blood viscosity is an issue with hypothermia, and hemodilution is always performed to maintain adequate CBF during cooling. pH management is also important because the cerebral vasculature is exquisitely sensitive to blood CO_2 levels. Generally, the preferred method of pH management during DHCA is the α-stat method, in which no correction is made for the patient's actual temperature and the oxygenator gas mixture and flows are adjusted to maintain a normothermic pH of 7.4 and a $Paco_2$ of 40 mmHg; in the pH-stat method, in contrast, co_2 gas is added to the oxygenator gas mixture. Therefore, it is generally accepted that, with α-stat management, there is relative alkalosis at low temperatures and flow-metabolism coupling is maintained. Other key anesthetic goals in the management of DHCA include profound muscle relaxation during the arrest period to minimize oxygen consumption; stress response attenuation; meticulous attention to glycemic control before, during, and after DHCA; and monitored suppression of metabolic and electrical activity in the brain. The neuroprotective effects of corticosteroids, mannitol, and barbiturates, as well as monitoring of JB oxygen saturation, have been well documented over the years. Detailed descriptions of retrograde perfusion and rewarming techniques are provided in Chap. 18; suffice it to say that, although mortality rates after procedures involving DHCA have decreased over the last few decades, the incidence of stroke has remained at approximately 8–10% at most centers. Slow and meticulous rewarming is mandatory because slow warming has been shown to decrease cerebral injury[53] and to slow JB desaturation.[107]

13.3.7 Total Body Hypothermia During Cardiopulmonary Resuscitation and Cardiovascular Collapse

Therapeutic total-body hypothermia has been used for neuroprotection in multiple forms over the years in both adult and pediatric populations. The benefits of this technique are apparent in cases of out-of-hospital cardiac arrest, in which total-body hypothermia has been shown to improve neurologic outcome. Additionally, therapeutic hypothermia has been suggested to improve outcomes in other situations, such as traumatic brain injury, neonatal asphyxia, cerebrovascular accident, and intracranial hypertension.[108]

In 1953, Bigelow and McBirnie[109] demonstrated the benefit of therapeutic hypothermia in a canine model in which, under deep hypothermia, the area of an experimentally induced neurologic injury showed less-than-normal rates of hemorrhage, cerebral edema, and leukocyte infiltration. In humans, the first successful use of therapeutic hypothermia was reported in 1959 by Benson et al.,[110] who cooled 12 patients after cardiac arrest. On the basis of published evidence, the Advanced Life Support Task Force of the International Liaison Committee on Resuscitation stated in November 2005 that therapeutic hypothermia should be used with unconscious adult patients with spontaneous circulation after out-of-hospital cardiac arrest.[111] The committee also recommended cooling such patients to 32–34°C for 12–24 h if the patient's initial cardiac rhythm was ventricular fibrillation.[111]

13.3.8 Impact of Hypothermia on Other Organ Systems

13.3.8.1 Cardiovascular System

The initial effects of hypothermia are associated with increased myocardial oxygen demand, cardiac output, systemic vascular resistance, central venous pressure, hypertension, and tachycardia secondary to catecholamine release. Further, hypothermia reduces metabolic rate, oxygen demand, heart rate, cardiac output, and blood pressure. Progressive reduction of temperature is associated with conduction abnormalities and arrhythmias and, when the temperature drops below 28°C, refractory ventricular fibrillation. A recent randomized, double-blind study by a group of investigators in Ottawa found that mild sustained hypothermia was not associated with a higher risk of perioperative myocardial infarction or postoperative atrial fibrillation.[18]

13.3.8.2 Respiratory System

Reduction in metabolic rate results in reduced co_2 production, necessitating adjustments in ventilatory settings to maintain adequate CBF. Hypothermia is associated with leftward shift of oxygen dissociation curve. Blood pH increases and $Paco_2$ reduces as temperature decreases. This physiologic response is the basis of the previously mentioned pH-stat (a "corrected" pH of 7.4 and a $Paco_2$ of 40 mmHg at the patient's current temperature) and α-stat (an "uncorrected" [relative to the patient's true temperature] pH of 7.4 and a $Paco_2$ of 40 mmHg at 37°C) management strategies. Hypothermic patients may have a higher risk of postoperative pneumonia. This is partly related to impaired immune function associated with induced hypothermia.

13.3.8.3 Renal System

Hypothermia is associated with cold diuresis, as well as lowered plasma potassium and magnesium concentrations. Intravascular volume depletion requires adequate fluid resuscitation and is one of the reasons that more vasopressor therapy is needed during hypothermia.

13.3.8.4 Gastrointestinal Function

Hypothermia is associated with decreased gastrointestinal motility. Serum amylase and liver enzymes are frequently elevated during hypothermia, resulting in reduced drug clearance, detoxification, and conjugation. Drug metabolism is also decreased, which prolongs the effects of volatile and intravenously administered anesthetic agents, as well as muscle relaxants. Minimal alveolar concentration is reduced by 5% for each degree of temperature drop. Hypothermia is associated with insulin resistance and decreased insulin release, which result in elevated glucose concentrations and poor glycemic control.

13.3.8.5 Hematologic Function

During hypothermia, hematologic function may be impaired secondary to platelet dysfunction and coagulopathy. However, two recent landmark studies concluded that deliberate perioperative hypothermia is not associated with increased risk of postoperative bleeding, blood product utilization, intubation time, hospital length of stay, or mortality in patients undergoing CABG surgery.[18,112]

13.3.9 Postoperative Hyperthermia and Induced Hypothermia

Postoperative hyperthermia occurs in at least 38% of patients and peaks with a bimodal distribution at means of 9 and 27 h after elective cardiac surgery requiring CPB (Fig. 13.6).[113] Grocott et al.[96] associated postoperative hyperthermia with cognitive dysfunction 6 weeks after CABG surgery. The same group of investigators reported that limiting rewarming during CPB and using surface rewarming after surgery minimize the risk of postoperative hypothermia.[114]

Frank stroke after cardiac surgery is a devastating complication with limited therapeutic options. Currently, there is no consensus about the best management strategy for perioperative stroke after cardiac surgery. Interestingly, some case reports have noted that early intra-arterial thrombolysis has been included in the treatment of acute ischemic stroke after cardiac surgery, with varying degrees of success.[115,116] Although these attempts constitute the first steps toward establishing the safety profile of intra-arterial thrombolysis in patients with recent cardiac surgery, it is too early to recommend this intervention for routine use in patients undergoing cardiac operations.

Another interesting strategy that has been instituted in the early postoperative period is to induce hypothermia to manage early postoperative stroke. Recently, Berger et al.[117] reported the case of a patient with a severe stroke syndrome who was treated with early moderate hypothermia but not thrombolysis. The authors used moderate hypothermia at 33°C for 72 h, followed by slow rewarming at a rate of 0.10°C per hour. Spontaneous recanalization occurred 3 days after stroke onset, and diffusion-weighted MRI showed significant reduction of the lesion. Further studies are required to establish whether induced moderate hypothermia results in improved functional recovery after perioperative stroke in cardiac surgical patients.

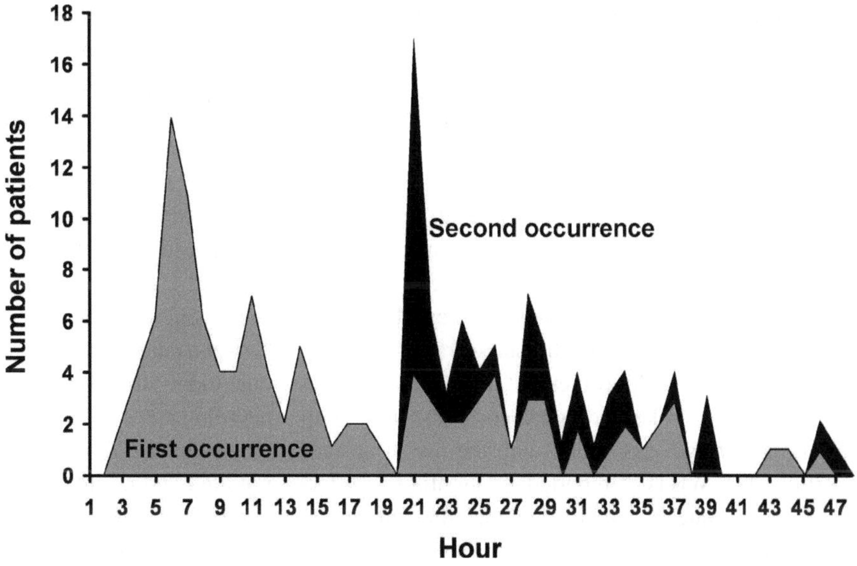

Fig. 13.6 Postoperative hyperthermia (Reprinted with permission of the Anesth Analg[113])

13.3.10 Treating Hyperthermia

It is best to take a multimodal approach to treating hyperthermia. The same techniques that are used to induce hypothermia can be applied to treat hyperthermia. In addition to the previously mentioned cooling blankets and endovascular cooling devices, other techniques may include the use of cooling caps or helmets, cold-water immersion, and additional invasive cooling techniques using nasogastric and rectal lavage, cold peritoneal lavage, CPB, ice water nasal lavage, cold carotid infusions, and single carotid artery perfusion with extracorporeal cooled blood.[118]

13.4 Studies of Temperature and Neuroprotection

13.4.1 Clinical Studies Assessing the Effect of Temperature on Neurologic Outcome in Cardiac Surgery

During the past 20 years, a significant number of prospective randomized clinical studies have assessed the effect of hypothermic versus normothermic CPB on neurologic outcome in cardiac surgery (Table 13.1). Conflicting and inconclusive results have been reported, mainly related to (1) differences in the patient population studied; (2) a wide range of temperature values used in cold, tepid, and warm groups; (3) various sites used for recording the temperature values; (4) differences in CPB techniques; (5) different temperature regimens used at critical CPB time points; (6) different myocardial protective techniques and surgical techniques; (7) different rates of rewarming; (8) different regimens for glucose control; and (9) lack of adequate postoperative control of hyperthermia.

Only two large, multicenter, randomized clinical trials[63,64] enrolled sufficient numbers of patients to provide adequate power to identify the stroke rate during the post-CABG period. Martin et al.[63] found a significant increase in the stroke rate in the normothermic group and no advantages associated with the use of normothermia. The WHTG[64] reported no significant differences in the rate of stroke or myocardial infarction. The difference in patient population enrolled in these studies – older and sicker patients in the first study versus younger and healthier in the second study – alone could explain these conflicting results. In addition, the WHTG used a wider range of temperature for the cold and warm groups. Whereas Martin et al.[63] actively cooled or rewarmed their patients to 28°C and 35°C, respectively, the WHTG allowed the temperatures of their subjects in the warm group to drift as low as 33°C. Thus, a greater variability in the $CMRo_2$ and CBF could have potentially occurred during the most physiologically critical periods of CPB, affecting the brain vulnerability and response to embolic and ischemic events. Moreover, plasma glucose levels varied significantly between the warm and cold groups in the study by Martin et al.[63] Higher glucose levels were achieved in the normothermic patients as a result of the use of continuous, dextrose-rich, warm, retrograde, blood cardioplegia in this particular group. Similarly high glucose levels were reported in both groups in the WHTG study, in which myocardial protection was achieved with cardioplegic solutions similar to those used by Martin et al. Finally, neither study provided information on postoperative temperature management. Postoperative hyperthermia is a common occurrence during the first 48 h after cardiac surgery, and it could have had a significant impact on the rate of adverse neurologic events.[96,113]

Four other smaller, randomized, controlled trials[22,54,119,120] involving a total 769 patients did not have sufficient power to demonstrate the beneficial effect of hypothermia on postoperative neurologic and neurocognitive function. Mora et al.,[66] in a subset of 138 patients from Martin et al.'s study, found that adverse neurologic outcomes occurred in 68 patients in the normothermic group and in none of the patients in the hypothermic group. The authors reported that the patients in the normothermic group were older, had a higher incidence of preexisting cerebrovascular disease, and had significantly higher blood glucose levels, which could potentially have influenced the results.

The use of tepid or mild hypothermia has also been tested in 4 studies[121–124] involving a total of 758 patients. Three out of four studies reported no relationship between temperature and neurologic outcome, whereas one study[122] found a trend toward an increase in adverse neurologic events in the cold group. Variables such as blood glucose levels and rate of rewarming were not reported and might have contributed to the confounding of the results. In addition, no information about the postoperative temperature management was provided.

Table 13.1 Temperature regimens and CNS outcomes in clinical studies

Investigator	Patients, no.	Study design	CPB temperatures	Temperature site	Glucose	Rewarming rate	Outcomes	
							Neurologic events	*Cognitive dysfunction*
Warm Heart Investigators[64]	1,732	Randomized (cold, warm)	Cold 25–30 °C Warm 33–37 °C	In-line venous	Not controlled	NR	NS	NI
McLean[120]	201	Randomized (cold, warm)	Cold ≤ 28 °C Warm > 34 °C	Nasopharyngeal	NR	NR	No relationship to temperature	No relationship to temperature
Martin[63]	1,001	Randomized[a]	28 °C, 35 °C	Nasopharyngeal	NR	NR	Higher in warm group	No relationship to temperature
Engelman[123]	51	Randomized (cold, tepid, warm)	20 °C, 32 °C, 37 °C	Nasopharyngeal Rectal	NR	NR	No relationship to temperature	NI
Engelman[122]	116	Randomized (cold, tepid, warm)	20 °C, 32 °C, 37 °C	Nasopharyngeal Rectal	NR	NR	Trend toward higher incidence in cold group	NI
Mora[66]	138	Randomized (cold/warm)	28 °C, 35 °C	Nasopharyngeal	Not controlled	NR	Higher in warm group	No relationship to temperature
Regragui[127]	96	Randomized (cold, tepid, warm)	28 °C, 32 °C, 37 °C	Nasopharyngeal	NR	Controlled	No relationship to temperature	Higher in warm group
Plourde[126]	62	Randomized (cold, warm)	28 °C, 36 °C	Nasopharyngeal	Controlled	NR	NI	No relationship to temperature
Heyer[119]	99	Randomized (cold/warm)	28 °C, 34 °C	Nasopharyngeal	NR	NR	No relationship to temperature	No relationship to temperature
Birdi[121]	300	Randomized (hypothermia, moderate hypothermia, normothermia)	20 °C, 32 °C, 37 °C	Nasopharyngeal	NR	Controlled	No relationship to temperature	NI
Engelman[124]	291	Randomized (cold, tepid, warm)	20 °C, 32 °C, 37 °C	N/A	NR	Controlled	No relationship to temperature	No relationship to temperature
Grigore[54]	300	Randomized (hypothermic, normothermic)	Hypothermic 28–30 °C Normothermic 35.5–36.5 °C	Nasopharyngeal	NR	Controlled	No relationship to temperature	No relationship to temperature

(continued)

Table 13.1 (continued)

Investigator	Patients, no.	Study design	CPB temperatures	Temperature site	Glucose	Rewarming rate	Outcomes	
							Neurologic events	*Cognitive dysfunction*
Nathan[55]	223	Randomized (all patients cooled to 32 °C)	Rewarmed to 34 °C Rewarmed to 37 °C	Nasopharyngeal	NR	NR	NI	Higher in warm group at 1 week and 3 months
Nathan[22]	223	Randomized (all patients cooled to 32 °C)	Rewarmed to 34 °C Rewarmed to 37 °C	Nasopharyngeal	NR	NR	NI	NS at 5 years
Boodhwani[18]	169	Randomized (hypothermic, normothermic)	Hypothermic 34 °C Normothermic 37 °C	Nasopharyngeal	NR	NR	No relationship to temperature	No relationship to temperature

[a]Systemic normothermia with continuous warm blood cardioplegia versus systemic hypothermia with intermittent cold crystalloid cardioplegia

NR refers to not reported; NI, not investigated; NS, not significant

A meta-analysis investigating the effect of hypothermia during CPB on neurologic and neurocognitive outcomes was recently published by Rees et al.[125] The authors reported an overall nonsignificant trend toward reduction of post-CABG strokes. This result was offset by a higher incidence of low-output syndrome in the hypothermic group and a trend toward a higher perioperative mortality and myocardial damage in the hypothermic group. The authors did not find a difference in the rate of overall adverse outcomes (stroke, perioperative death, myocardial infarction, low-output syndrome, or use of an intra-aortic balloon pump).

Controversy continues about whether the use of hypothermia preserves cognitive function after cardiac surgery. Most studies have shown no benefit with the use of hypothermic CPB in this regard.[54,120,124,126] Although Regragui et al.[127] showed better cognitive outcomes with the use of tepid CPB (32°C), as compared with the use of warm CPB (37°C), the use of cold CPB (28°C) did not yield any additional benefits. Additionally, a recent landmark study by Nathan et al.[55] found that patients who were separated from CPB at 34°C versus 37°C performed better on neurocognitive tests 1 week and 3 months after CABG surgery. However, a more recent study by the same group of investigators found that, in the absence of rewarming and cerebral hyperthermia, sustained mild hypothermia did not improve cognitive outcome.[18] These controversial results might have been influenced by the use of different rates of rewarming or no rewarming. The rate of rewarming is known to have an impact on postoperative cognitive performance, particularly in elderly and diabetic patients.[53,128] Grocott et al.[96] reported worsened neurocognitive outcomes in the setting of postoperative hyperthermia. Unreported and uncontrolled temperature regimens during the first 48 h after surgery might have played a significant role in the confounding reported results.

13.4.2 Recommendations for Perioperative Temperature Management

Thus, despite the numerous clinical trials that have been conducted on temperature and neurologic outcome, we can conclude only that hypothermia might provide additional neurologic protection and reduce the rate of strokes, an effect that is offset by an increase in perioperative mortality and myocardial damage. We cannot draw any conclusions about the effect of mild hypothermic or tepid CPB on brain function, nor can we form conclusions about the relationship between temperature and postoperative neurocognitive performance.

The well-known and well-demonstrated physiologic and pathophysiologic neuroprotective effects of hypothermia on ischemic brain insult, as well as clinically proven hypothermic neuroprotection in stroke, neurosurgical, and cardiac-arrest patient populations, are not obvious in the clinical settings of CPB. Such a noteworthy discrepancy can only be clarified by conducting large, randomized, prospective, national trials that are well controlled for all of the previously mentioned variables and, perhaps, that involve tepid CPB.

Our current perioperative recommendations for temperature management in cardiac operations include (1) monitoring nasopharyngeal and arterial inflow temperatures; (2) maintaining mild hypothermia (34–35°C), particularly in patients at high risk for developing a CNS injury, as has been previously described; (3) rewarming the patient slowly; (4) avoiding cerebral hyperthermia; (5) considering weaning from CPB at (34–35°C), particularly in high-risk patients; and (6) avoiding postoperative hyperthermia.

Acknowledgment The authors thank Mrs. Catherine Friederich Murray and Mr. Steve Palmer for their help with the preparation of this manuscript.

References

1. Cottrell JE, Smith DS. *Anesthesia and Neurosurgery*. 4th ed. St. Louis: Mosby; 2001.
2. Michenfelder JD, Milde JH. The relationship among canine brain temperature, metabolism, and function during hypothermia. *Anesthesiology*. 1991;75:130-136.
3. Klementavicius R, Nemoto EM, Yonas H. The Q10 ratio for basal cerebral metabolic rate for oxygen in rats. *J Neurosurg*. 1996;85:482-487.
4. Hoffman WE, Albrecht RF, Miletich DJ. Regional cerebral blood flow changes during hypothermia. *Cryobiology*. 1982;19:640-645.
5. Govier AV, Reves JG, McKay RD, et al. Factors and their influence on regional cerebral blood flow during nonpulsatile cardiopulmonary bypass. *Ann Thorac Surg*. 1984;38: 592-600.
6. Schwartz AE, Sandhu AA, Kaplon RJ, et al. Cerebral blood flow is determined by arterial pressure and not cardiopulmonary bypass flow rate. *Ann Thorac Surg*. 1995;60:165-169.

7. Woodcock TE, Murkin JM, Farrar JK, Tweed WA, Guiraudon GM, McKenzie FN. Pharmacologic EEG suppression during cardiopulmonary bypass: cerebral hemodynamic and metabolic effects of thiopental or isoflurane during hypothermia and normothermia. *Anesthesiology*. 1987;67:218-224.
8. Dreyer WJ, Phillips SC, Lindsey ML, et al. Interleukin 6 induction in the canine myocardium after cardiopulmonary bypass. *J Thorac Cardiovasc Surg*. 2000;120:256-263.
9. Qing M, Vazquez-Jimenez JF, Klosterhalfen B, et al. Influence of temperature during cardiopulmonary bypass on leukocyte activation, cytokine balance, and post-operative organ damage. *Shock*. 2001;15:372-377.
10. Vazquez-Jimenez JF, Qing M, Hermanns B, et al. Moderate hypothermia during cardiopulmonary bypass reduces myocardial cell damage and myocardial cell death related to cardiac surgery. *J Am Coll Cardiol*. 2001;38:1216-1223.
11. Frangogiannis NG, Mendoza LH, Lindsey ML, et al. IL-10 is induced in the reperfused myocardium and may modulate the reaction to injury. *J Immunol*. 2000;165:2798-2808.
12. Meldrum DR, Meng X, Dinarello CA, et al. Human myocardial tissue TNFalpha expression following acute global ischemia in vivo. *J Mol Cell Cardiol*. 1998;30:1683-1689.
13. Selnes OA, Goldsborough MA, Borowicz LM, McKhann GM. Neurobehavioural sequelae of cardiopulmonary bypass. *Lancet*. 1999;353:1601-1616.
14. Newman MF, Mathew JP, Grocott HP, et al. Central nervous system injury associated with cardiac surgery. *Lancet*. 2006;368:694-703.
15. Newman MF, Kirchner JL, Phillips-Bute B, et al. Longitudinal assessment of neurocognitive function after coronary-artery bypass surgery. *N Engl J Med*. 2001;344:395-402.
16. Silbert BS, Scott DA, Evered LA, et al. A comparison of the effect of high- and low-dose fentanyl on the incidence of postoperative cognitive dysfunction after coronary artery bypass surgery in the elderly. *Anesthesiology*. 2006;104:1137-1145.
17. Jensen BO, Hughes P, Rasmussen LS, Pedersen PU, Steinbruchel DA. Cognitive outcomes in elderly high-risk patients after off-pump versus conventional coronary artery bypass grafting: a randomized trial. *Circulation*. 2006;113:2790-2795.
18. Boodhwani M, Rubens F, Wozny D, Rodriguez R, Nathan HJ. Effects of sustained mild hypothermia on neurocognitive function after coronary artery bypass surgery: a randomized, double-blind study. *J Thorac Cardiovasc Surg*. 2007;134:1443-1450.
19. Djaiani G, Fedorko L, Borger MA, et al. Continuous-flow cell saver reduces cognitive decline in elderly patients after coronary bypass surgery. *Circulation*. 2007;116:1888-1895.
20. Rubens FD, Boodhwani M, Mesana T, Wozny D, Wells G, Nathan HJ. The cardiotomy trial: a randomized, double-blind study to assess the effect of processing of shed blood during cardiopulmonary bypass on transfusion and neurocognitive function. *Circulation*. 2007;116:I89-I97.
21. Selnes OA, Royall RM, Grega MA, Borowicz LM Jr, Quaskey S, McKhann GM. Cognitive changes 5 years after coronary artery bypass grafting: is there evidence of late decline? *Arch Neurol*. 2001;58:598-604.
22. Nathan HJ, Rodriguez R, Wozny D, et al. Neuroprotective effect of mild hypothermia in patients undergoing coronary artery surgery with cardiopulmonary bypass: five-year follow-up of a randomized trial. *J Thorac Cardiovasc Surg*. 2007;133:1206-1211.
23. Bokesch PM, Izykenova GA, Justice JB, Easley KA, Dambinova SA. NMDA receptor antibodies predict adverse neurological outcome after cardiac surgery in high-risk patients. *Stroke*. 2006;37:1432-1436.
24. Bucerius J, Gummert JF, Borger MA, et al. Predictors of delirium after cardiac surgery delirium: effect of beating-heart (off-pump) surgery. *J Thorac Cardiovasc Surg*. 2004;127:57-64.
25. Djaiani G, Fedorko L, Borger M, et al. Mild to moderate atheromatous disease of the thoracic aorta and new ischemic brain lesions after conventional coronary artery bypass graft surgery. *Stroke*. 2004;35:e356-e358.
26. McKhann GM, Grega MA, Borowicz LM, et al. Encephalopathy and stroke after coronary artery bypass grafting. *Arch Neurol*. 2002;59:1422-1428.
27. Borger MA, Ivanov J, Weisel RD, Rao V, Peniston CM. Stroke during coronary bypass surgery: principal role of cerebral macroemboli. *Eur J Cardiothorac Surg*. 2001;19:627-632.
28. Nussmeier NA. A review of risk factors for adverse neurologic outcome after cardiac surgery. *J Extra Corpor Technol*. 2002;34:4-10.
29. Bucerius J, Gummert JF, Borger MA, et al. Stroke after cardiac surgery: a risk factor analysis of 16, 184 consecutive adult patients. *Ann Thorac Surg*. 2003;75:472-478.
30. Karkouti K, Djaiani G, Borger M, et al. Low hematocrit during cardiopulmonary bypass is associated with increased risk of perioperative stroke in cardiac surgery. *Ann Thorac Surg*. 2005;80:1381-1387.
31. McKhann GM, Grega MA, Borowicz LM Jr, Baumgartner WA, Selnes OA. Stroke and encephalopathy after cardiac surgery: an update. *Stroke*. 2006;37:562-571.
32. Selim M. Perioperative stroke. *N Engl J Med*. 2007;356:706-713.
33. Choudhary SK, Bhan A, Sharma R, et al. Aortic atherosclerosis and perioperative stroke in patients undergoing coronary artery bypass: role of intra-operative transesophageal echocardiography. *Int J Cardiol*. 1997;61:31-38.
34. Newman MF, Wolman R, Kanchuger M, et al. Multicenter preoperative stroke risk index for patients undergoing coronary artery bypass graft surgery. *Circulation*. 1996;94(Suppl II):II-74-II-80.
35. Roach GW, Kanchuger M, Mangano CM, et al. Adverse cerebral outcomes after coronary bypass surgery. Multicenter Study of Perioperative Ischemia Research Group and the Ischemia Research and Education Foundation Investigators. *New Engl J Med*. 1996;335:1857-1863.
36. McKhann GM, Goldsborough MA, Borowicz LM Jr, et al. Predictors of stroke risk in coronary artery bypass patients. *Ann Thorac Surg*. 1997;63:516-521.
37. Borger MA, Ivanov J, Weisel RD, et al. Decreasing incidence of stroke during valvular surgery. *Circulation*. 1998;98:II137-II143.
38. Hogue CW Jr, Murphy SF, Schechtman KB, Davila-Roman VG. Risk factors for early or delayed stroke after cardiac surgery. *Circulation*. 1999;100:642-647.
39. Puskas F, Grocott HP, White WD, Mathew JP, Newman MF, Bar-Yosef S. Intraoperative hyperglycemia and cognitive decline after CABG. *Ann Thorac Surg*. 2007;84:1467-1473.

40. Goto T, Baba T, Honma K, et al. Magnetic resonance imaging findings and postoperative neurologic dysfunction in elderly patients undergoing coronary artery bypass grafting. *Ann Thorac Surg*. 2001;72:137-142.
41. Davila-Roman VG, Barzilai B, Wareing TH, Murphy SF, Schechtman KB, Kouchoukos NT. Atherosclerosis of the ascending aorta: prevalence and role as an independent predictor of cerebrovascular events in cardiac patients. *Stroke*. 1994;25:2010-2016.
42. van der Linden J, Hadjinikolaou L, Bergman P, Lindblom D. Postoperative stroke in cardiac surgery is related to the location and extent of atherosclerotic disease in the ascending aorta. *J Am Coll Cardiol*. 2001;38:131-135.
43. Djaiani G. Aortic arch atheroma: stroke reduction in cardiac surgical patients. *Semin Cardiothorac Vasc Anesth*. 2006;10: 143-157.
44. Bainbridge D. Aortic assessment for cardiac surgical procedures. *Semin Cardiothorac Vasc Anesth*. 2006;10:158-161.
45. Hogue CW Jr, Selnes OL, McKhann GM. Should all patients undergoing cardiac surgery have preoperative psychometric testing: a brain stress test? *Anesth Analg*. 2007; 104:1012-1014.
46. Filsoufi F, Rahmanian PB, Castillo JG, Bronster D, Adams DH. Incidence, topography, predictors and long-term survival after stroke in patients undergoing coronary artery bypass grafting. *Ann Thorac Surg*. 2008;85:862-871.
47. Grocott HP, White WD, Morris RW, et al. Genetic polymorphisms and the risk of stroke after cardiac surgery. *Stroke*. 2005;36:1854-1858.
48. Mathew JP, Podgoreanu MV, Grocott HP, et al. Genetic variants in P-selectin and C-reactive protein influence susceptibility to cognitive decline after cardiac surgery. *J Am Coll Cardiol*. 2007;49:1934-1942.
49. Ozatik MA, Gol MK, Fansa I, et al. Risk factors for stroke following coronary artery bypass operations. *J Card Surg*. 2005;20:52-57.
50. Hammon JW, Stump DA, Butterworth JF, et al. Single cross-clamp improves 6 month cognitive outcome in high-risk coronary bypass patients: the effect of reduced aortic manipulation. *J Thorac Cardiovasc Surg*. 2006;131:114-121.
51. Zingone B, Rauber E, Gatti G, et al. The impact of epiaortic ultrasonographic scanning on the risk of perioperative stroke. *Eur J Cardiothorac Surg*. 2006;29:720-728.
52. Boodhwani M, Rubens FD, Wozny D, et al. Predictors of early neurocognitive deficits in low-risk patients undergoing on-pump coronary artery bypass surgery. *Circulation*. 2006;114:I461-I466.
53. Grigore AM, Grocott HP, Mathew JP, et al. The rewarming rate and increased peak temperature alter neurocognitive outcome after cardiac surgery. *Anesth Analg*. 2002;94:4-10.
54. Grigore AM, Mathew J, Grocott HP, et al. Prospective randomized trial of normothermic versus hypothermic cardiopulmonary bypass on cognitive function after coronary artery bypass graft surgery. *Anesthesiology*. 2001;95:1110-1119.
55. Nathan HJ, Wells GA, Munson JL, Wozny D. Neuroprotective effect of mild hypothermia in patients undergoing coronary artery surgery with cardiopulmonary bypass: a randomized trial. *Circulation*. 2001;104:I85-I91.
56. Libman RB, Wirkowski E, Neystat M, Barr W, Gelb S, Graver M. Stroke associated with cardiac surgery: determinants, timing, and stroke subtypes. *Arch Neurol*. 1997;54:83-87.
57. Likosky DS, Leavitt BJ, Marrin CA, et al. Intra- and postoperative predictors of stroke after coronary artery bypass grafting. *Ann Thorac Surg*. 2003;76:428-434.
58. Likosky DS, Marrin CA, Caplan LR, et al. Determination of etiologic mechanisms of strokes secondary to coronary artery bypass graft surgery. *Stroke*. 2003;34:2830-2834.
59. Boivie P, Edstrom C, Engstrom KG. Side differences in cerebrovascular accidents after cardiac surgery: a statistical analysis of neurologic symptoms and possible implications for anatomic mechanisms of aortic particle embolization. *J Thorac Cardiovasc Surg*. 2005;129:591-598.
60. Ritzl A, Meisel S, Wittsack HJ, et al. Development of brain infarct volume as assessed by magnetic resonance imaging (MRI): follow-up of diffusion-weighted MRI lesions. *J Magn Reson Imaging*. 2004;20:201-207.
61. Paparella D, Galeone A, Venneri MT, et al. Activation of the coagulation system during coronary artery bypass grafting: comparison between on-pump and off-pump techniques. *J Thorac Cardiovasc Surg*. 2006;131:290-297.
62. Frank SM, Fleisher LA, Breslow MJ, et al. Perioperative maintenance of normothermia reduces the incidence of morbid cardiac events: a randomized clinical trial. *Jama*. 1997;277:1127-1134.
63. Martin TD, Craver JM, Gott JP, et al. Prospective, randomized trial of retrograde warm blood cardioplegia: myocardial benefit and neurologic threat. *Ann Thorac Surg*. 1994;57:298-302.
64. The Warm Heart Trials Group. Normothermic vs hypothermic blood cardioplegia for coronary bypass surgery: a randomized trial in 1732 patients. *Lancet*. 1994;343:559-563.
65. Ali MS, Harmer M, Vaughan RS, et al. Changes in cerebral oxygenation during cold (28 degrees C) and warm (34 degrees C) cardiopulmonary bypass using different blood gas strategies (alpha-stat and pH-stat) in patients undergoing coronary artery bypass graft surgery. *Acta Anaesthesiol Scand*. 2004;48:837-844.
66. Mora CT, Henson MB, Weintraub WS, et al. The effect of temperature management during cardiopulmonary bypass on neurologic and neuropsychologic outcomes in patients undergoing coronary revascularization. *J Thorac Cardiovasc Surg*. 1996;112:514-522.
67. Ginsberg MD, Busto R. Combating hyperthermia in acute stroke: a significant clinical concern. *Stroke*. 1998;29:529-534.
68. Polderman KH. Keeping a cool head: how to induce and maintain hypothermia. *Crit Care Med*. 2004;32:2558-2560.
69. Polderman KH. Application of therapeutic hypothermia in the ICU: opportunities and pitfalls of a promising treatment modality. Part I: Indications and evidence. *Intensive Care Med*. 2004;30:556.
70. Azzimondi G, Bassein L, Nonino F, et al. Fever in acute stroke worsens prognosis. A prospective study. *Stroke*. 1995;26:2040-2043.
71. Wang Y, Lim LL, Levi C, Heller RF, Fisher J. Influence of admission body temperature on stroke mortality. *Stroke*. 2000;31:404-409.
72. Reith J, Jorgensen HS, Pedersen PM, et al. Body temperature in acute stroke: relation to stroke severity, infarct size, mortality, and outcome. *Lancet*. 1996;347:422-425.
73. Kammersgaard LP, Jorgensen HS, Rungby JA, et al. Admission body temperature predicts long-term mortality after acute stroke: the Copenhagen Stroke Study. *Stroke*. 2002;33:1759-1762.

74. Kasner SE, Wein T, Piriyawat P, et al. Acetaminophen for altering body temperature in acute stroke: a randomized clinical trial. *Stroke*. 2002;33:130-134.
75. Mayer SA, Kowalski RG, Presciutti M, et al. Clinical trial of a novel surface cooling system for fever control in neurocritical care patients. *Crit Care Med*. 2004;32:2508-2515.
76. Shann KG, Likosky DS, Murkin JM, et al. An evidence-based review of the practice of cardiopulmonary bypass in adults: a focus on neurologic injury, glycemic control, hemodilution, and the inflammatory response. *J Thorac Cardiovasc Surg*. 2006;132:283-290.
77. Hogue CW Jr, Palin CA, Arrowsmith JE. Cardiopulmonary bypass management and neurologic outcomes: an evidence-based appraisal of current practices. *Anesth Analg*. 2006; 103:21-37.
78. Prakash O, Jonson B, Bos E, Meij S, Hugenholtz PG, Hekman W. Cardiorespiratory and metabolic effects of profound hypothermia. *Crit Care Med*. 1978;6:340-346.
79. Berger C, Schabitz WR, Georgiadis D, Steiner T, Aschoff A, Schwab S. Effects of hypothermia on excitatory amino acids and metabolism in stroke patients: a microdialysis study. *Stroke*. 2002;33:519-524.
80. Berger C, Schabitz WR, Wolf M, Mueller H, Sommer C, Schwab S. Hypothermia and brain-derived neurotrophic factor reduce glutamate synergistically in acute stroke. *Exp Neurol*. 2004;185:305-312.
81. Fischer S, Renz D, Wiesnet M, Schaper W, Karliczek GF. Hypothermia abolishes hypoxia-induced hyperpermeability in brain microvessel endothelial cells. *Brain Res Mol Brain Res*. 1999;74:135-144.
82. Huet O, Kinirons B, Dupic L, et al. Induced mild hypothermia reduces mortality during acute inflammation in rats. *Acta Anaesthesiol Scand*. 2007;51:1211-1216.
83. Kimura A, Sakurada S, Ohkuni H, Todome Y, Kurata K. Moderate hypothermia delays proinflammatory cytokine production of human peripheral blood mononuclear cells. *Crit Care Med*. 2002;30:1499-1502.
84. Xu L, Yenari MA, Steinberg GK, Giffard RG. Mild hypothermia reduces apoptosis of mouse neurons in vitro early in the cascade. *J Cereb Blood Flow Metab*. 2002;22:21-28.
85. Zhao H, Wang JQ, Shimohata T, et al. Conditions of protection by hypothermia and effects on apoptotic pathways in a rat model of permanent middle cerebral artery occlusion. *J Neurosurg*. 2007;107:636-641.
86. Kovesdi E, Czeiter E, Tamas A, et al. Rescuing neurons and glia: is inhibition of apoptosis useful? *Prog Brain Res*. 2007;161:81-95.
87. Bernard SA, Gray TW, Buist MD, et al. Treatment of comatose survivors of out-of-hospital cardiac arrest with induced hypothermia. *N Engl J Med*. 2002;346:557-563.
88. Hypothermia After Cardiac Arrest Study Group. Mild therapeutic hypothermia to improve the neurologic outcome after cardiac arrest. *N Engl J Med*. 2002;346:549-556.
89. Bernard SA, Buist MD. Induced hypothermia in critical care medicine: a review. *Crit Care Med*. 2003;31:2041-2051.
90. Marion DW. Controlled normothermia in neurologic intensive care. *Crit Care Med*. 2004;32:S43-S45.
91. Polderman KH. Application of therapeutic hypothermia in the intensive care unit: opportunities and pitfalls of a promising treatment modality. Part 2: Practical aspects and side effects. *Intensive Care Med*. 2004;30:757-769.
92. Polderman KH, Ely EW, Badr AE, Girbes AR. Induced hypothermia in traumatic brain injury: considering the conflicting results of meta-analyses and moving forward. *Intensive Care Med*. 2004;30:1860-1864.
93. Crowder CM, Tempelhoff R, Theard MA, Cheng MA, Todorov A, Dacey RG Jr. Jugular bulb temperature: comparison with brain surface and core temperatures in neurosurgical patients during mild hypothermia. *J Neurosurg*. 1996;85:98-103.
94. Nussmeier NA, Cheng W, Marino M, et al. Temperature during cardiopulmonary bypass: the discrepancies between monitored sites. *Anesth Analg*. 2006;103:1373-1379.
95. Nathan HJ, Lavallee G. The management of temperature during hypothermic cardiopulmonary bypass: I. Canadian survey. *Can J Anaesth*. 1995;42:669-671.
96. Grocott HP, Mackensen GB, Grigore AM, et al. Postoperative hyperthermia is associated with cognitive dysfunction after coronary artery bypass graft surgery. *Stroke*. 2002;33:537-541.
97. Safar P. Mild hypothermia in resuscitation: a historical perspective. *Ann Emerg Med*. 2003;41:887-888. author reply 8.
98. Safar PJ, Kochanek PM. Therapeutic hypothermia after cardiac arrest. *N Engl J Med*. 2002;346:612-613.
99. Wagner KR, Zuccarello M. Local brain hypothermia for neuroprotection in stroke treatment and aneurysm repair. *Neurol Res*. 2005;27:238-245.
100. Bigelow WG, Lindsay WK, Greenwood WF. Hypothermia; its possible role in cardiac surgery: an investigation of factors governing survival in dogs at low body temperatures. *Ann Surg*. 1950;132:849-866.
101. Bigelow WG, Callaghan JC, Hopps JA. General hypothermia for experimental intracardiac surgery; the use of electrophrenic respirations, an artificial pacemaker for cardiac standstill and radio-frequency rewarming in general hypothermia. *Ann Surg*. 1950;132:531-539.
102. Bigelow WG, Callaghan JC, Hopps JA. General hypothermia for experimental intracardiac surgery; the use of electrophrenic respirations, an artificial pacemaker for cardiac standstill, and radio-frequency rewarming in general hypothermia. *Trans Meet Am Surg Assoc*. 1950;68: 211-219.
103. Simpson RE, Walter GA, Phillis JW. The effects of hypothermia on amino acid neurotransmitter release from the cerebral cortex. *Neurosci Lett*. 1991;124:83-86.
104. Sano T, Drummond JC, Patel PM, Grafe MR, Watson JC, Cole DJ. A comparison of the cerebral protective effects of isoflurane and mild hypothermia in a model of incomplete forebrain ischemia in the rat. *Anesthesiology*. 1992;76: 221-228.
105. Griepp RB, Ergin MA, McCullough JN, et al. Use of hypothermic circulatory arrest for cerebral protection during aortic surgery. *J Card Surg*. 1997;12:312-321.
106. McCullough JN, Zhang N, Reich DL, et al. Cerebral metabolic suppression during hypothermic circulatory arrest in humans. *Ann Thorac Surg*. 1999;67:1895-1899. discussion 919-21.
107. Kawahara F, Kadoi Y, Saito S, Goto F, Fujita N. Slow rewarming improves jugular venous oxygen saturation during rewarming. *Acta Anaesthesiol Scand*. 2003; 47:419-424.

108. Alzaga AG, Cerdan M, Varon J. Therapeutic hypothermia. *Resuscitation*. 2006;70:369-380.
109. Bigelow WG, McBirnie JE. Further experiences with hypothermia for intracardiac surgery in monkeys and groundhogs. *Ann Surg*. 1953;137:361-365.
110. Benson DW, Williams GR Jr, Spencer FC, Yates AJ. The use of hypothermia after cardiac arrest. *Anesth Analg*. 1959;38:423-428.
111. Nolan JP, Morley PT, Hoek TL, Hickey RW. Therapeutic hypothermia after cardiac arrest. An advisory statement by the Advancement Life support Task Force of the International Liaison committee on Resuscitation. *Resuscitation*. 2003;57:231-235.
112. Nathan HJ, Parlea L, Dupuis JY, et al. Safety of deliberate intraoperative and postoperative hypothermia for patients undergoing coronary artery surgery: a randomized trial. *J Thorac Cardiovasc Surg*. 2004;127:1270-1275.
113. Thong WY, Strickler AG, Li S, et al. Hyperthermia in the forty-eight hours after cardiopulmonary bypass. *Anesth Analg*. 2002;95:1489-1495.
114. Bar-Yosef S, Mathew JP, Newman MF, Landolfo KP, Grocott HP. Prevention of cerebral hyperthermia during cardiac surgery by limiting on-bypass rewarming in combination with post-bypass body surface warming: a feasibility study. *Anesth Analg*. 2004;99:641-646.
115. Fukuda I, Imazuru T, Osaka M, Watanabe K, Meguro K, Wada M. Thrombolytic therapy for delayed, in-hospital stroke after cardiac surgery. *Ann Thorac Surg*. 2003;76:1293-1295.
116. Moazami N, Smedira NG, McCarthy PM, et al. Safety and efficacy of intraarterial thrombolysis for perioperative stroke after cardiac operation. *Ann Thorac Surg*. 2001;72.1933-1937.
117. Berger C, Schramm P, Schwab S. Reduction of diffusion-weighted MRI lesion volume after early moderate hypothermia in ischemic stroke. *Stroke*. 2005;36:e56-e58.
118. Sterz F, Holzer M, Roine R, et al. Hypothermia after cardiac arrest: a treatment that works. *Curr Opin Crit Care*. 2003;9:205-210.
119. Heyer EJ, Adams DC, Delphin E, et al. Cerebral dysfunction after coronary artery bypass grafting done with mild or moderate hypothermia. *J Thorac Cardiovasc Surg*. 1997;114:270-277.
120. Mclean RF, Wong BI, Naylor CD, et al. Cardiopulmonary bypass, temperature, and central nervous system dysfunction. *Circulation*. 1994;90:250-255.
121. Birdi I, Regragui I, Izzat MB, Bryan AJ, Angelini GD. Influence of normothermic systemic perfusion during coronary artery bypass operations: a randomized prospective study. *J Thorac Cardiovasc Surg*. 1997;114:475-481.
122. Engelman RM, Pleet AB, Rousou JA, et al. What is the best perfusion temperature for coronary revascularization? *J Thorac Cardiovasc Surg*. 1996;112:1622-1632. discussion 32-3.
123. Engelman RM, Pleet AB, Rousou JA, et al. Does cardiopulmonary bypass temperature correlate with postoperative central nervous system dysfunction? *J Card Surg*. 1995;10:493-497.
124. Engelman RM, Pleet AB, Rousou JA, et al. Influence of cardiopulmonary bypass perfusion temperature on neurologic and hematologic function after coronary artery bypass grafting. *Ann Thorac Surg*. 1999;67:1547-1555. discussion 56.
125. Rees K, Beranek-Stanley M, Burke M, Ebrahim S. Hypothermia to reduce neurological damage following coronary artery bypass surgery. *Cochrane Database Syst Rev*. 2001:CD002138.
126. Plourde G, Leduc AS, Morin JE, et al. Temperature during cardiopulmonary bypass for coronary artery operations does not influence postoperative cognitive function: a prospective, randomized trial. *J Thorac Cardiovasc Surg*. 1997;114:123-128.
127. Regragui I, Birdi I, Izzat MB, et al. The effects of cardiopulmonary bypass temperature on neuropsychologic outcome after coronary artery operations: a prospective randomized trial. *J Thorac Cardiovasc Surg*. 1996;112:1036-1045.
128. Newman MF, Kramer D, Croughwell ND, et al. Differential age effects of mean arterial pressure and rewarming on cognitive dysfunction after cardiac surgery. *Anesth Analg*. 1995;81:236-242.

Studies of Nonpharmacological Interventions to Reduce Brain Injury

14

Aaron M. Ranasinghe and Timothy J. Jones

14.1 Introduction

Since the inception of cardiac surgery, the majority of operations have benefited from advances in anesthetic, surgical, and perfusion techniques to reduce both morbidity and mortality. Perhaps, one of the most feared complications for both patients and relatives following cardiac surgery is brain injury (BI). Following cardiac surgery, BI is not only associated with an increase in mortality, but also physical and mental disability as well as related emotional and financial consequences. These costs are not only borne by the patient, but place significant demands on relatives, carers, and healthcare systems. It has been estimated that the financial cost of stroke is between $90,000 and $228,000 over a patient's life.[1]

14.2 Definitions of Brain Injury Following Cardiac Surgery

BI is a spectrum of injury ranging from death and major physical impairment to subtle neuropsychological and mood changes. For ease of categorization, brain injury has traditionally been divided into three categories[2]:

- Type I or focal BI
- Type II or global BI
- Neuropsychological deficit (NPD)

The spectrum of disorders that are categorized by type I and II BI are detailed in Table 14.1.[3] However, in the clinical setting, the picture of BI that the patient presents with is not as clear cut, and in reality, BI is not an easily classifiable entity with patients presenting with a combination of some or all of these features.

14.3 Incidence of Brain Injury Following Cardiac Surgery

There are a wide range of outcome measures that can be examined to look at BI following cardiac surgery; however, there is no single "gold standard" test that can elucidate as to whether a patient has BI. At present, there are two widely accepted clinical outcome measures relating BI

1. Type I injury or "stroke" – determined by neurological dysfunction on clinical examination and usually radiologically confirmed
2. Type II injury – determined by clinical assessment
3. NPD – determined by sophisticated postoperative neuropsychometric testing

The true incidence of BI following cardiac surgery is difficult to define. For patients undergoing coronary artery bypass graft surgery (CABG), the incidence of type I and II neurological deficits are quoted as being between 0.9% to 5.4%[3–5] and 3.0% to 10%, respectively.[3,6] Occurrence of either type I or II injury is associated with an increase in patient mortality tenfold for type I and fivefold for type II.[3]

The reported incidence of NPD following such surgery varies even more widely being reported as 28–79% in the immediate post-operative period[7,8] with an incidence of 19–57% persisting at 6 months following surgery.[9,10] The variability in reporting of BI is related to a number of factors.

A.M. Ranasinghe (✉)
Department of Cardiovascular Medicine,
University of Birmingham, Birmingham, UK
e-mail: a.m.ranasinghe@bham.ac.uk

R.S. Bonser et al. (eds.), *Brain Protection in Cardiac Surgery*,
DOI: 10.1007/978-1-84996-293-3_14, © Springer-Verlag London Limited 2011

Table 14.1 Type 1 and 2 neurological injuries

Type I neurological injury (focal)	Fatal injury
	Stroke
	Coma
	TIA
Type II neurological injury (global)	New deterioration intellectual function
	Confusion
	Agitation
	Disorientation
	Memory deficit
	Seizure without focal injury

Formal neurological examination following cardiac surgery is associated with a number of problems. Such an examination attempts to locate the site of the injury rather than quantifying it.[11] In the postoperative period, patients may not be physically fit enough to cooperate fully with a detailed neurological examination. In addition, patients who have had a complicated postoperative course with long periods of sedation and intensive care treatment will not be able to undergo formal examination and lesions may be missed at a later date. There is a 13% incidence of peripheral nerve lesions following CABG.[12] These relate mainly to traction injuries of the brachial plexus and tend to resolve in the short term,[13,14] but they still need to be differentiated from BI as they may well have an influence on the detection of type I BI. Visual examination is also mandatory for a complete examination in these patients as neuro-ophthalmological defects have been detected in up to 25% of patients following CPB.[15]

NPD requires a more subtle battery of tests to elicit its presence. The full battery of neuropsychometric (NP) tests available would be inappropriate for patients undergoing cardiac surgery as they take several hours to perform. To avoid mental exhaustion and nonparticipation, a battery of tests that check the main cognitive domains are employed. The international consensus on the extent and type of NP assessment considered optimal for the measurement of brain injury following CPB[16] has published guidelines. Appropriate tests and the domains they test are detailed in Table 14.2. The tests examine the cognitive domains of memory (verbal, visual, and general), sustained attention and concentration, executive functioning and fine motor skills. It is not possible to predict where CPB-related BI will occur and therefore which cognitive domains will be affected, the test battery is designed to examine as broad a range of functions as possible without being prohibitively time-consuming and tiring. This limited range of tests is unable to provide a fully comprehensive NP assessment (and is not intended to) but provides a tool with which it is possible to measure a change in performance between pre- and postintervention assessments.

The quoted incidence of NPD varies widely according to the timing of test, batteries of tests used, patient characteristics as well as the way in which the NPD is defined. Two commonly used definitions of NPD are a

Table 14.2 A typical battery of neuropsychometric tests and domains assessed by individual tests

Neuropsychometric test	Domain tested	Scores yielded
Folstein mini-mental status examination (MMSE)	General memory function	Total correct of possible 30
Trails making tests (A and B)	Attention and concentration	Time to completion (seconds)
Letter cancellation test (LCT)	Sustained concentration and attention	Time to completion and number of errors
Symbol digit modalities test (SDMT)	Sustained concentration and attention	Time to completion and number correct of possible 50
Grooved pegboard (GPB)	Manual dexterity and fine motor control	Time to completion – Dominant and nondominant hands
Finger tapping	Manual dexterity and fatigability	Time to completion – Dominant and nondominant hands
Rey auditory verbal learning test (RAVLT)	Immediate verbal memory and retention	Number recalled (15 words, 7 readings)
Nonverbal memory test (NVM)	Visual memory	Time to completion and number correct of possible 20

20% decline or a greater than one standard deviation decline in two or more tests. Both these are accepted methods for characterizing NPD following cardiac surgery.[17] The main problem with applying a single case definition such as this is the phenomenon of regression to the mean. This describes a statistical phenomenon in which extreme scores tend to become less extreme after repeated examinations (although a "real" change has not actually occurred). Therefore, those who score high to begin with may be seen as deteriorating and conversely those with low scores may be seen to improve even though there is no true difference. The precise interpretation of these deteriorations in NPD is unclear. However, this does not imply that measuring NPD following cardiac surgery is not of benefit. A one standard deviation drop in some tests can equate to the difference in performance between a 40- and a 60-year-old.[6]

14.4 Factors Predisposing to Brain Injury Post Cardiac Surgery

There are a number of factors that relate to the relative risk of patients suffering BI following cardiac surgery. Some factors predispose for the different categories of injury, type I, type II, and NPD although there is an obvious overlap between the groups. Risk factors can also be subdivided into those related to the patient, type of operation, and CPB protocols. These risk factors are[3,6,18]:

- Age
- Proximal aortic atheroma
- Diabetes
- Hypertension
- Use of IABP
- Unstable angina
- Pulmonary disease
- Excessive alcohol intake
- Baseline intellectual function
- Baseline functional status

14.5 Cerebral Physiology and Metabolism

At normothermia in an awake subject, the human brain receives approximately 14% of the cardiac output (750 mL min^{-1}); this accounts for approximately 20% of the total body oxygen consumption. However, during hypothermic CPB with an alpha stat regimen, the brain receives only 5–7% of cardiac output.

Cerebral blood flow (CBF) is maintained at a relatively constant rate by autoregulation. Total CBF is influenced by a number of factors. The process of autoregulation allows for CBF to be maintained at around 45–60 m1.100 g^{-1} brain tissue min^{-1}. This is in spite of variations in cerebral perfusion pressure (CPP), which is determined by mean arterial blood pressure minus intracranial pressure. Autoregulation is well maintained within the range of CPP of 50–150 mmHg. Outside of this range, this phenomenon is lost.

14.5.1 *Effects of Blood Gas and Temperature Management on Cerebral Vasculature*

Physiological variables such as pH, temperature, and hematocrit (all of which can be controlled during CPB) have important effects on cerebral perfusion.

Carbon dioxide (CO_2) is the main determinant of reactivity of the cerebral vasculature. Hypercapnia leads to vasodilatation and conversely hypocapnia leads to vasoconstriction. Management of CO_2 levels and therefore cerebral vascular reactivity while on CPB has been the subject of much research. The solubility of CO_2 is temperature dependent. Reductions in body temperature lead to increased solubility of CO_2 within the blood. Therefore, despite an unchanged total CO_2 level, the measured concentration of arterial carbon dioxide ($PaCO_2$) is reduced. At normothermia (37°C), normal acid–base balance is a pH of 7.40 with a $PaCO_2$ of 40 mmHg. There are two strategies during CPB for management of acid–base, pH stat, and alpha stat. In brief, pH stat involves maintaining $PaCO_2$ at 40 mmHg by addition of CO_2 as body temperature is reduced. During alpha stat management, nontemperature corrected blood gas management is employed. This allows for autoregulation to be maintained. With the use of pH stat management, autoregulation is lost and therefore changes in CPP relate directly to changes in CBF. The relative uses of these two methods of arterial blood gas management during CPB will be discussed in more detail later in this chapter.

The effect of temperature on the cerebral vasculature depends upon CO_2 management as detailed above. During episodes of deep hypothermia (15–20°C), autoregulation does not occur, regardless of acid–base management.

Management of hematocrit levels during CPB can lead to alterations in CBF. During cooling, the viscosity of blood increases and consequently CBF is reduced. This led to a vogue for hemodiluting patients undergoing cardiac surgery with profound hypothermia. However, animal studies have suggested that maintaining a higher hematocrit (30% vs. 10%) does not impair cerebral microcirculation and severe hemodilution leads to impaired cerebral oxygenation during the cooling phase of CPB.[19]

14.5.2 Cerebral Metabolism

Cerebral metabolic demand is the most important determinant of CBF. The relationship between the two is termed "flow metabolism coupling." Metabolic demand is determined by calculation of cerebral oxygen consumption ($CMRO_2$). As the brain has no oxygen stores, $CMRO_2$ is a true reflection of brain metabolic activity and can be calculated using the following equation (where a-jvD02 is the cerebral arteriovenous oxygen content difference):

$$CMRO_2 = CBF \times a - jvD02$$

CBF and $CMRO_2$ are not uniform throughout the brain and change with the metabolic demands placed on a region. During periods of CPB with alpha stat management, this relationship is preserved and as oxygen utilization increases so does CBF. However, with pH stat management, this relationship is lost.[20]

14.6 Intraoperative Monitoring of Brain Injury During Cardiac Surgery

There is currently no gold standard for assessing and measuring cerebral physiological variables during cardiac surgery. There are a number of techniques, which may be utilized. As with any method of monitoring, ideally these techniques need to be practical, noninvasive, and acceptable to both medical staff and the patients.

14.6.1 Noninvasive Methods

14.6.1.1 Transcranial Doppler

Transcranial Doppler (TCD) provides a measure of cerebral blood velocity. It may also be used to detect emboli. The TCD is placed over the temporal bone and focused on the middle cerebral artery. This enables for a quantitative assessment of cerebral perfusion. Changes in TCD velocity mirror changes in CBF but do not provide a direct measurement of CBF.[21] TCD is a continuous noninvasive, portable, and inexpensive tool. Interpretation of velocity and embolic signals does, however, require technical skill.

Using TCD in a randomized controlled study of 100 patients, those that received cardiac surgery with a 40-μm arterial line filter had a reduced incidence of NPD (8%) versus those that did not (27%).[22] In this study, Pugsley demonstrated not only a reduction in NPD but also a correlation between the number of emboli and the incidence of postoperative NPD. Patients with embolic counts of >1,000 had a 43% incidence of NPD compared with those with embolic counts of <200 who had an 8.6% incidence.

The type of information provided by TPD with regard to real-time episodes of embolization allows surgeons to modify and refine their individual techniques in attempts to reduce embolic load.

14.6.1.2 Echocardiography

Transesophageal echocardiography (TEE) has been used to both assess aortic atheroma and demonstrate embolic phenomenon during cardiac surgery. TEE is a useful monitoring tool and has been used to demonstrate the presence of gaseous emboli during and after CPB.[23–25] However, TEE is operator-dependent and, although in the UK its use is becoming more widespread, there still remain issues over TEE availability. The use of TEE is further limited by its relatively poorer ability to visualize the distal ascending aorta, which is the prime site for aortic cannulation and cross-clamp application. This area is also the most significantly affected by atherosclerosis.[26,27]

14.6.1.3 Epiaortic Ultrasound Scanning

Direct intra-operative scanning of the aorta during surgery allows for more accurate detection of aortic atheroma. It is noninvasive, portable reproducible, and easy to use.[28] Epiaortic ultrasound scanning has been demonstrated to be superior to digital palpation, which only detects between 50% and 70% of atherosclerotic plaques[29,30] and allows for modification of surgical technique to minimize plaque disruption. Furthermore, epiaortic ultrasound has an advantage over TEE because it is better able to visualize the distal ascending aorta and proximal aortic arch.

Zigone et al. in a consecutive cohort of over 2,000 patients demonstrated that epiaortic ultrasound influences change in surgical strategies when performed on a regular basis.[31] The most common changes included alteration in aortic cannulation and aortic cross-clamp sites. Furthermore, use of epiaortic scanning within this study either on a selected population or on all patients led to a reduction in stroke rate versus a consecutive historical cohort that had not undergone epiaortic scanning. Not performing epiaortic scanning and extracardiac arteriopathy was independently associated with an increased risk of early stroke.

14.6.1.4 Electroencephalogram

The electroencephalogram (EEG) represents electrical activity within the cerebral cortex. In noncardiac surgery, it has been demonstrated to be both a sensitive and specific means of detecting cerebral hypoperfusion and ischemia.[32–34]

Two studies have reported improvements in neurological outcomes associated with the use of EEG in cardiac surgery. The first of these reported improvements in postoperative NPD (reduced from 44% to 5%) with alterations in either $PaCO_2$ or perfusion pressure based on EEG changes.[35] The other study reported a reduction in postoperative disorientation from 29 to 4% when blood pressure was increased in response to EEG evidence of cerebral hypoperfusion.[36] There are, however, a number of other studies with conflicting results.[37,38]

Although the EEG is portable, noninvasive, and continuous, there are a number of problems associated with its use and interpretation, related to electrical artifact, depth of anesthesia, hypothermia, hemodilution, and changes in $PaCO_2$.

14.6.1.5 Near-Infrared Spectroscopy

The principle of near-infrared spectroscopy (NIRS) is very similar to that of pulse oximetry. There are a number of devices available to measure cerebral cortex oxygen saturations. These devices monitor changes in regional cerebral oxygen saturation ($rCSO_2$) within samples of blood in the cerebral cortex. Measurements are achieved in a noninvasive continuous fashion and are obtained by passing near-infrared light from the forehead into the cerebral cortex. Changes in the intensity of reflected near-infrared light represent changes in concentrations of oxy- and deoxyhemoglobin as well as various cytochromes. This allows for measurement of intravascular and intracellular oxygenation. The majority of the blood in the region of the cortex monitored is venous blood. Therefore, changes in $rCSO_2$ obtained are influenced by arterial oxygen delivery and cerebral oxygen consumption. Therefore, imbalances in either oxygen supply or consumption are reflected by changes in $rCSO_2$. It is of particular use in cardiac surgery as it can provide continuous real-time assessment of brain oxygen levels. It can also be utilized in situations of nonpulsatile or no-flow such as CPB or hypothermic circulatory arrest (HCA).

Lower baseline levels of $rCSO_2$ are associated with increased peri-operative mortality in children undergoing correction of congenital heart defects.[39] Real-time monitoring with NIRS to detect episodes of cerebral hypoxia is a controversial issue. The data obtained in the form of $rCSO_2$ needs to be interpreted with caution as they are subject to a number of intrinsic and extrinsic factors. Variables that are known to affect $rSCO_2$ include hemoglobin concentration, arterial blood pressure, temperature, and systemic oxygen saturations.[40] These variables need to be corrected to accurately interpret results obtained from NIRS. Furthermore, there is a lack of predefined values for warning or intervention associated with changes in $rCSO_2$ obtained with NIRS. It has been reported that levels of $rCSO_2$ reductions of greater than 20% from baseline or $rCSO_2$ levels less than 40–50% are associated with hypoxic ischemic neuronal injury.[41,42] Clinically, it may be more relevant to monitor trends in $rCSO_2$ rather than look at absolute values.[40,43]

A recent randomized controlled trial (200 patients) studying the effects of intervention on changes in $rCSO_2$ in patients undergoing CABG demonstrated that monitoring of $rCSO_2$ avoids cerebral desaturation and is associated with a reduction of major organ dysfunction. The control group of patients had $rCSO_2$ monitoring but without intervention. In the intervention group that most commonly falls in $rCSO_2$ was corrected by increased pump flow, increased mean arterial pressure, or normalization of CO_2. A significantly greater number of patients in the control group experienced a composite end point of major organ morbidity or mortality. Control patients also had longer periods of cerebral desaturation and longer intensive care unit stay as well as a trend towards increased overall increase in length of hospitalization. Patients with major organ morbidity or mortality had lower baseline and mean $rCSO_2$, more episodes of cerebral desaturation, and longer intensive care and hospital stay. Although not powered to assess the incidence of stroke, less patients in the intervention group (1% vs. 4%) experienced stroke.[44]

14.6.2 *Invasive Methods*

14.6.2.1 Jugular Venous Oxygen Saturation

Jugular venous oxygen saturation ($SjVO_2$) allows for monitoring of cerebral venous oxygen content. Reduction in $SjVO_2$ implies an imbalance between CBF and $CMRO_2$. To achieve $SjVO_2$ desaturation, either CBF must be reduced or $CMRO_2$ increased. $SjVO_2$ does not correlate well with mixed venous oxygen saturations.[45] To measure $SjVO_2$, a cannula is passed retrogradely through the internal jugular vein and positioned in the jugular bulb. Measurements of $SjVO_2$ can then be obtained either continuously or intermittently.[46,47] $SjVO_2$ allows for measurement of global oxygenation but does not provide more specific regional information; therefore, it may not detect focal events. In a study by Croughwell[48] observing 255 patients undergoing cardiac surgery, they reported a relationship between NPD and $SjVO_2$, demonstrating that desaturation results from increased oxygen extraction due to inadequate oxygen delivery.

$SjVO_2$ monitoring allows for continuous global monitoring during surgery. However, it is an invasive form of monitoring. The anatomical drainage of the internal jugular vein where the catheter is sited is not entirely intracerebral; therefore, it does not provide a 100% true reflection of cerebral oxygen consumption, but is nonetheless still used as a measure. To date, there are no randomized controlled trials examining $SjVO_2$ and outcome.

14.7 Prevention of Brain Injury

14.7.1 *Reduction of Embolic Load*

Embolization of foreign and native material during CPB is a known complication and much research has been performed on this area. Historically, emboli were classified according to size, either micro or macro emboli. The definition of size of emboli is a somewhat arbitrary measure. The basis of this classification is related to the ability of an embolus to obstruct a 200-μm vessel.[49] Perhaps, a more useful classification is one based on the nature of the emboli, defining them as biological (blood borne), nonbiological (foreign to the host), or gaseous.[50] These are defined in Table 14.3. The attraction of this system of classification of emboli is that it allows us to formulate strategies to reduce their incidence.

14.7.1.1 Arterial Line Filters

Arterial line filters attempt to deal with the problems associated with particulate debris during CPB. They

Table 14.3 Characterization of emboli reported during CPB

Biological	Nonbiological	Gaseous
Atheroma	PVC fragments	Air
Calcium	Aluminum debris	Oxygen
Fibrin	Silicone	Nitrogen
Platelet aggregates	Bone wax	Carbon dioxide
Red cell aggregates	Glove powder	Nitrous oxide
Neutrophil aggregates	Cotton fibers	
Chylomicrons		
Lipids		

have been demonstrated to remove micro-emboli.[51] The presence of a micropore filter within the arterial line portion of the CPB circuit reduces both the number of emboli in the arterial line downstream from the filter and the number of emboli detected within the middle cerebral artery.[52,53] In a randomized controlled study, Pugsley[22] demonstrated a reduction in NPD by using a 40-μm filter as well as a correlation between the number of emboli and the incidence of postoperative NPD.

Other methods of arterial filtration include intra-aortic filters such as the Embol-X intra-aortic filter (Embol-X, Mountain View, CA) and the cobra™ catheter (Cardeon, USA).

In a trial of 1,289 patients utilizing an Embol-X intra-aortic filter, particulate emboli were identified in 96.8% of filters successfully deployed. There was no difference detected in the rate of stroke, TIA, or death. However, the study was not powered to detect a difference in outcome, but rather to assess the safety and efficacy of the Embol-X in capturing emboli. Use of the Embol-X filter reduced a composite endpoint of neurological deficit, renal dysfunction, myocardial infarction, gastrointestinal complications, peripheral embolism, or death (24% vs. 36%).[54]

The cobra™ catheter delivers differential perfusion temperatures to the brain and body, thereby attempting to minimize the negative effects of hypothermia to the body while maintaining the beneficial effects of hypothermia to the brain. In addition, the catheter has an inflatable baffle to potentially prevent emboli from entering the cerebral circulation. In a small randomized controlled trial ($n = 60$) by Kaukuntla et al., the cobra catheter was able to achieve differential perfusion temperatures. The study was not powered to detect neurological outcomes and no difference was demonstrated in either the number of emboli detected by TCD or in NP assessment at 1 and 8 weeks.[55]

14.7.1.2 Perfusion Intervention

The incidence and prevention of embolization with regard to arterial line filters has already been dealt with in this chapter. It has been demonstrated that perfusion interventions during cardiac surgery are associated with increased emboli.[56–58] Perfusion interventions have been demonstrated to provoke micro-embolization when patients are monitored using TCD. Mean rates of emboli are greatest during administration of drugs and blood sampling (drug administration leading to the greatest proportion of emboli) even when compared with surgical events such as administration and removal of the aortic cross-clamp.[56] These micro-emboli are gaseous in nature and enter the venous reservoir on injection of drugs into the circuit. These bubbles are then able to traverse the arterial filter and lead to gaseous micro-embolization.

14.7.1.3 Oxygenators

Membrane oxygenators produce less micro-emboli than bubble oxygenators and are used almost exclusively throughout the western world. Blauth and colleagues also demonstrated an increase in NPD with the use of bubble versus membrane oxygenators.[59,60]

14.7.1.4 Aortic Manipulation

Postmortem studies have demonstrated that the single-most important cause of stroke following cardiac surgery is from embolization of atheromatous material, presumably from the aorta.[3,61] While aortic atheroma relates to the incidence of stroke, it has not been demonstrated to be a significant risk factor for NPD.[62] The risk of embolization is present at several points during an operation. Maneuvers that risk aortic embolization include cannulation and placement of aortic clamps either for administration of cardioplegia or side biting clamps to allow placement of proximal anastomoses. Advanced aortic atheroma is associated with increased incidence of stroke.[63–65]

There are two popular methods of grading aortic atheroma based on ultrasound findings. The first is normal, mild, moderate, and severe depending on the degree of intimal thickening and other related factors.[29] The full classification is given in Table 14.4.[29,67] In a study of 1,500 patients undergoing cardiac surgery all with epiaortic ultrasound scanning, Beribeau and colleagues demonstrated the incidence of aortic atheroma to be 16% normal, 57% mild, 19% moderate, and 8% severe within their population. There was an associated increase in both stroke rate and mortality associated with increasing severity of atheroma, with stroke rates of 1.2%, 2.5%, 3.5%, and 10.0% and mortality rates of 2.8%, 3.6%, 6.0%, and 8.0% for normal aorta, mild, moderate, and severe atheroma, respectively.[66]

Table 14.4 Grading and characteristics of aortic atheroma

Grade of aortic atheroma	Characteristics
a	
Normal	No identifiable intimal thickening
Mild	Increased intimal echo density with thickening
Moderate	Increased intimal echo density with atheroma > 5 mm
Severe	Atheroma > 5 mm with one of the following mobile/ulcerating lesions, extensive calcification, large protruding atheromatous debris or thrombus, porcelain aorta
b	
Grade I	Normal or mild intimal thickening
Grade II	Severe intimal thickening without protruding atheroma
Grade III	Atheroma protruding < 5 mm
Grade IV	Atheroma protruding > 5 mm
Grade V	Any size atheroma with mobile component

In the second classification system,[67] aortic atheroma is graded from grade I (least severe) to grade V (most severe); the criteria for grading of aortic atheroma by this method are listed in Table 14.4.[29,67] In a study of 189 patients undergoing CABG surgery with aortic assessment by TEE, increasing grades of aortic atheroma were predictors of stroke and death at 6 months postoperatively. At 1-week post-operatively, no patients with grade I/II atheroma had experienced a stroke (0/123). Incidence of stroke for grade III, IV, and V aortic atheroma were significantly greater, 5.5% (2/36), 10.5% (2/19), and 45.5% (5/11), respectively.[65]

In patients who are suspected to or are known to have significant atheroma, the risk of stroke may be minimized by avoiding repeated manipulation of the aorta. Intra-operative imaging of the aorta with either TEE or epiaortic ultrasound will provide a useful adjunct to manual palpation and allow for more appropriate cannulation and clamp placement to minimize embolic events.

Hammon et al. reported a trial in patients undergoing CABG examining the effects of reduced aortic manipulation. They randomized 237 patients to a "traditional" technique of multiple aortic cross-clamping (MAC – cross-clamping for distal anastomoses and partial occlusion for proximal anastomoses) versus a single clamp (SAC) technique (all anastomoses during a single period of cross-clamping) with an aortic cross-clamp that exerted less stress on the aortic wall. A third group of patients ($n=68$) undergoing off pump CABG were also consented for NP testing and included in the analysis. Patients underwent NP testing pre-operatively and at three time points in the postoperative period (3–7 days, 3–6 weeks, and 6 months). There was no difference in the incidence of stroke. There was no significant difference in the incidence of immediate post-operative NPD. At 6 weeks following surgery, there was a significant difference in NPD detected for SAC vs. MAC (31.8% vs. 51.0%) and a similar finding at 6 months for SAC vs. MAC (29.7% vs. 57.1%). Also of note was the fact that patients who underwent MAC did not have a significant reduction in NPD over a 5-month period, whereas in both the SAC and off pump group, rates of NPD progressively reduced, perhaps suggesting a less permanent injury in those groups. It should be remembered that in this study, the off-pump patients were not randomized to this intervention but chosen due to favorable anatomy and cardiac function. Nonetheless, there was no difference detected in the rate of NPD between off-pump and SAC groups.[68]

In a study performed by Borger,[69] site of cannulation of the aorta was demonstrated to be important in reducing embolic load. Thirty four patients undergoing CABG with an SAC technique were randomized to either conventional ascending aortic cannulation or distal arch cannulation with placement of the cannula tip distal to the left subclavian artery. Cerebral embolic load as assessed by TCD was significantly reduced in the distal arch cannulation group and this was found to be especially so during times of perfusion intervention. Although the technique of distal arch cannulation may be more technically demanding, it should be borne in mind particularly in patients with large amounts of atheroma as a potential technique to reduce cerebral embolic load.

14.7.1.5 Off-Pump Coronary Artery Bypass Graft Surgery

Off-pump coronary artery bypass grafting (OPCAB) can potentially minimize aortic manipulation. Performing OPCAB means that there is no need to cannulate the ascending aorta or apply an aortic cross-clamp to deliver cardioplegia. This removes two of the potential points in CABG surgery when aortic atheroma may embolize. Furthermore, if OPCAB is performed using a "Y-graft" technique from a pedicled left internal mammary artery graft, this further reduces the need to place an aortic side biting clamp for proximal coronary anastomosis. In a consecutive series of 700 patients[70] undergoing OPCAB, patients who had a "no touch" aortic procedure with Y-grafts versus those who underwent OPCAB with proximal anastomoses performed with a side-biting aortic clamp demonstrated a significant reduction in the incidence of stroke 0.2% vs. 2.2% for no-touch vs. side-biting clamp, respectively. In a logistic regression analysis, application of side-biting aortic clamp was the only independent predictor of stroke in this group of patients (odds ratio 28.5). OPCAB has been demonstrated to have a lower but not significant rate of postoperative stroke in a series of over 1,000 patients (1.8% vs. 2.5%).[71] There are a number of studies that have been performed looking at NPD following OPCAB. Of the randomized controlled trials, the study by Van Dijk et al. in 2002[72] recruited the greatest number of patients (281) and followed this group up over a 12-month period using a standard ten test battery. At 3 months following surgery, 29% of patients in the conventional and 21% in the OPCAB had an NPD (not statistically significant). At 12 months, 34% and 31% of patients had an NPD in the conventional and OPCAB groups, respectively (again not statistically significant). Recent 5-year data published from this trial suggest that there is no long-term difference in NCD for conventional versus OPCAB.[73] A smaller study by Zamvar[74] suggested that there is a reduction in NPD in patients undergoing OPCAB at 1 and 10 weeks following surgery 27% vs. 63% and 10% vs. 40% for OPCAB versus conventional surgery, respectively. However, this is not in keeping with other published literature on NCD following OPCAB[75,76] and the data from Van Dijk's much larger trial.

Although theoretically it would seem that OPCAB could reduce BI following cardiac surgery, the literature does not fully support this. Perhaps, the greatest potential for OPCAB in reducing BI is in those patients who undergo this surgery with a strict no-touch aortic technique.

14.7.1.6 Lipid Emboli

The occurrence of fat or lipid emboli during CPB has been documented. A major source of lipid emboli is from mediastinal blood returned to the CPB circuit via cardiotomy suction.[77] Moody and colleagues have demonstrated the presence of many thousands of small capillary and arteriolar dilatations or SCADs in the brains of dogs and humans who have undergone CPB.[78] They represent lipid emboli[79] and an association has been made with their presence and the direct return of mediastinal blood to the CPB circuit.[80] Use of cardiotomy suction is a widespread practice throughout the UK and provides a source of blood for transfusion for patients in the peri- and postoperative period. The commonly used micropore filters in the CPB are not effective at dealing with lipid emboli. These emboli are not only restricted to the brain but other end-organs.[81] Cell salvage systems collect blood from the operative field via suction and mix it with heparinized saline. The blood is then processed via centrifugation to separate the red blood cells from the plasma and debris. The red cells are washed with saline to remove further cellular debris, plasma, lipids, free hemoglobin, and coagulation factors before being stored in a re-infusion bag prior to use. The ability of cell salvage systems to reduce nonemulsified fat, cholesterol, and triglyceride has been demonstrated in vitro[82] and substantiated by animal work.[83] Cell salvage has been demonstrated to safely reduce transfusion requirements in patients undergoing CABG.[84,85] Cell salvage has been demonstrated to reduce a combined end-point of stroke, arrhythmia, renal failure, and myocardial infarction.[86] Although there are no randomized controlled trials to date on neurological outcomes in relation to utilization of cell salvage, a recent trial has demonstrated a reduction in serum markers of BI in patients undergoing CABG[87] it would seem intuitive that reduction of lipid emboli would reduce BI.

14.7.2 Temperature Management

Temperature management plays a vital role in cardiac surgical procedures. Hypothermia provides both myocardial and neurological protection. Cardiac surgical procedures such as CABG and valve surgery are commonly performed in the current era with only moderate systemic hypothermia (cooling to 28–34°C).

Animal studies have demonstrated a reduction in histopathological cerebral damage to rodents with mild hypothermia.[88] In CABG surgery, there is conflicting data as to the neurological benefits of mild systemic hypothermia. In a study of over 1,000 patients receiving either systemic normothermia (35°C) or mild systemic hypothermia (28°C), Martin et al.[89] reported a significant reduction in both total neurological events (4.5% vs. 1.4%) and acute stroke (3.1% vs. 1.0%) for normothermia vs. hypothermia, respectively. In a study of over 1,700 patients from Toronto[90] randomized to either normothermia (33–37°C) vs. hypothermia (25–30°C), there was no reported difference in the incidence of stroke 1.6% vs. 1.5% for normothermia vs. hypothermia. Differences in outcomes between the studies may relate to differences in study and temperature management protocols.

CPB and the use of an external heat exchanger to independently control blood temperature results in large temperature gradients between blood and body tissues, particularly during periods of active cooling and rewarming. Cerebral hyperthermia is likely to occur when the arterial blood inflow temperature exceeds 37.5°C. In a survey of UK perfusion practices, McGuirk et al.[91] reported that a maximal arterial inflow temperature of 38–39°C was used during rewarming by 60% of surgeons. In practice, the adequacy of rewarming is assessed by achieving a predetermined regional body temperature such as a nasopharyngeal temperature of 37°C. However, during rewarming, peripheral temperature measurement underestimates brain temperature, and caution is therefore required to avoid hyperthermic arterial inflow, which may inadvertently result in cerebral hyperthermia.[92] Cerebral hyperthermia may increase the severity and extent of neurological injury following stroke.[93,94] Postoperative hyperthermia in the intensive care has also been demonstrated to be associated with increased NPD. However, it remains unclear as to whether hyperthermia is the primary cause of the poorer outcome or is it the event that leads to NPD that is associated with hyperthermia.[95] In an attempt to shorten CPB time, the rate of rewarming is fast relying on a high arterial inflow temperature (38–39°C) resulting in the creation of significant temperature gradients within and between organs. Grigore et al.[96] prospectively studied the effects of different rewarming strategies in patients undergoing moderate hypothermic CPB. Patients who were rewarmed slowly, maintaining a temperature gradient of less than 2°C between nasopharyngeal and arterial inflow temperature, had better cognitive performance at 6 weeks postsurgery compared to patients who were rewarmed conventionally with a gradient of 4–6°C. To enable rewarming, a temperature gradient must be maintained between the arterial blood and the tissues, but the practice of maintaining an arterial inflow temperature of 39°C during rewarming must be questioned. Reducing the arterial blood inflow temperature will prolong the rewarming time and consequently CPB time, but it will probably facilitate more uniform rewarming, potentially reducing tissue temperature gradients and the occurrence of postoperative hypothermia. It may also reduce the incidence of inadvertent cerebral hyperthermia. In a study performed by Nathan et al.,[97] 144 CABG patients were randomized to have their intra-operative temperature maintained at either normothermia (37°C) or hypothermia (34°C) with no rewarming before arrival on intensive care. There was no difference in blood loss, intubation time, postoperative stay, myocardial infarction, or mortality between groups. It has previously been demonstrated by this group that patients undergoing this strategy of temperature management of mild hypothermia without further rewarming have a reduction in immediate postoperative NPD.[98] In long-term follow-up of this group, those patients who had greater NPD immediately following surgery had poorer performance at 5 years. The early benefits of hypothermia in relation to NPD were not apparent at 5 years.[99] It therefore appears that mild peri-operative hypothermia is safe and may well have benefit in terms of reducing early BI following CABG.

14.7.3 Blood Gas Management

The strategy employed for acid–base balance during CPB, either alpha- or pH-stat, has a major influence on CBF.

Alpha stat management allows for variation in pH with hypothermia. This results in a relative alkalosis and preserves CBF: $CMRO_2$ during cooling until the temperature at which autoregulation becomes uncoupled (approximately 22°C). There are several studies that suggest that alpha stat management in adults leads to equivalent[100] or superior neurological outcomes versus pH stat management.[101,102] These studies were conducted in patients undergoing moderate hypothermia. This is the main strategy employed in adults undergoing hypothermic CPB.

The alternative strategy is pH stat management (this is the technique employed by hibernating animals).

This strategy maintains pH during cooling by addition of CO_2. This means that autoregulation is uncoupled and CBF varies as a direct relation of CPP. Addition of CO_2 leads to cerebral vasodilatation and increased cerebral blood flow.

A number of animal studies by the Boston Children's Hospital on piglets suggested that pH strategies protect the brain better than alpha stat during periods of HCA.[103,104] In a clinical study of 182 infants undergoing cardiac surgery from the Boston group randomized to either alpha or pH stat, those in the pH stat group had a tendency to reduced evidence of both clinical and EEG seizures as well as earlier return of EEG activity and reductions in other morbidities.[105,106] In a follow-up study, the group did not find a significant difference in development or neurological outcome at 1, 2, or 4 years between groups.[107] Currently, pH stat is the management strategy of choice in pediatric patients undergoing surgery with HCA. There is, however, concern that suppression of cellular function with pH stat results in delayed cerebral metabolic recovery following HCA. This has led some groups to use a strategy of pH stat during cooling with conversion to alpha stat prior to circulatory arrest and subsequent rewarming in order to enhance cerebral cooling and subsequently improve metabolic recovery.[108]

There are no randomized trials as yet comparing alpha stat and pH stat strategies in adults undergoing surgery with HCA. The concern raised over pH stat management in adults is the theoretical possibility of increased cerebral embolization from an atheromatous aorta during associated periods of increased CBF. The optimal clinical strategy at present remains unclear.

14.7.4 Deep Hypothermic Circulatory Arrest

More complex procedures such as surgery involving the aortic arch in which cerebral blood flow may be interrupted as well as in complex congenital procedures when a bloodless field is required to facilitate operative techniques may require a period of hypothermic circulatory arrest (HCA). This technique employs profound hypothermia with cooling to 15–20°C. Cooling to such temperatures leads to a reduction in both CBF and $CMRO_2$.

Hypothermia leads to a reduction in tissue metabolic demands. For every 10°C reduction in temperature, $CMRO_2$ falls by a factor of 2-4.[109] This is known as the Q_{10}. In clinical and experimental models, times of 30–45 min are tolerated and other factors other than just hypothermia may play a role in neuroprotection at such degrees of hypothermia.[50] There is evidence that the Q_{10} is higher for infants[109] secondary to an increased basal metabolic rate, implying that they may be able to tolerate longer periods of HCA.

The current method of cooling to such temperatures is to provide a slow period of cooling on CPB.[110] This allows uniform cooling of all areas of the brain. Application of topical head ice packs during the period of cooling and maintained in position during the period of HCA are employed to prevent inadvertent cerebral rewarming. Aortic arch surgery utilizing HCA as a method of neuroprotection has a risk of stroke of 5–7%, an incidence of transient neurological deficit as high as 20% with most patients being at risk of some form of NPD.[111–116] The most important determinant of neurological outcome following HCA is the duration of HCA. Arrest times greater than 25 min are associated with an increased risk of transient neurological deficit; arrest times greater than 40 min are associated with an increased risk of stroke; and mortality increases substantially if HCA is prolonged over 65 min.[117] In pediatric surgery, the Boston circulatory arrest trial examined the effects of HCA in children undergoing d-transposition of the great arteries. One hundred and fifty-five children underwent neurological testing at 8 years of age. Children who had periods of HCA versus those who had periods of low-flow CPB had significantly greater deficits on tests of motor function, and HCA durations of greater than 41 min were associated with adverse neurodevelopmental outcomes.[107,118]

14.7.5 Cerebral Perfusion

It is possible to perfuse the brain during periods of HCA. This may be achieved either retrogradely by placement of a cannula in the superior vena cava or antegradely by cannulation of the innominate and left carotid arteries. These techniques are used as adjuncts to HCA in order to attempt to prolong safe arrest duration and reduce BI. There are a number of unanswered questions with regard to these techniques including optimal delivery conditions and constitution of perfusate.[110]

14.7.5.1 Retrograde Cerebral Perfusion

Retrograde cerebral perfusion (RCP) is a technique that has been employed as a possible method of cerebral protection during aortic arch surgery. The theoretical benefits of RCP include maintenance of cerebral hypothermia, provision of cerebral metabolites, flushing of emboli, and removal of breakdown products of metabolism. Disadvantages include potential cerebral edema worsening BI.[119] Recent randomized controlled trials have cast doubt over the benefits of RCP. These studies demonstrated that RCP did not attenuate metabolic changes associated with HCA or reduce the incidence of neurological injury.[112,119,120]

14.7.5.2 Selective Antegrade Cerebral Perfusion

Selective antegrade cerebral perfusion (SACP) is the preferred adjunct to HCA. It is achieved by direct selective cannulation of either the innominate or left common carotid arteries or both. In a prospective randomized controlled trial of SACP and HCA vs. HCA alone in aortic arch surgery, use of SACP as an adjunct to HCA has been demonstrated to attenuate the metabolic changes observed after HCA.[121] Other large studies have also demonstrated that the use of SACP is associated with low mortality and excellent neurological outcomes with published rates of permanent neurological deficit of 2.4–3.8% and temporary neurological deficit of 4.2–5.6%.[122,123]

SACP is now currently the most widely used adjunct to neurological protection for surgery requiring HCA. However, there are still a number of issues that need to be answered with randomized controlled trials with regard to SACP. These include route of delivery, optimal flow rate, perfusate temperate, cooling and rewarming protocols, blood-gas management, and optimal monitoring. A possible strategy for the management of these variables has recently been published by Harrington et al.[110] and is detailed in Table 14.5.

A number of groups have advocated moving away from deep hypothermia and suggested the possibility of moderate hypothermia (2–28°C) with SACP as the primary method of neuroprotection.[124,125] Reasons for implication of such a strategy include reduced metabolic and cellular homeostatic derangement and coagulopathy. Kamiyama and colleagues in a retrospective review of patients undergoing aortic arch repair with

Table 14.5 A suggested protocol for conduct and monitoring during SACP (From Harrington et al.[110] reproduced with permission of Elsevier)

Monitoring
Bilateral radial artery pressure monitoring
Jugular bulb temperature and O_2 saturation monitoring
In-cannula SACP pressure monitoring
Trans-cranial Doppler middle cerebral artery velocity monitoring
Cooling
Cannulation: distal arch or axillary (redo)
Temperature gradient: ≤7°C
Perfusion flow: 2.2–2.4 L min^{-1} min^{-2}
Cooling duration > 50 min
Nasopharyngeal temperature at arrest: 15°C for > 5 min
Jugular bulb O_2 saturation at arrest: ≥95%
Pretreatment: mannitol 1 g kg^{-1}; dexamethasone 100 mg (20 min prearrest)
Hematocrit: 20–30%
pH management: alpha-stat
Glucose management: insulin sliding scale (WBG < 10 mmol L^{-1})
Arrest period
Position: Trendelenberg 15°
HCA for anticipated arrest times ≤ 20 min
SACP for other cases
SACP
Cannulation: balloon perfusion cannulae via innominate and left carotid arteries
Left subclavian artery: occlusion with embolectomy catheter
Perfusate temperature 15°C
Hematocrit: 20–30%
Flow rate 10 mL kg^{-1} min^{-1}
Perfusion pressure 30–50 mmHg
Reperfusion
Rigorous arch airdrill
Perfusion flow: 2.2–2.4 L min^{-1} min^{-2}
Reperfusion temperature 15°C for 5 min
Rewarming
Temperature gradient: ≤7°C
Perfusion flow: 2.2–2.4 L min^{-1} min^{-2}

Table 14.5 (continued)

Nasopharyngeal temperature maximum: 36.5°C
Arterial outflow temperature maximum: 37°C
Rewarming duration: nasopharyngeal temperature 36.5°C + 10–20 min
Hematocrit: 20–30%
pH management: alpha-stat
Glucose management: insulin sliding scale (WBG < 10 mmol L^{-1})

HCA and SACP[124] subdivided patients into those undergoing surgery with moderate (25–28°C) and deep (20–24.9°C) hypothermia. They did not demonstrate any significant difference in re-exploration for bleeding rates in either the entire cohort or in propensity-matched pairs. Pacini and colleagues were also unable to demonstrate any difference in re-exploration for bleeding in patients undergoing aortic arch surgery at<25°C or≥25°C.[125] In a subgroup analysis of patients with HCA times greater than 60 min, no patients in the deep hypothermia group experienced paraplegia, whereas 2/11 (18.2%) in the moderate group experienced paraplegia (not statistically significant), with a trend toward increased mortality in the deep vs. moderate hypothermia groups, 3/11 (27.3%) vs. 2/16 (12.5%), respectively.

Historically, paraplegia has not been viewed as a major concern in aortic arch surgery. However, due to recent trends in moving away from deep hypothermia, Etz and colleagues have demonstrated in an animal model the potential safety issues associated with the use of moderate hypothermia and SACP in relation to spinal cord injury.[126] Initially, Strauch[127] as part of the same group demonstrated that the tolerance of the spinal cord to ischemia in a porcine model at normothermia (36.5°C) was 20 min but after 25 min led to paraplegia. At mild hypothermia (32°C), the safe period was 50 min with delayed developing after 60 min of clamping associated with development of delayed paraplegia. Etz extrapolated this data and suggested that with moderate hypothermia (28°C) and SACP, an ischemic time of 90 min would be safe and up to 120 min detrimental. Paraparesis occurred in two out of five animals in the 90-min SACP group and paraplegia in all animals in the 120-min SACP group. This suggests that the margins of safety for spinal cord injury with moderate hypothermia are not as great as has been readily assumed.

14.8 Conclusions

BI following cardiac surgery is a real and devastating complication. There are a number of nonpharmacological methods attempting to reduce BI following cardiac surgery and these strategies relate to interventions employed by surgeons, anesthetists, and perfusionists as well as specific procedure-related interventions. While none of these strategies provide a total reduction in BI, any reduction in this most devastating of complication is of utmost importance.

References

1. Eagle KA, Guyton RA, Davidoff R, et al. ACC/AHA guidelines for coronary artery bypass graft surgery: a report of the American College of Cardiology/American Heart Association task force on Practice Guidelines (Committee to revise the 1991 Guidelines for Coronary Artery Bypass Graft Surgery). *J Am Coll Cardiol.* 1999;34:1262-1347.
2. Roach G, Kanchuger M, Mangano C, et al. Adverse cerebral outcomes after coronary bypass surgery. *NEJM.* 1996;335: 1857-1863.
3. Roach GW, Kanchuger M, Mangano CM, Newman M, Nussmeier N, Wolman R, Aggarwal A, Marschall K, Graham SH, Ley C, Ozanne G, Mangano DT, Herskowitz A, Katseva V, Sears R, The Multicenter Study of Perioperative Ischemia Research G, the Ischemia R, Education Foundation I. Adverse Cerebral Outcomes after Coronary Bypass Surgery. N Engl J Med. 1996;335:1857-1864.
4. Tuman KJ, McCarthy RJ, Najafi H, Ivankovich AD. Differential effects of advanced age on neurologic and cardiac risks of coronary artery operations. *J Thorac Cardiovasc Surg.* 1992;104:1510-1517.
5. Shaw PJ, Bates D, Cartlidge NE, Heaviside D, Julian DG, Shaw DA. Early neurological complications of coronary artery bypass surgery. *Br Med J (Clin Res Ed).* 1985;291:1384-1387.
6. Taggart DP, Westaby S. Neurological and cognitive disorders after coronary artery bypass grafting. *Curr Opin Cardiol.* 2001;16:271-276.
7. Savageau JA, Stanton BA, Jenkins CD, Klein MD. Neuropsychological dysfunction following elective cardiac operation I. Early assessment. *J Thorac Cardiovasc Surg.* 1982;84:585-594.
8. Shaw PJ, Bates D, Cartlidge NE, et al. Early intellectual dysfunction following coronary bypass surgery. *QJ Med.* 1986; 58:59-68.

9. Savageau JA, Stanton BA, Jenkins CD, Frater RW. Neuropsychological dysfunction following elective cardiac operation II. A six-month reassessment. *J Thorac Cardiovasc Surg*. 1982;84:595-600.
10. Shaw PJ, Bates D, Cartlidge NE, et al. Long-term intellectual dysfunction following coronary artery bypass graft surgery: a six month follow-up study. *QJ Med*. 1987;62:259-268.
11. Heyer EJ, Delphin E, Adams DC, et al. Cerebral dysfunction after cardiac operations in elderly patients. *Ann Thorac Surg*. 1995;60:1716-1722.
12. Lederman RJ, Breuer AC, Hanson MR, et al. Peripheral nervous system complications of coronary artery bypass graft surgery. *Ann Neurol*. 1982;12:297-301.
13. Morin JE, Long R, Elleker MG, Eisen AA, Wynands E, Ralphs-Thibodeau S. Upper extremity neuropathies following median sternotomy. *Ann Thorac Surg*. 1982;34:181-185.
14. Roy RC, Stafford MA, Charlton JE. Nerve injury and musculoskeletal complaints after cardiac surgery: influence of internal mammary artery dissection and left arm position. *Anesth Analg*. 1988;67:277-279.
15. Shaw PJ, Bates D, Cartlidge NE, et al. Neuro-ophthalmological complications of coronary artery bypass graft surgery. *Acta Neurol Scand*. 1987;76:1-7.
16. Murkin JM, Newman SP, Stump DA, Blumenthal JA. Statement of consensus on assessment of neurobehavioral outcomes after cardiac surgery. *Ann Thorac Surg*. 1995;59: 1289-1295.
17. Blumenthal JA, Mahanna EP, Madden DJ, White WD, Croughwell ND, Newman MF. Methodological issues in the assessment of neuropsychologic function after cardiac surgery. *Ann Thorac Surg*. 1995;59:1345-1350.
18. Arrowsmith JE, Grocott HP, Reves JG, Newman MF. Central nervous system complications of cardiac surgery. *Br J Anaesth*. 2000;84:378-393.
19. Duebener L, Sakamoto T, Hatsuoka S, et al. Effects of hematocrit on cerebral microcirculation and tissue oxygenation during deep hypothermic bypass. *Circulation*. 2001;104:260-264.
20. Murkin JM, Farrar JK, Tweed WA, McKenzie FN, Guiraudon G. Cerebral autoregulation and flow/metabolism coupling during cardiopulmonary bypass: the influence of PaCO2. *Anesth Analg*. 1987;66:825-832.
21. Trivedi UH, Patel RL, Turtle MRJ, Venn GE, Chambers DJ. Relative Changes in Cerebral Blood Flow During Cardiac Operations Using Xenon-133 Clearance Versus Transcranial Doppler Sonography. *Ann Thorac Surg*. 1997;63:167-174.
22. Pugsley W, Klinger L, Paschalis C, Treasure T, Harrison M, Newman S. The impact of microemboli during cardiopulmonary bypass on neuropsychological functioning. *Stroke*. 1994;25:1393-1399.
23. Oka Y, Moriwaki KM, Hong Y, et al. Detection of air emboli in the left heart by M-mode transesophageal echocardiography following cardiopulmonary bypass. *Anesthesiology*. 1985;63:109-113.
24. Oka Y, Inoue T, Hong Y, Sisto DA, Strom JA, Frater RW. Retained intracardiac air. Transesophageal echocardiography for definition of incidence and monitoring removal by improved techniques. *J Thorac Cardiovasc Surg*. 1986;91:329-338.
25. Duff HJ, Buda AJ, Kramer R, Strauss HD, David TE, Berman ND. Detection of entrapped intracardiac air with intraoperative echocardiography. *Am J Cardiol*. 1980;46:255-260.
26. Tobler H, Edwards J. Frequency and location of atherosclerotic plaques in the ascending aorta. *J Thorac Cardiovasc Surg*. 1988;96:304-306.
27. Konstadt S, Reich D, Quintana C,ML. The ascending aorta: how much does transesophageal echocardiography see? *Anesth Analg*. 1994;78:240-244.
28. Davila-Roman V, Phillips K, Daily B, Davila R, Kouchoukos N, Barzilai B. Intraoperative transesophageal echocardiography and epiaortic ultrasound for assessment of atherosclerosis of the thoracic aorta. *J Am Coll Cardiol*. 1996;28:942-947.
29. Wareing TH, Davila-Roman VG, Barzilai B, Murphy SF, Kouchoukos NT. Management of the severely atherosclerotic ascending aorta during cardiac operations. A strategy for detection and treatment. *J Thorac Cardiovasc Surg*. 1992;103:453-462.
30. Katz E, Tunick P, Rusinek H, Ribakove G, Spencer F, Kronzon I. Protruding aortic atheromas predict stroke in elderly patients undergoing cardiopulmonary bypass: experience with intraoperative transesophageal echocardiography. *J Am Coll Cardiol*. 1992;20:70-77.
31. Zingone B, Rauber E, Gatti G, et al. The impact of epiaortic ultrasonographic scanning on the risk of perioperative stroke. *Eur J Cardiothorac Surg*. 2006;29:720-728.
32. Sharbrough FW, Messick JM Jr, Sundt TM Jr. Correlation of continuous electroencephalograms with cerebral blood flow measurements during carotid endarterectomy. *Stroke*. 1973;4:674-683.
33. Sundt TM Jr, Sharbrough FW, Piepgras DG, Kearns TP, Messick JM Jr, O'Fallon WM. Correlation of cerebral blood flow and electroencephalographic changes during carotid endarterectomy: with results of surgery and hemodynamics of cerebral ischemia. *Mayo Clin Proc*. 1981;56:533-543.
34. Messick JM Jr, Casement B, Sharbrough FW, Milde LN, Michenfelder JD, Sundt TM Jr. Correlation of regional cerebral blood flow (rCBF) with EEG changes during isoflurane anesthesia for carotid endarterectomy: critical rCBF. *Anesthesiology*. 1987;66:344-349.
35. Arom KV, Cohen DE, Strobl FT. Effect of intraoperative intervention on neurological outcome based on electroencephalographic monitoring during cardiopulmonary bypass. *Ann Thorac Surg*. 1989;48:476-483.
36. Edmonds HL Jr, Griffiths LK, van der Laken J, Slater AD, Shields CB. Quantitative electroencephalographic monitoring during myocardial revascularization predicts postoperative disorientation and improves outcome. *J Thorac Cardiovasc Surg*. 1992;103:555-563.
37. Toner I, Taylor KM, Lockwood G, Newman S, Smith PL. EEG changes during cardiopulmonary bypass surgery and postoperative neuropsychological deficit: the effect of bubble and membrane oxygenators. *Eur J Cardiothorac Surg*. 1997;11:312-319.
38. Bashein G, Nessly ML, Bledsoe SW, et al. Electroencephalography during surgery with cardiopulmonary bypass and hypothermia. *Anesthesiology*. 1992;76:878-891.
39. Fenton KN, Freeman K, Glogowski K, Fogg S, Duncan KF. The significance of baseline cerebral oxygen saturation in children undergoing congenital heart surgery. *Am J Surg*. 2005;190:260-263.
40. Schwarz G, Litscher G, Delgado PA, Klein GE. An NIRS matrix for detecting and correcting cerebral oxygen desatu-

ration events during surgery and neuroendovascular procedures. *Neurol Res*. 2005;27:423-428.

41. Andropoulos DB, Stayer SA, Diaz LK, Ramamoorthy C. Neurological monitoring for congenital heart surgery. *Anesth Analg*. 2004;99:1365-1375.
42. Levy WJ, Levin S, Chance B. Near-infrared measurement of cerebral oxygenation. Correlation with electroencephalographic ischemia during ventricular fibrillation. *Anesthesiology*. 1995;83:738-746.
43. Schwarz G, Litscher G. Transcranial cerebral oximetry, transcranial Doppler sonography, and heart rate variability: useful neuromonitoring tools in anaesthesia and intensive care? *Eur J Anaesthesiol*. 2002;19:543-549.
44. Murkin JM, Adams SJ, Novick RJ, et al. Monitoring brain oxygen saturation during coronary bypass surgery: a randomized, prospective study. *Anesth Analg*. 2007;104: 51-58.
45. Croughwell ND, White WD, Smith LR, et al. Jugular bulb saturation and mixed venous saturation during cardiopulmonary bypass. *J Card Surg*. 1995;10:503-508.
46. Croughwell ND, Frasco P, Blumenthal JA, Leone BJ, White WD, Reves JG. Warming during cardiopulmonary bypass is associated with jugular bulb desaturation. *Ann Thorac Surg*. 1992;53:827-832.
47. Nakajima T, Kuro M, Hayashi Y, Kitaguchi K, Uchida O, Takaki O. Clinical evaluation of cerebral oxygen balance during cardiopulmonary bypass: on-line continuous monitoring of jugular venous oxyhemoglobin saturation. *Anesth Analg*. 1992;74:630-635.
48. Croughwell ND, Newman MF, Blumenthal JA, et al. Jugular bulb saturation and cognitive dysfunction after cardiopulmonary bypass. *Ann Thorac Surg*. 1994;58: 1702-1708.
49. Stump DA, Rorie KD, Jones TJ. Does off-pump coronary artery bypass surgery reduce the risk of brain injury? *Heart Surg Forum*. 2001;4(Suppl 1):S14-S18.
50. Gravlee GP, Davis RF, Stammers A, Ungerleider RM. *Cardiopulmonary Bypass: Principles and Practice*. 2nd ed. New York: Lippincott Williams and Wilkins; 2000.
51. Mejak BL, Stammers A, Rauch E, Vang S, Viessman T. A retrospective study on perfusion incidents and safety devices. *Perfusion*. 2000;15:51-61.
52. Loop FD, Szabo J, Rowlinson RD, Urbanek K. Events related to microembolism during extracorporeal perfusion in man: effectiveness of in-line filtration recorded by ultrasound. *Ann Thorac Surg*. 1976;21:412-420.
53. Padayachee TS, Parsons S, Theobold R, Gosling RG, Deverall PB. The effect of arterial filtration on reduction of gaseous microemboli in the middle cerebral artery during cardiopulmonary bypass. *Ann Thorac Surg*. 1988;45:647-649.
54. Banbury MK, Kouchoukos NT, Allen KB, et al. Emboli capture using the Embol-X intraaortic filter in cardiac surgery: a multicentered randomized trial of 1,289 patients. *Ann Thorac Surg*. 2003;76:508-515. discussion 515.
55. Kaukuntla H, Walker A, Harrington D, Jones T, Bonser RS. Differential brain and body temperature during cardiopulmonary bypass – a randomised clinical study. *Eur J Cardiothorac Surg*. 2004;26:571-579.
56. Taylor RL, Borger MA, Weisel RD, Fedorko L, Feindel CM. Cerebral microemboli during cardiopulmonary bypass: increased emboli during perfusionist interventions. *Ann Thorac Surg*. 1999;68:89-93.
57. Borger MA, Feindel CM. Cerebral emboli during cardiopulmonary bypass: effect of perfusionist interventions and aortic cannulas. *J Extra Corpor Technol*. 2002;34:29-33.
58. Rodriguez RA, Williams KA, Babaev A, Rubens F, Nathan HJ. Effect of perfusionist technique on cerebral embolization during cardiopulmonary bypass. *Perfusion*. 2005; 20:3-10.
59. Blauth C, Smith P, Newman S, et al. Retinal microembolism and neuropsychological deficit following clinical cardiopulmonary bypass: comparison of a membrane and a bubble oxygenator. A preliminary communication. *Eur J Cardiothorac Surg*. 1989;3:135-138.
60. Blauth CI, Smith PL, Arnold JV, Jagoe JR, Wootton R, Taylor KM. Influence of oxygenator type on the prevalence and extent of microembolic retinal ischemia during cardiopulmonary bypass Assessment by digital image analysis. *J Thorac Cardiovasc Surg*. 1990;99:61-69.
61. Blauth CI, Cosgrove DM, Webb BW, et al. Atheroembolism from the ascending aorta. An emerging problem in cardiac surgery. *J Thorac Cardiovasc Surg*. 1992;103:1104-1111, discussion 1111-1102.
62. Bar-Yosef S, Anders M, Mackensen GB, Ti LK, Mathew JP, Phillips-Bute B, Messier RH, Grocott HP, The Neurological Outcome Research G, Center CIotDH. Aortic Atheroma Burden and Cognitive Dysfunction after Coronary Artery Bypass Graft Surgery. Ann Thorac Surg. 2004;78: 1556-1562.
63. Kapetanakis EI, Stamou SC, Dullum MK, et al. The impact of aortic manipulation on neurologic outcomes after coronary artery bypass surgery: a risk-adjusted study. *Ann Thorac Surg*. 2004;78:1564-1571.
64. Barbut D, Lo YW, Hartman GS, et al. Aortic atheroma is related to outcome but not numbers of emboli during coronary bypass. *Ann Thorac Surg*. 1997;64:454-459.
65. Hartman GS, Yao FS, Bruefach M III, et al. Severity of aortic atheromatous disease diagnosed by transesophageal echocardiography predicts stroke and other outcomes associated with coronary artery surgery: a prospective study. *Anesth Analg*. 1996;83:701-708.
66. Beribeau Y, Westbrook B. Intraoperative epiaortic ultrasound. In: *Echocardiography in Adult Cardiac Surgery*. 2007 www.nhheart.com/Epiaortic.pdf.
67. Ribakove GH, Katz ES, Galloway AC, et al. Surgical implications of transesophageal echocardiography to grade the atheromatous aortic arch. *Ann Thorac Surg*. 1992;53:758-761.
68. Hammon JW, Stump DA, Butterworth JF, et al. Single cross-clamp improves 6-month cognitive outcome in high-risk coronary bypass patients: the effect of reduced aortic manipulation. *J Thorac Cardiovasc Surg*. 2006;131:114-121.
69. Borger MA, Taylor RL, Weisel RD, et al. Decreased cerebral emboli during distal aortic arch cannulation: a randomized clinical trial. *J Thorac Cardiovasc Surg*. 1999;118: 740-745.
70. Lev-Ran O, Braunstein R, Sharony R, et al. No-touch aorta off-pump coronary surgery: the effect on stroke. *J Thorac Cardiovasc Surg*. 2005;129:307-313.
71. Biancari F, Mosorin M, Rasinaho E, et al. Postoperative stroke after off-pump versus on-pump coronary artery bypass surgery. *J Thorac Cardiovasc Surg*. 2007;133:169-173.

72. van Dijk D, Jansen EW, Hijman R, et al. Cognitive outcome after off-pump and on-pump coronary artery bypass graft surgery: a randomized trial. *JAMA*. 2002;287:1405-1412.
73. van Dijk D, Spoor M, Hijman R, et al. Cognitive and cardiac outcomes 5 years after off-pump vs on-pump coronary artery bypass graft surgery. *JAMA*. 2007;297:701-708.
74. Zamvar V, Williams D, Hall J, et al. Assessment of neurocognitive impairment after off-pump and on-pump techniques for coronary artery bypass graft surgery: prospective randomised controlled trial. *BMJ*. 2002;325:1268.
75. Taggart DP, Browne SM, Halligan PW, Wade DT. Is cardiopulmonary bypass still the cause of cognitive dysfunction after cardiac operations? *J Thorac Cardiovasc Surg*. 1999; 118:414-420, discussion 420-411.
76. Lloyd CT, Ascione R, Underwood MJ, Gardner F, Black A, Angelini GD. Serum S-100 protein release and neuropsychologic outcome during coronary revascularization on the beating heart: a prospective randomized study. *J Thorac Cardiovasc Surg*. 2000;119:148-154.
77. Liu JF, Su ZK, Ding WX. Quantitation of particulate microemboli during cardiopulmonary bypass: experimental and clinical studies. *Ann Thorac Surg*. 1992;54:1196-1202.
78. Moody DM, Brown WR, Challa VR, Stump DA, Reboussin DM, Legault C. Brain microemboli associated with cardiopulmonary bypass: a histologic and magnetic resonance imaging study. *Ann Thorac Surg*. 1995;59:1304-1307.
79. Brown WR, Moody DM, Stump DA, Deal DD, Anderson RL. Dog model for cerebrovascular studies of the proximal-to-distal distribution of sequentially injected emboli. *Microvasc Res*. 1995;50:105-112.
80. Brooker RF, Brown WR, Moody DM, et al. Cardiotomy suction: a major source of brain lipid emboli during cardiopulmonary bypass. *Ann Thorac Surg*. 1998;65:1651-1655.
81. Bronden B, Dencker M, Allers M, Plaza I, Jonsson H. Differential distribution of lipid microemboli after cardiac surgery. *Ann Thorac Surg*. 2006;81:643-648.
82. Booke M, Fobker M, Fingerhut D, Storm M, Mortlemans Y, Van Aken H. Fat elimination during intraoperative autotransfusion: an in vitro investigation. *Anesth Analg*. 1997;85:959-962.
83. Kincaid EH, Jones TJ, Stump DA, et al. Processing scavenged blood with a cell saver reduces cerebral lipid microembolization. *Ann Thorac Surg*. 2000;70:1296-1300.
84. Murphy GJ, Allen SM, Unsworth-White J, Lewis CT, Dalrymple-Hay MJ. Safety and efficacy of perioperative cell salvage and autotransfusion after coronary artery bypass grafting: a randomized trial. *Ann Thorac Surg*. 2004;77:1553-1559.
85. Niranjan G, Asimakopoulos G, Karagounis A, Cockerill G, Thompson M, Chandrasekaran V. Effects of cell saver autologous blood transfusion on blood loss and homologous blood transfusion requirements in patients undergoing cardiac surgery on- versus off-cardiopulmonary bypass: a randomised trial. *Eur J Cardiothorac Surg*. 2006; 30:271-277.
86. McGill N, O'Shaughnessy D, Pickering R, Herbertson M, Gill R. Mechanical methods of reducing blood transfusion in cardiac surgery: randomised controlled trial. *BMJ*. 2002;324:1299.
87. Carrier M, Denault A, Lavoie J, Perrault LP. Randomized controlled trial of pericardial blood processing with a cell-saving device on neurologic markers in elderly patients undergoing coronary artery bypass graft surgery. *Ann Thorac Surg*. 2006;82:51-55.
88. Busto R, Dietrich WD, Globus MY, Valdes I, Scheinberg P, Ginsberg MD. Small differences in intraischemic brain temperature critically determine the extent of ischemic neuronal injury. *J Cereb Blood Flow Metab*. 1987;7: 729-738.
89. Martin TD, Craver JM, Gott JP, et al. Prospective, randomized trial of retrograde warm blood cardioplegia: myocardial benefit and neurologic threat. *Ann Thorac Surg*. 1994;57:298-302. discussion 302-294.
90. The Warm Heart Investigators. Randomised trial of normothermic versus hypothermic coronary bypass surgery. *Lancet*. 1994;343:559-563.
91. McGuirk SP, Jones TJ, Graham TR, Bonser RS, Stump DA. What is "standard" perfusion practice in the United Kingdom and Ireland. Abstract presented at the Society of Cardiothoracic Surgeons of Great Britain and Ireland Annual Meeting, 2005.
92. Kaukuntla H, Harrington D, Bilkoo I, Clutton-Brock T, Jones T, Bonser R. Temperature monitoring during cardiopulmonary bypass - do we undercool or overheat the brain? Eur J Cardiothorac Surg. 2004;26:580-585.
93. Dietrich WD, Busto R, Valdes I, Loor Y. Effects of normothermic versus mild hyperthermic forebrain ischemia in rats. Stroke. 1990;21:1318-1325.
94. Minamisawa H, Smith ML, Siesjo BK. The effect of mild hyperthermia and hypothermia on brain damage following 5, 10, and 15 minutes of forebrain ischemia. Ann Neurol. 1990;28:26-33.
95. Grocott HP, Mackensen GB, Grigore AM, et al. Postoperative hyperthermia is associated with cognitive dysfunction after coronary artery bypass graft surgery. Stroke. 2002;33:537-541.
96. Grigore AM, Grocott HP, Mathew JP, et al. The rewarming rate and increased peak temperature alter neurocognitive outcome after cardiac surgery. Anesth Analg. 2002;94:4-10, table of contents.
97. Nathan HJ, Parlea L, Dupuis JY, et al. Safety of deliberate intraoperative and postoperative hypothermia for patients undergoing coronary artery surgery: a randomized trial. J Thorac Cardiovasc Surg. 2004;127:1270-1275.
98. Nathan HJ, Wells GA, Munson JL, Wozny D. Neuroprotective effect of mild hypothermia in patients undergoing coronary artery surgery with cardiopulmonary bypass: a randomized trial. Circulation. 2001;104: I85-I91.
99. Nathan HJ, Rodriguez R, Wozny D, et al. Neuroprotective effect of mild hypothermia in patients undergoing coronary artery surgery with cardiopulmonary bypass: five-year follow-up of a randomized trial. *J Thorac Cardiovasc Surg*. 2007;133:1206-1211.
100. Bashein G, Townes BD, Nessly ML, et al. A randomized study of carbon dioxide management during hypothermic cardiopulmonary bypass. *Anesthesiology*. 1990;72: 7-15.
101. Patel RL, Turtle MR, Chambers DJ, James DN, Newman S, Venn GE. Alpha-stat acid-base regulation during cardiopulmonary bypass improves neuropsychologic outcome in patients undergoing coronary artery bypass grafting. *J Thorac Cardiovasc Surg*. 1996;111:1267-1279.
102. Stephan H, Weyland A, Kazmaier S, Henze T, Menck S, Sonntag H. Acid-base management during hypothermic cardiopulmonary bypass does not affect cerebral metabolism

but does affect blood flow and neurological outcome. *Br J Anaesth*. 1992;69:51-57.
103. Kirshbom PM, Skaryak LR, DiBernardo LR, et al. pH-stat cooling improves cerebral metabolic recovery after circulatory arrest in a piglet model of aortopulmonary collaterals. *J Thorac Cardiovasc Surg*. 1996;111:147-155.
104. Priestley MA, Golden JA, O'Hara IB, McCann J, Kurth CD. Comparison of neurologic outcome after deep hypothermic circulatory arrest with alpha-stat and pH-stat cardiopulmonary bypass in newborn pigs. *J Thorac Cardiovasc Surg*. 2001;121:336-343.
105. Du Plessis A, Jonas R, Wypij D, et al. Perioperative effects of alpha-stat versus pH-stat strategies for deep hypothermic cardiopulmonary bypass in infants. *J Thorac Cardiovasc Surg*. 1997;114:991-1001.
106. Wypij D, Newburger JW, Rappaport LA, et al. The effect of duration of deep hypothermic circulatory arrest in infant heart surgery on late neurodevelopment: the Boston circulatory arrest trial. *J Thorac Cardiovasc Surg*. 2003;126: 1397-1403.
107. Bellinger DC, Wypij D, du Plessis AJ, et al. Developmental and neurologic effects of alpha-stat versus pH-stat strategies for deep hypothermic cardiopulmonary bypass in infants. *J Thorac Cardiovasc Surg*. 2001;121:374-383.
108. Skaryak LA, Chai PJ, Kern FH, Greeley WJ, Ungerleider RM. Blood gas management and degree of cooling: effects on cerebral metabolism before and after circulatory arrest. *J Thorac Cardiovasc Surg*. 1995;110:1649-1657.
109. Greeley W, Kern F, Ungerleider R, et al. The effect of hypothermic cardiopulmonary bypass and total circulatory arrest on cerebral metabolism in neonates, infants, and children. *J Thorac Cardiovasc Surg*. 1991;101:783-794.
110. Harrington DK, Fragomeni F, Bonser RS. Cerebral perfusion. *Ann Thorac Surg*. 2007;83:S799-S804.
111. Hagl C, Ergin M, Galla J, et al. Neurologic outcome after ascending aorta-aortic arch operations: effect of brain protection technique in high-risk patients. *J Thorac Cardiovasc Surg*. 2001;121:1107-1121.
112. Harrington DK, Bonser M, Moss A, Heafield MT, Riddoch MJ, Bonser RS. Neuropsychometric outcome following aortic arch surgery: a prospective randomized trial of retrograde cerebral perfusion. *J Thorac Cardiovasc Surg*. 2003; 126:638-644.
113. Immer F, Barmettler H, Berdat P, et al. Effects of deep hypothermic circulatory arrest on outcome after resection of ascending aortic aneurysm. *Ann Thorac Surg*. 2002; 74:422-425.
114. Czerny M, Fleck T, Zimpfer D, et al. Risk factors of mortality and permanent neurologic injury in patients undergoing ascending aortic and arch repair. *J Thorac Cardiovasc Surg*. 2003;126:1296-1301.
115. Ehrlich M, Ergin M, McCullough J, et al. Predictors of adverse outcome and transient neurological dysfunction after ascending aortic/hemiarch replacement. *Ann Thorac Surg*. 2000;69:1755-1763.
116. Reich D, Uysal S, Sliwinski M, et al. Neuropsychologic outcome after deep hypothermic circulatory arrest in adults. *J Thorac Cardiovasc Surg*. 1999;117:156-163.
117. Svensson LG, Crawford ES, Hess KR, et al. Deep hypothermia with circulatory arrest. Determinants of stroke and early mortality in 656 patients. *J Thorac Cardiovasc Surg*. 1993;106:19-28.
118. Bellinger DC, Wypij D, duDuplessis AJ, et al. Neurodevelopmental status at eight years in children with dextrotransposition of the great arteries: the Boston Circulatory Arrest Trial. *J Thorac Cardiovasc Surg*. 2003; 126: 1385-1396.
119. Wong CH, Bonser RS. Does retrograde cerebral perfusion affect risk factors for stroke and mortality after hypothermic circulatory arrest? *Ann Thorac Surg*. 1999;67: 1900-1903.
120. Bonser R, Wong C, Harrington D, et al. Failure of retrograde cerebral perfusion to attenuate metabolic changes associated with hypothermic circulatory arrest. *J Thorac Cardiovasc Surg*. 2002;123:943-950.
121. Harrington DK, Walker AS, Kaukuntla H, et al. Selective antegrade cerebral perfusion attenuates brain metabolic deficit in aortic arch surgery: a prospective randomized trial. *Circulation*. 2004;110:II231-II236.
122. Kazui T, Yamashita K, Washiyama N, et al. Usefulness of antegrade selective cerebral perfusion during aortic arch operations. *Ann Thorac Surg*. 2002;74:S1806-S1809.
123. Di Eusanio M, Schepens M, Morshuis W, et al. Brain protection using antegrade selective cerebral perfusion: a multicenter study. *Ann Thorac Surg*. 2003;76:1181-1189.
124. Kamiya H, Hagl C, Kropivnitskaya I, et al. The safety of moderate hypothermic lower body circulatory arrest with selective cerebral perfusion: a propensity score analysis. *J Thorac Cardiovasc Surg*. 2007;133:501 509.
125. Pacini D, Leone A, Di ML, et al. Antegrade selective cerebral perfusion in thoracic aorta surgery: safety of moderate hypothermia. *Eur J Cardiothorac Surg*. 2007;31:618-622.
126. Etz CD, Luehr M, Kari FA, Lin HM, Kleinman G, Zoli S, Plestis KA, Griepp RB. Selective cerebral perfusion at 28°C - is the spinal cord safe? Euro J Cardiothorac Surg. In Press, Corrected Proof. *Eur J Cardiothorac Surg*. 2009;36:946-55.
127. Strauch JT, Lauten A, Spielvogel D, et al. Mild hypothermia protects the spinal cord from ischemic injury in a chronic porcine model. *Eur J Cardiothorac Surg*. 2004;25: 708-715.

Pharmacological Studies to Reduce Brain Injury in Cardiac Surgery

15

Deborah K. Harrington, Vamsidhar B. Dronavalli, and Robert S. Bonser

15.1 Introduction

An array of drugs have been used both experimentally and clinically as putative "neuroprotective agents" in an attempt to reduce the incidence of brain injury following cardiac surgery. Many have been used empirically with relatively little hard evidence supporting their use. Recently however, an increased understanding of the pathophysiology of ischemic brain injury has led to a more scientific approach and the introduction of many more possible therapeutic agents. Experimental trials are underway in several areas and there are real possibilities of future pharmacological neuroprotective drugs for use as adjuncts in cardiac surgery. Many of the studies have been conducted in models of hypothermic circulatory arrest (HCA) because of the higher incidence of brain injury observed in patients undergoing surgery utilizing HCA than in conventional cardiac surgery.[1,2] This chapter aims to summarize the agents most commonly described so far and the evidence available for their use.

15.2 Glutamate Receptor Blockers

Glutamate excitotoxicity is the major underlying mechanism by which hypoxia and ischemia lead to neuronal cell death and has been reviewed in detail elsewhere.[3] Glutamate is the major excitatory amino acid in the brain and has been shown to have potent neurotoxicity in conditions of metabolic stress such as hypoxia and ischemia. Excessive synaptic accumulation of glutamate can cause neuronal overactivation and precipitate a cascade of events ultimately leading to cell death (Fig. 15.1). Glutamate receptors are divided into N-methyl-D-aspartate (NMDA) and non-NMDA subtypes. A number of receptor blockers of both types have been investigated as potential neuroprotective agents and a summary of the major NMDA receptor antagonist studies is shown in Table 15.1.

In a series of blinded, canine HCA experiments, a selective NMDA glutamate receptor antagonist, Dizocilpine or MK 801[4,5] or placebo vehicle was administered intravenously. Treatment began pre-arrest and continued up to 20 h postoperatively. Results revealed significantly better neurological function in terms of behavioral scores and less neuronal injury on histological examination in the treated animals. Unfortunately, MK801 clinical trials were later abandoned when high doses were found to cause necrosis in cultured rat neurones.[6]

Another NMDA receptor antagonist, Memantine,[7] is a well-tolerated drug already used in the treatment of disorders such as Parkinson's and Alzheimer's disease, though experimental studies have shown conflicting results. In a prospective randomized porcine study, Memantine or placebo was given intravenously prior to HCA. Behavioral and histological outcomes were similar suggesting no neuroprotective effect in this scenario.

Other NMDA receptor antagonists, Dextrorphan[8] and Dextromethorphan, reduce neurological damage in small animal models of spinal cord ischemia but have potent neurological side-effects including nausea and vomiting, ataxia, nystagmus, and hallucinations.[9] Riluzole is better tolerated but has shown no benefit in human stroke studies.[6]

D.K. Harrington (✉)
Department of Cardiothoracic Surgery, Queen Elizabeth Hospital, University Hospital Birmingham NHS Trust, Edgbaston, Birmingham, UK
e-mail: dkharrington@hotmail.com

R.S. Bonser et al. (eds.), *Brain Protection in Cardiac Surgery*,
DOI: 10.1007/978-1-84996-293-3_15, © Springer-Verlag London Limited 2011

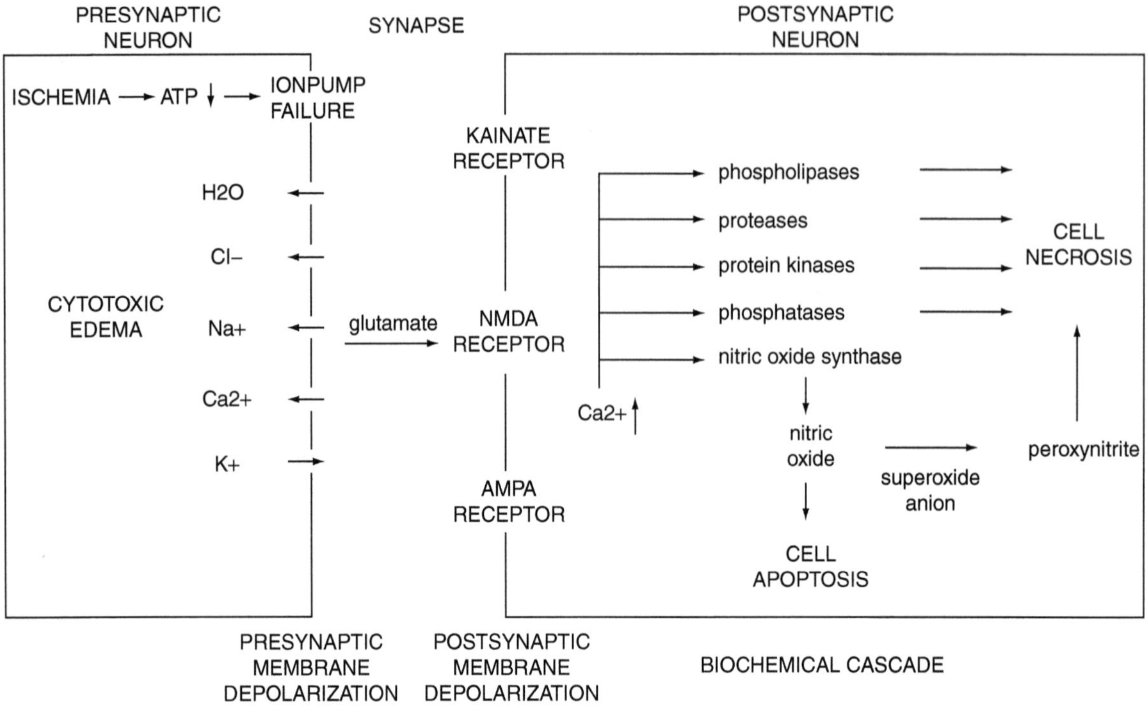

Fig. 15.1 Simplified pathway of glutamate excitotoxicity

Table 15.1 Major studies involving NMDA receptor antagonists

Drug	Type of study	Outcome	Limitations
Dizocilpine (MK 801)	Randomized, canine	Better neurological and histological outcome	Necrosis in cultured rat neurons
Memantine	Randomized, porcine	No benefit, neurological or histological	Well tolerated, no benefit
Dextrorphan	Small animal	Reduced neurological damage in spinal cord models	Potent neurological side-effects
Dextromethorphan	Small animal	Reduced neurological damage in spinal cord models	Potent neurological side-effects
Riluzole	Human stroke studies	No neurological benefit	Well tolerated, no benefit
Remacemide	Prospective randomized trial, humans	Possible neuropsychometric benefit	Side-effects, dizziness, drowsiness, ataxia

The NMDA receptor antagonist, Remacemide, was tested in a prospective randomized trial in 171 patients undergoing coronary artery bypass surgery.[10] There was no difference between groups in the primary end-point of decline in neuropsychometric performance of one standard deviation or more in two or more tests. Although the primary end-point was not attained, treated patients demonstrated significantly greater improvement in overall neuropsychometric change (Z-score) and changes in three individual tests. Reported side-effects included dizziness, drowsiness, and ataxia. To our knowledge, no further cardiac surgical clinical studies are planned.

The effects of the non-NMDA glutamate receptor antagonists such as the selective AMPA (α (alpha)-amino-3-hydroxy-5-methyl-4-isoxazolepropionic acid) receptor antagonist 6-nitro-7-sulfamoyl-benzo(f) quinoxaline-2,3-dione (NBQX),[5,11] have been studied in a canine model of HCA. Drug or placebo was given for 5 h after HCA. Once again, treated animals had a significantly better outcome in terms of behavioral score and histopathology than the nontreated controls.

The limiting factor for most of the agents described above is their unpleasant neurological and cardiovascular side–effects, which remain an obstacle to their clinical use.[6]

15.3 Nitric Oxide Synthase Inhibitors

Nitric oxide (NO) has also been implicated in glutamate excitotoxicity and is known in certain circumstances to mediate neuronal cell death.[12] NO is produced by activation of NO synthase (NOS) when calcium enters NMDA glutamate channels, is a potent free radical, and triggers DNA damage. The NOS inhibitor L-nitroarginine methyl ester (L-NAME) has been studied by several investigators of neuroprotection in experimental studies with conflicting results. In dogs undergoing HCA,[5] the usually enhanced activity of nitric oxide synthase in the basal ganglia, can be blocked by L-NAME. In a neonatal piglet study,[13] animals were divided into four groups. One received L-NAME before CPB, another received L-arginine to enhance nitric oxide synthesis pre-CPB and continuing post-HCA, another received both drugs and the final group received neither drug. The results showed that L-NAME increased cerebrovascular resistance and reduced recovery of high-energy phosphates and pH, but L-arginine increased cerebral blood flow, and recovery of high-energy phosphates. In the group that received both drugs, L-arginine did not completely reverse the effects of L-NAME. The overall effect of NO was thought to be beneficial possibly due to its vasodilatory actions. The fact that L-arginine only partially reversed the effects of L-NAME suggests that mechanisms other than NOS inhibition were contributing to neurotoxicity.

Similar results were obtained in another series of neonatal pig studies.[14] In one study, pigs received L-NAME after HCA and were compared to a control group, and in another study they received L-arginine after HCA and were again compared to a control group. L-NAME resulted in reduced cerebral blood flow and cerebral metabolic rate, whereas L-arginine improved recovery of cerebral blood flow and cerebral metabolic rate postarrest.

Contrasting results were found in another randomized pig study,[15] where a much lower dose of L-NAME was administered after circulatory arrest during reperfusion. NO levels were significantly lower in the treatment group, but there were no differences observed in terms of cerebral blood flow, lactate, or cerebral tissue water content. Recovery of somatosensory-evoked potentials was significantly better in the treatment group leading the authors to conclude that L-NAME could potentially mitigate against cerebral reperfusion injury. Conclusions from these studies are limited by the large variation in dosages and timings of drug administration.

Further studies have investigated the effects of specific neuronal NOS (nNOS) inhibitors on different mechanisms of cell death after HCA.[12,16] In the first study, dogs received the nNOS inhibitor 7-nitroindazole, or placebo, intraperitoneally, starting pre-arrest and continuing every 2 h until sacrifice 8 h postoperatively. Histological examination revealed significant inhibition of early neuronal apoptosis in the animals treated with 7-nitroindazole. In the second study, dogs were given another nNOS inhibitor 17477AR, or placebo, intravenously, 2 h after HCA and then every 12 h until 24 h postoperatively. Treated animals were found to have reduced levels of NO production by intracerebral microdialysis, and reduced neuronal necrosis on histological examination. They also had superior neurological function in terms of behavior, level of consciousness, motor, and sensory function. The group, therefore, concluded that NO plays a significant role in both neuronal apoptosis and necrosis after HCA, and that specific inhibition of nNOS could prove an effective neuroprotective strategy. Clinical evaluation of nNOS inhibitors thus requires further study.

15.4 Barbiturates

Barbiturates remain the most commonly administered drug used as a neuroprotective agent in surgery utilizing HCA in the UK.[17] Although they have several potential benefits, they also have significant side-effects and the clinical evidence for their use remains largely anecdotal. From laboratory studies, the main mechanism of action of barbiturates is believed to be enhancement of cerebral metabolic suppression but they are also thought to act as free radical scavengers.[18,19] High-dose barbiturates may largely abolish electro-cerebral activity and inhibit seizure development, which might otherwise exacerbate cerebral ischemia and lead to further injury. Barbiturates have also been shown to improve the outcome of focal cerebral ischemic insults in animal models of stroke, but evidence is conflicting after global ischemic insults.

The first prospective randomized controlled trial of barbiturate use in cardiac surgery was performed in 182 patients undergoing open heart operations requiring cardiopulmonary bypass (CPB).[20] Patients in the treatment group received enough thiopental to maintain EEG silence prior to aortic cannulation and until the end of CPB. The outcome measures were neuropsychiatric dysfunction, which included a neurological examination, psychiatric assessment, and performance of one neuropsychometric test, on days 1 and 10 postoperatively. There were no differences between the groups on day 1, but the barbiturate-treated patients had significantly less postoperative neuropsychiatric dysfunction than control patients on day 10. However, they also had a greater inotrope requirement, prolonged awakening times, and longer times to extubation. The limitations of this study included the heterogeneous mix of patients and operation types and that neuropsychometric evaluation was limited to a single test.

Another prospective randomized thiopentone study was conducted in coronary artery bypass surgery.[21] Three hundred patients were allocated to either thiopentone to produce an isoelectric EEG, or saline placebo, from administration of heparin to decannulation. The primary outcome measure was postoperative stroke and this was not significantly different between the groups. Again, barbiturate-treated patients had significantly longer awakening times and a greater requirement for inotropic support. The study was underpowered to detect a difference in stroke rate and did not have cognitive outcome assessment.

Additional concerns regarding barbiturate use arose following an HCA study in sheep in which phosphocreatine/adenosine triphosphate ratios (PCr/ATP ratio) were measured as a marker of cerebral tissue energy state throughout CPB and arrest.[22] Sodium thiopental was administered at the start of CPB until HCA. PCr/ATP ratio was significantly lower in the treated animals than nontreated controls throughout cooling, HCA, and reperfusion. This is in contrast to the maintenance of PCr/ATP ratio normally demonstrated during hypothermia and implied that barbiturates may be detrimental to cerebral function. However, the treated animals in this study also received dopamine to counteract the potentially negatively inotropic effects of thiopentone and this may have been a confounding factor.

A retrospective clinical study comparing low (15 mg/kg) and high (30 mg/kg) dose thiopentone usage in HCA has also been reported.[23] The observed fall of jugular venous pO_2 during HCA was less with the higher dose, suggesting a neuroprotectant effect due to suppressed cerebral oxygen consumption. The study was retrospective and there were no differences in clinical outcome between the two dosage groups.

Thus, although their use remains widespread, the evidence for barbiturate neuroprotection remains indeterminate and increasingly the risks of prolonged awakening and increased inotropic support are now thought by many to outweigh any potential benefits.

15.5 Propofol

A widely used anesthetic agent, propofol has also been investigated as a potential neuroprotective agent. Propofol is a sterically hindered phenol with a very short acting anesthetic effect and a safe side-effect profile. It has been demonstrated to have free radical scavenging and anti-inflammatory properties..[24] A randomized study of 30 patients undergoing CPB,[25] either with propofol or a control anesthetic measured cerebral blood flow using ^{133} Xenon clearance and cerebral oxygen consumption. Propofol reduced cerebral blood flow and cerebral oxygen consumption compared to controls. However, no differences in clinical outcome were demonstrable[26] In a randomized study of 225 patients undergoing heart valve replacement, propofol-treated patients did no better in terms of neuropsychometric dysfunction, depression, or anxiety postoperatively. A small observational study performed in patients undergoing cardiopulmonary bypass and hypothermic circulatory arrest for cerebral aneurysm surgery confirmed the lack of myocardial depression and short awakening times associated with propofol usage but failed to demonstrate any neuroprotective effect.[27] Thus, propofol has definite advantages over barbiturates in terms of myocardial depression and awakening times, but any neuroprotective effects are as yet clinically unproven.

15.6 Volatile Anesthetics

Volatile anesthetics provide improvement in outcome in laboratory studies of both focal and global ischemia.[24,28] In rat models of focal cerebral ischemia, the inhalational agents' halothane, isoflurane, and sevoflurane have all been demonstrated to reduce cortical infarct volume. Desflurane has also been shown to produce improved neurological outcome in a piglet model of low flow cardiopulmonary bypass when compared to fentanyl-based anesthetic.[29]

Most studies evaluate neurological injury after only short recovery periods, up to a few days, but a more sustained benefit up to 4 weeks after ischemia has also been shown. In global ischemia, a transient improvement in outcome with volatile agents has been demonstrated and the potential mechanisms for neuroprotection include suppression of energy requirements, reduction of glutamate excitotoxicity, regulation of postischemic intracellular calcium responses, and a preconditioning effect.

Many experimental and clinical studies have demonstrated an improved outcome using volatile anesthetics in terms of myocardial outcome,[30] but as yet no clinical studies of volatile agents as neuroprotectants have been performed.

15.7 Steroids

The rationale for the use of steroids in cardiac surgery is largely based on their potential to reduce the inflammatory response associated with CPB. Their mechanisms of action are complex, but include the inhibition of membrane phospholipid breakdown, the reduction of edema formation, and free radical scavenging. High-dose methylprednisolone has also been shown to have a direct neuroprotective effect against lipid peroxidation,[31] a final common pathway in DNA damage and cell death.

Steroids are known to reduce cerebral edema although their use following trauma or ischemic stroke remains controversial.[32] Steroid administration is frequently performed prior to HCA and there are now several experimental studies providing evidence for a potential benefit. However, the optimal timing, dosage, and route of administration remain unclear.

To ascertain the cerebral effects of steroids in relation to HCA, Langley et al.[32] performed a randomized study in piglets. Treatment animals were given high-dose methylprednisolone prior to induction of anesthesia. Recovery of both cerebral blood flow and metabolism post HCA was significantly greater in the steroid-treated animals suggesting attenuation of the normal cerebral response to ischemia.

Two further studies also used high-dose methylprednisolone in piglets undergoing HCA.[33,34] The first study compared systemic steroid treatment pre-operatively, to steroids as part of the CPB pump prime solution. The systemic steroid group had significantly less total body edema, as well as evidence of reduced cerebrovascular leak and improved immunohistochemical markers of neuroprotection. The second study compared preoperative systemic steroids, steroids in the pump prime, and a control no steroid group. The preoperative systemic steroid group had a significantly reduced inflammatory response; however, the pump prime group and control group demonstrated no significant differences.

Another study examining the timing of steroid administration was performed by Lodge and coworkers,[35] also in piglets. In this study, inflammatory markers were measured in a control group, a group receiving high-dose methylprednisolone pre-operatively, and a group receiving high-dose methylprednisolone in the CPB prime solution. Outcomes were significantly better in the preoperative treatment group, though the authors did conclude that receiving steroid in the pump prime was better than receiving no steroid at all.

Clinical studies have also demonstrated a reduction in the inflammatory response to CPB using steroids.[36,37] A small randomized study of coronary artery bypass patients gave intravenous methylprednisolone before CPB and intravenous dexamethasone up to 24 h postoperatively. Steroids produced a significant reduction in cytokine and interleukin levels. A further randomized study in children undergoing open heart surgery compared a bolus of dexamethasone pre-CPB to placebo. The steroid group not only demonstrated a reduction in cytokine levels, but also significantly required less fluid and shorter mechanical ventilation periods postoperatively.

Thus, evidence suggests a possible neuroprotective effect of steroids, particularly in high doses, and preoperative administration is likely to be more beneficial than peri-operative but further clinical studies are indicated. One area of concern regarding steroid use is the associated development of hyperglycemia. This has been shown to be detrimental in an animal model of global ischemia but not corroborated clinically.[24]

15.8 Free Radical Scavengers

Oxygen free radicals such as NO are released as a result of glutamate excitotoxicity induced by hypoxia and ischemia, and are mediators of subsequent neuronal cell death. Several drugs have been investigated as neuroprotectants because of their free radical scavenging mechanism. One such drug is the xanthine oxidase inhibitor allopurinol, which has been shown to both scavenge and inhibit production of oxygen free radicals. Reduced cerebral edema and improved histological outcome was demonstrated in a rat model of hypoxic-ischemic injury.[38] In a prospective randomized study of 169 coronary artery bypass patients, two doses of allopurinol or placebo were given preoperatively.[39] Treated patients had a lower mortality and better indices of cardiac performance, suggesting benefits as a myocardial protectant. The potential neuroprotective effects of allopurinol were investigated in a clinical study of infant heart surgery and HCA.[40] A randomized placebo-controlled trial of 318 patients was performed and the drug was administered intravenously pre-operatively, during and after surgery. There were no differences between groups in terms of the primary endpoint, which was a combination of death, seizures, and coma. However, there were significantly fewer seizures in children with hypoplastic left heart syndrome treated with allopurinol. Thus, certain high-risk patient subsets may benefit from such treatment.

Another free radical scavenger investigated as a potential neuroprotectant is α (alpha)-phenyl-*tert*-butyl nitrone otherwise known as PBN. PBN had previously been shown to protect cerebellar neurons and reduce cortical infarct size in rat models of ischemic stroke.[41] It was then studied by Langley et al. in their piglet model of HCA.[42] Animals who received PBN had significantly greater recovery of cerebral blood flow and metabolism post HCA than control animals. Clinical studies using the drug though are awaited.

Antivasospastic substance (1,2-bis[nicotinamido]–propene) is also a free radical scavenger thought to act by suppressing the increased influx of water and sodium across the blood–brain barrier during the formation of cerebral edema. It was used as a pharmacological adjunct in a dog study of HCA,[43] compared to mannitol and a control group. Animals treated with antivasospastic substance had significantly lower cerebrovascular resistance, intracranial pressure, and brain tissue water content than the untreated controls.

15.9 Mannitol

Mannitol is often used peri-operatively in cardiac surgery as it is a known osmotic diuretic, preserves water in the vascular lumen, and may thus prevent the development of ischemic brain edema.[17,44] It may also have a role as a free radical scavenger, enhancing the protective effect on brain tissue.[19] Mannitol was studied in the above experiments by Yoshimura and colleagues[43] and was found to have similar effects to those described above relating to antivasospastic substance. However, despite its widespread use, there are no randomized trials using mannitol either experimentally or clinically in cardiac surgery.

15.10 Calcium Channel Blockers

Calcium channel blockers have been proposed as a potential neuroprotective adjunct for two main reasons. First, the influx of intracellular calcium is instrumental in the processes leading to cell death, and second, the vasodilatory effects of calcium channel blockers could be beneficial during periods of reduced cerebral blood flow.[45] In experimental studies of focal and global ischemia, the calcium channel blocker nimodipine has been demonstrated to increase cerebral blood flow in ischemic areas.[19] A prospective randomized clinical study in acute ischemic stroke found improved mortality in patients treated with nimodipine. However, in cardiac surgery, the use of calcium channel blockers was largely abandoned in this context since the early termination of a randomized clinical trial of nimodipine conducted in valve replacement patients.[46] The trial was ended prematurely due to a significant increase in both mortality and major bleeding in the nimodipine group, without any beneficial neuroprotective effects having been demonstrated. Since then, no further clinical trials of calcium channel blockers in cardiac surgery have been reported. However, nimodipine remains in widespread use as a treatment for vasospasm following subarachnoid hemorrhage.[47] Its exact mechanisms of action in this circumstance are incompletely understood though it is likely to be due to vasodilation and improvement in cerebral blood flow.

15.11 Beta-Adrenergic Receptor Antagonists

The β (beta) blocker propranolol was suggested as a possible neuroprotective agent after unexpected observations during experiments on lambs undergoing HCA.[48] In a randomized trial, treated animals were given intravenous propranolol on induction, and EEG monitoring was performed continuously throughout the operation. The propranolol group had a significantly shorter time until reappearance of the EEG signal after HCA. The authors speculated that this may have been due to blunting of the catecholamine response to HCA or a membrane stabilizing effect by the propranolol.

A single-center observational analysis of 2,575 elective coronary artery bypass patients[49] was performed to study neurological outcome in patients taking pre- or peri-operative β (beta) blockers versus those taking none. The outcomes measured were stroke, coma, and transient ischemic attack (TIA). The β (beta) blocker group had significantly better neurological outcome in terms of the combined endpoints of stroke, coma, and TIA, and for stroke and coma combined. However, this was not a randomized study and the drug protocols were not standardized. Nevertheless, the data suggest that further studies regarding the neuroprotective effects of β (beta) blockers are warranted.

15.12 Aprotinin

Aprotinin is a nonspecific serine protease inhibitor involved in many hemostatic and inflammatory pathways and until recently enjoyed widespread use in cardiac surgery as a hemostatic adjunct.[50] Aprotinin has been proven to reduce the requirement for peri-operative blood transfusion in cardiac surgery and experimentally had also been identified as a possible neuroprotective agent. Recently, a direct neuroprotective effect of aprotinin against glutamate excitotoxicity in mice neurones has been demonstrated.[51] A meta-analysis of previous randomized clinical trials involving aprotinin in coronary artery bypass surgery[52] suggested that while it significantly reduced transfusion requirements, it did not affect mortality, myocardial infarction, or renal failure rates and its use was associated with a reduced risk of stroke. A further combined analysis of prospective randomized studies of aprotinin in coronary artery bypass surgery[53] also found that full-dose aprotinin was associated with a lower risk of adverse cerebrovascular outcomes without affecting the risk of death or perioperative myocardial infarction. A pilot prospective randomized study assessing aprotinin neuroprotection was also performed in 36 patients undergoing coronary artery bypass surgery using a neurocognitive test battery assessment pre-operatively and at 4 days and 6 weeks postoperatively. In this study, the aprotinin group had significantly better neurocognitive outcome at both time points postoperatively.[54]

The recent publication of the BART study, together with some other heavily debated reports,[55] has now largely removed aprotinin from the cardiac surgical pharmacopeia. The prospective randomized blinded BART trial compared aprotinin, tranexamic acid, and aminocaproic acid in high-risk cardiac surgery patients and was terminated early due to excess mortality in the aprotinin group. At the time of writing, concerns over the safety of aprotinin have been sufficient to suspend or abandon its use in the majority of cases.

15.13 Anticonvulsants

The sodium channel blocker lamotrigine is used as an antiepileptic agent and is generally well tolerated with few side-effects. Small animal studies have shown it to improve brain protection after ischemia.[56] It was also found to attenuate cortical glutamate release during cerebral ischemia in a normothermic porcine model of cardiopulmonary bypass.[57] In a series of experiments in a chronic porcine model of HCA,[58,59] lamotrigine-treated animals had significantly improved outcome in terms of EEG recovery, behavioral outcome, and histopathological scores.

The anticonvulsant sodium valproate has also been studied in a canine model of hypothermic circulatory arrest.[60] Treated animals demonstrated significantly better neurological and histological outcome than untreated controls.

Other anticonvulsants such as the sodium channel blocker phenytoin and the drug felbamate have additionally been identified as possible neuroprotectants. Studies have suggested a beneficial effect in small animal models of ischemia, but no clinical cardiac surgical studies have yet been performed.[61,62]

15.14 Lidocaine

Lidocaine is a sodium channel blocking local anesthetic and class Ia anti-arrhythmic agent that may also have neuroprotectant properties. When used intravenously, in high doses, lidocaine can produce electrocerebral silence and reduce cerebral metabolic rate.[19] Blockade of sodium potassium ATPase channels abolishes synaptic electrical activity and reduces ion leakage (sodium influx and potassium efflux), thereby reducing energy requirement and decreasing cellular oxygen consumption. In rodent models, lidocaine improves recovery from transient focal ischemia,[63] and in canine studies, significantly improves behavioral outcome versus placebo when administered pre- and post-HCA.[64] Two prospective randomized clinical studies using lidocaine have been performed in conventional cardiac surgery patients. In the first,[65] the study group comprised 65 left-sided valve surgery patients, some of whom underwent concomitant coronary artery surgery. The treatment group received a 48-h infusion of lidocaine from anesthetic induction. Neuropsychometric testing, performed pre-operatively, 10 days and 10 weeks postoperatively, demonstrated worse outcomes in the placebo group at both time points. Deficits were defined as a deterioration in ≥ 1 test. The lidocaine group also had improved results in certain individual test scores. However, the study was limited by heterogeneity in the patient population, a variability in anesthetic management, and a lower than accepted threshold for defining a modest neuropsychometric change as significant.

The second study[66] studied cognitive dysfunction in 118 patients undergoing coronary artery bypass surgery. Patients received lidocaine or placebo pre-bypass, continued until the end of the operation. Neuropsychometric testing was performed pre-operatively and at 9 days postoperatively. Treated patients had a significantly lower incidence of neurocognitive decline measured as a one standard deviation decline in two or more tests. (18.6% compared to 40% in the placebo group). This study again lacked a completely standard anesthetic protocol. Nevertheless, lidocaine appears safe and clearly warrants further study as a neuroprotective agent.

15.15 Calcineurin Inhibitors

The immunosuppressive agent cyclosporine A has been demonstrated to protect against reperfusion–reperfusion injury in rat brains.[67] The Mount Sinai group has now published several reports on the use of the immunosuppressant as a neuroprotective agent prior to HCA.[68,69] Its mechanism of action in this role is unclear,[70] but in porcine studies, treated animals showed better recovery of visual evoked potentials and behavioral recovery.[69] The authors speculated that there may be further as yet undetermined anti-inflammatory actions of the drug, which deserve further investigation.

15.16 GM_1-Ganglioside

GM_1-ganglioside is a nonspecific neuroprotectant whose mechanism of action is still unclear. Studies suggest an effect similar to glutamate receptor blockers, and it has also been shown to limit excitatory amino acid neurotoxicity as well as have an effect on NO metabolism. Its actions were further investigated[5,71] in canine studies of HCA. Results revealed a significantly better neurological outcome in treated animals as well as significantly less selective neuronal necrosis on histological examination.

15.17 Fructose-1,6-Bisphosphate

Fructose-1,6-bisphosphate (F1BP) is a high-energy intermediate in anaerobic glycolysis. It preserves cellular ATP and prevents intracellular calcium ion accumulation. There are conflicting reports of a neuroprotective effect. F1BP has been shown to have a beneficial effect in small animals studies,[72] but not necessarily in larger species.[73] However, in one chronic porcine model HCA study,[74] animals received either two infusions of F1BP, just before and just after 75 min of HCA or a placebo. Treated animals had significantly better behavioral scores and histological outcomes as well as better fluid balance and lower intracranial pressures. Brain glucose, pyruvate, and lactate levels were also higher in the treatment group suggesting supportive effects on cerebral metabolism.

15.18 Glucose Insulin Potassium Solutions

Glucose insulin potassium (GIK) solutions have been used as substrate support to enhance hemodynamic performance and reduce myocardial injury following cardiac surgery.[75] Glucose is the major energy source for aerobic metabolism and anaerobic glycolysis by the brain during periods of ischemia.[76] Insulin has been shown to reduce neurological injury in animal models of both focal and global ischemia.[77,78] Thus theoretically, the combination of glucose and insulin may have neuroprotective effects; however, the use of GIK solutions could also result in periods of hyperglycemia.[79]

There is a degree of evidence that hyperglycemia may be associated with brain injury in various settings. It is associated with a worse outcome in brain-injured patients;[80] adult diabetics show poorer neurological recovery after cerebral ischemic stroke than their non-diabetic counterparts;[81] and in intensive care patients, hyperglycemia is associated with poorer outcome.[82]

Hyperglycemia causes increased intracellular acidosis and a lower pH, and has been demonstrated to accelerate neuronal necrosis in certain regions of the brain in a study of newborn dogs undergoing HCA.[83] In clinical studies, a correlation between the marker of cerebral ischemia, creatine phosphokinase BB, and blood glucose was demonstrated in infants undergoing HCA[84] though this was not associated with any detrimental clinical outcome. Other studies have yielded conflicting results between hyperglycemia and adverse neurological outcome.[85–88]

In clinical studies of GIK in cardiac surgery, no differences in terms of neurological or neuropsychometric outcome have as yet been demonstrated though this may be due to studies being underpowered to detect such endpoints.[75,89] Further studies probably using multicenter trials are warranted.

15.19 Diazoxide

A novel approach to neuroprotection has been introduced by the use of ischemic preconditioning. Brief episodes of ischemia protect against subsequent lethal ischemia, an effect known as ischemic preconditioning, which is not only often used in myocardial protection[90] but has also been demonstrated experimentally in neurological protection.[91] The process can be induced pharmacologically by potassium channel openers acting on the inner mitochondrial membrane. This is known as pharmacological preconditioning and one such drug is diazoxide. Baumgartner's group performed two animal studies[92,93]comparing those receiving diazoxide and those without. There was a significant improvement both in terms of neurological outcome and brain histology in the diazoxide-treated animals, thus indicating its potential as a neuroprotective agent.

15.20 Gene Therapy (Nuclear Factor κ(kappa)B Decoy)

Nuclear factor-κ(kappa)B(NF-κ(kappa)B) is a transcriptional factor of many genes whose expression is related to reperfusion–reperfusion injury, including cytokines, interleukins, and adhesion molecules. Inhibitors of NF-κ (kappa) B such as aspirin have been shown to block ischemic injury in neurons.[94] Previous studies have demonstrated that the transfection of decoy oligodeoxynucleotides (ODNs) would block activation of cytokines and adhesion molecules.[95] Ueno et al.[96] hypothesized that transfection of NF-κ (kappa) B ODNs into neurones could form a new cerebroprotective strategy. They demonstrated effective inhibition of tumor necrosis factor α (alpha), interleukin 1β (beta), and intracellular adhesion molecule 1 as well as the attenuation of neuronal damage using the above technique in a rat model of global ischemia.

15.21 Erythropoietin

Erythropoietin (EPO) has been shown to have a number of effects other than its hematopoietic one, including possible neuroprotective effects. The mechanisms for this are unclear; they may include modulation of the inflammatory response, protection from NMDA receptor-mediated glutamate excitotoxicity, alterations to NO metabolism, or effects on calcium channels.[97] Recombinant human erythropoietin was demonstrated to decrease NO formation after brain ischemia in gerbils, and was also associated with reduced cerebral edema and increased survival. EPO receptors are found in neurones and stroke model studies have shown evidence of a neuroprotective effect.[98] In a stroke model of hypertensive rats, infusion of EPO supported neurone survival and prevented cerebrocortical infarction enlarging after occlusion of the middle cerebral artery. However, a large animal study of EPO or placebo[99] failed to demonstrate a neuroprotective effect. Pigs were randomized to intravenous recombinant human EPO or saline prior to HCA, and results revealed an increased EPO concentration in the cerebrospinal fluid of treated animals along with lower brain tissue concentrations of glutamate, but no significant differences in terms of EEG, behavioral outcome, or brain histology. Neuroprotection may still be achieved though with different dosages or timings of EPO administration.

15.22 Summary

In summary, despite many studies and ongoing work, there remains little firm evidence for the use of pharmacological adjuncts to cardiac surgery. However, a significant increase in the understanding of brain injury, along with the development of drugs specifically targeted according to this pathophysiology, will surely lead to newer and better neuroprotectants. Many more drugs other than the ones mentioned above are being investigated, though the evidence remains as yet indeterminate.[19] The likely limiting factor of any neuroprotective agent is its side-effects, and these have been prohibitive in a number of instances so far.[6] Until such time, as clear evidence is available many will continue to use "best guess" neuroprotectants, particularly in high-risk cases such as those utilizing hypothermic circulatory arrest.

References

1. Svensson L, Crawford E, Hess K, et al. Deep hypothermia with circulatory arrest. Determinants of stroke and early mortality in 656 patients. *J Thorac Cardiovasc Surg*. 1993; 106:19-31.
2. Ergin M, Galla J, Lansman S, et al. Hypothermic circulatory arrest in operations on the thoracic aorta: Determinants of operative mortality and outcome. *J Thorac Cardiovasc Surg*. 1994;107:788-799.
3. Olney J, Ho O, Rhee V, et al. Neurotoxic effects of glutamate. *N Engl J Med*. 1973;289:1374-1375.
4. Redmond J, Gillinov A, Zehr K, et al. Glutamate excitotoxicity: a mechanism of neurologic injury associated with hypothermic circulatory arrest. *J Thorac Cardiovasc Surg*. 1994;107:776-786.
5. Baumgartner W, Redmond M, Brock M, et al. Pathophysiology of cerebral injury and future management. *J Card Surg*. 1997;12:300-311.
6. Muir K, Lees K. Clinical experience with excitatory amino acid antagonist drugs. *Stroke*. 1995;26:503-513.
7. Rimpilainen J, Pokela M, Kiviluoma K, et al. The N-methyl-D-aspartate antagonist memantine has no neuroprotective effect during hypothermic circulatory arrest: a study in the chronic porcine model. *J Thorac Cardiovasc Surg*. 2001;121:957-970.
8. Terada H, Kazui T, Takinami M, et al. Reduction of ischemic spinal cord injury by dextrorphan: comparison of several methods of administration. *J Thorac Cardiovasc Surg*. 2001;122:979-985.
9. George C, Goldberg M, Choi D, et al. Dextromethorphan reduces neocortical ischemic neuronal damage in vivo. *Brain Res*. 1988;440:375-379.
10. Arrowsmith J, Harrison M, Newman M, et al. Neuroprotection of the brain during cardiopulmonary bypass: a randomized trial of remacemide during coronary artery bypass in 171 patients. *Stroke*. 1998;29:2357-2362.
11. Redmond J, Zehr K, Blue M, et al. AMPA glutamate receptor antagonism reduces neurologic injury after hypothermic circulatory arrest. *Ann Thorac Surg*. 1995;59:579-584.
12. Tseng E, Brock M, Lange M, et al. Neuronal nitric oxide synthase inhibition reduces neuronal apoptosis after hypothermic circulatory arrest. *Ann Thorac Surg*. 1997;64:1639-1647.
13. Hiramatsu T, Jonas R, Miura T, et al. Cerebral metabolic recovery from deep hypothermic circulatory arrest after treatment with arginine and nitro-arginine methyl ester. *J Thorac Cardiovasc Surg*. 1996;112:698-707.
14. Tsui S, Kirshbom P, Davies M, et al. Nitric oxide production affects cerebral perfusion and metabolism after deep hypothermic circulatory arrest. *Ann Thorac Surg*. 1996;61:1699-1707.
15. Segawa D, Hatori N, Yoshizu H, et al. The effect of nitric oxide synthase inhibitor on reperfusion injury of the brain under hypothermic circulatory arrest. *J Thorac Cardiovasc Surg*. 1998;115:925-930.
16. Tseng E, Brock M, Lange M, et al. Nitric oxide mediates neurologic injury after hypothermic circulatory arrest. *Ann Thorac Surg*. 1999;67:65-71.
17. Dewhurst A, Moore S, Liban J. Pharmacological agents as cerebral protectants during deep hypothermic circulatory

arrest in adult thoracic aortic surgery. *Anesthesia*. 2002; 57:1016-1021.
18. Shapiro H. Barbiturates in brain ischemia. *B J Anesthesia*. 1985;57:82-95.
19. Hall R, Murdoch J. Brain protection: physiological and pharmacological considerations. Part II: the pharmacology of brain protection. *Can J Anaesth*. 1990;37:762-777.
20. Nussmeier N, Arlund C, Slogoff S. Neuropsychiatric complications after cardiopulmonary bypass: cerebral protection by a barbiturate. *Anesthesiology*. 1985;64:165-170.
21. Zaidan J, Klochany A, Martin W, et al. Effect of thiopental on neurologic outcome following coronary artery bypass grafting. *Anesthesiology*. 1991;74:406-411.
22. Siegman M, Anderson R, Balaban R, et al. barbiturates impair cerebral metabolism during hypothermic circulatory arrest. *Ann Thorac Surg*. 1992;54:1131-1136.
23. Hirotani T, Kameda T, Kumamoto T, et al. Protective effect of thiopental against cerebral ischemia during circulatory arrest. *Thorac Cardiovasc Surg*. 1999;47:223-228.
24. Fukuda S, Warner D. Cerebral protection. *B J Anesthesia*. 2007;99(1):10-17.
25. Newman M, Murkin J, Roach G, et al. Cerebral physiologic effects of burst suppression doses of propofol during non-pulsatile cardiopulmonary bypass. *Anesth Analg*. 1995;81:452-457.
26. Roach G, Newman M, Murkin J, et al. Ineffectiveness of burst suppression therapy in mitigating perioperative cerebrovascular dysfunction. *Anesthesiology*. 1999;90:1255-1264.
27. Stone J, Young W, Marans Z, et al. Consequences of electroencephalographic-suppressive doses of propofol in conjunction with deep hypothermic circulatory arrest. *Anesthesiology*. 1996;85:497-501.
28. Kawaguchi M, Furuya H, Patel P. Neuroprotective effects of anesthetic agents. *J Anesth*. 2005;19:150-156.
29. Loepke A, Priestley M, Schultz S, et al. Desflurane improves neurologic outcome after low-flow cardiopulmonary bypass in newborn pigs. *Anesthesiology*. 2002;97:1521-1527.
30. Landoni G, Biondi-Zoccai G, Zangrillo A, et al. Desfurane and sevoflurane in cardiac surgery: a meta-analysis of randomized clinical trials. *J Cardiothorac Vasc Anes*. 2007;21(4):502-511.
31. Chumas P, Del Bigio M, Drake J, et al. A comparison of the protective effect of dexamethasone to other potential prophylactic agents in a neonatal rat model of cerebral hypoxia-ischemia. *J Neurosurg*. 1993;79:414-420.
32. Langley S, Chai P, Jaggers J, et al. Preoperative high dose methylprednisolone attenuates the cerebral response to deep hypothermic circulatory arrest. *Eur J Cardiothorac Surg*. 2000;17:279-286.
33. Shum-Tim D, Tchervenkov C, Jamal A, et al. Systemic steroid pretreatment improves cerebral protection after circulatory arrest. *Ann Thorac Surg*. 2001;72:1465-1472.
34. Shum-Tim D, Tchervenkov C, Laliberte E, et al. Timing of steroid treatment is important for cerebral protection during cardiopulmonary bypass and circulatory arrest: minimal protection of pump prime methylprednisolone. *Eur J Cardiothorac Surg*. 2003;24:125-132.
35. Lodge A, Chai P, Daggett C, et al. Methylprednisolone reduces the inflammatory response to cardiopulmonary bypass in neonatal piglets: timing of dose is important. *J Thorac Cardiovasc Surg*. 1999;117:515-522.
36. Engelman R, Rousou J, Flack J III, et al. Influence of steroids on complement and cytokine generation after cardiopulmonary bypass. *Ann Thorac Surg*. 1995;60:801-804.
37. Bronicki R, Backer C, Baden H, et al. Dexamethasone reduces the inflammatory response to cardiopulmonary bypass in children. *Ann Thorac Surg*. 2000;69:1490-1495.
38. Palmer C, Vannucci R, Towfighi J. Reduction of perinatal hypoxic-ischemic brain damage with allopurinol. *Pediatr Res*. 1990;27(4):332-336.
39. Johnson W, Kayser K, Brenowitz J, et al. A randomized controlled trial of allopurinol in coronary bypass surgery. *Am Heart J*. 1991;121:20-24.
40. Clancy R, McGaurn S, Goin J, et al. Allopurinol neurocardiac protection trial in infants undergoing heart surgery using deep hypothermic circulatory arrest. *Pediatrics*. 2001;108:61-70.
41. Cao X, Phillis J. A-Phenyl-tert-butyl-nitrone reduces cortical infarct and edema in rats subjected to focal ischemia. *Brain Res*. 1994;644:267-272.
42. Langley S, Chai P, Jaggers J, et al. The free radical spin trap a-phenyl-tert-butyl nitrone attenuates the cerebral response to deep hypothermic ischemia. *J Thorac Cardiovasc Surg*. 2000;119:305-313.
43. Yoshimura N, Okada M, Ota T, et al. Pharmacologic intervention for ischemic brain edema after retrograde cerebral perfusion. *J Thorac Cardiovasc Surg*. 1995; 109:1173-1181.
44. Hirotani T, Kameda T, Kumamoto T, et al. Aortic arch repair using hypothermic circulatory arrest technique associated with pharmacological brain protection. *Eur J Cardiothorac Surg*. 2000;18:545-549.
45. Griepp E, Griepp R. Cerebral consequences of hypothermic circulatory arrest in adults. *J Card Surg*. 1992;7(2):134-155.
46. Legault C, Furberg C, Wagenknecht L, et al. Nimodipine neuroprotection in cardiac valve replacement. *Stroke*. 1996;27:593-598.
47. Keyrouz S, Diringer M. Clinical review: prevention and therapy of vasospasm in subarachnoid hemorrhage. *Crit Care*. 2007;11(4):220-237.
48. Azariades M, Firmin R, Lincoln C, et al. The effect of propanolol on the cerebral electrical response to deep hypothermia and total circulatory arrest in lambs. *J Thorac Cardiovasc Surg*. 1990;99:1030-1037.
49. Amory D, Grigore A, Amory J, et al. Neuroprotection is associated with b-adrenergic receptor antagonists during cardiac surgery: evidence from 2,575 patients. *J Cardiothorac Vasc Anes*. 2002;16(3):270-277.
50. Murkin J. Postoperative cognitive dysfunction: aprotinin, bleeding and cognitive testing. *Can J Anaesth*. 2004;51: 957-962.
51. Iwata Y, Nicole O, Okamura T, et al. Aprotinin confers neuroprotection by reducing excitotoxic cell death. *J Thorac Cardiovasc Surg*. 2008;135:573-578.
52. Sedrakyan A, Treasure T, Elefteriades J. Effect of aprotinin on clinical outcomes in coronary artery bypass graft surgery: a systemic review and meta-analysis of randomized clinical trials. *J Thorac Cardiovasc Surg*. 2004;128:442-448.
53. Royston D, Levy J, Fitch J, et al. Full-dose aprotinin use in coronary artery bypass graft surgery: an analysis of perioperative pharmacotherapy and patient outcomes. *Anesth Analg*. 2006;103:1082-1088.

54. Harmon D, Ghori K, Eustace N, et al. Aprotinin decreases the incidence of cognitive deficit following CABG and cardiopulmonary bypass: a pilot randomized controlled study. *Can J Anaesth*. 2004;51(10):1002-1009.
55. Fergusson D, Hebert P, Mayer C, et al. A comparison of aprotinin and lysine analogues in high-risk cardiac surgery. *N Engl J Med*. 2008;358(22):2319-2331.
56. Bacher A, Zornow M. Lamotrigine inhibits extracellular glutamate accumulation during transient global cerebral ischemia in rabbits. *Anesthesiology*. 1997;86:459-463.
57. Conroy B, Black D, Lin C, et al. Lamotrigine attenuates cortical glutamate release during global cerebral ischemia in pigs on cardiopulmonary bypass. *Anesthesiology*. 1999;90: 844-854.
58. Anttila V, Rimpilainen J, Pokela M, et al. Lamotrigine improves cerebral outcome after hypothermic circulatory arrest: a study in a chronic porcine model. *J Thorac Cardiovasc Surg*. 2000;120:247-255.
59. Rimpilainen J, Romsi P, Pokela M, et al. Lamotrigine plus leukocyte filtration as a neuroprotective strategy in experimental hypothermic circulatory arrest. *Ann Thorac Surg*. 2002;73:163-172.
60. Williams J, Barreiro C, Nwakanma L, et al. Valproic acid prevents brain injury in a canine model of hypothermic circulatory arrest: a promising new approach to neuroprotection during cardiac surgery. *Ann Thorac Surg*. 2006; 81:2235-2242.
61. Weber M, Taylor C. Damage from oxygen and glucose deprivation in hippocampal slices is prevented by tetrodotoxin, lidocaine and phenytoin without blockade of action potentials. *Brain Res*. 1994;664:167-177.
62. Shuaib A, Waqaar T, Ijaz M, et al. Neuroprotection with felbamate: a 7- and 28-day study in transient forebrain ischemia in gerbils. *Brain Res*. 1996;727:65-70.
63. Lei B, Cottrell J, Kass I. Neuroprotective effect of low-dose lidocaine in a rat model of transient focal cerebral ischemia. *Anesthesiology*. 2001;95:445-451.
64. Zhou Y, Wang D, Du M, et al. Lidocaine prolongs the safe duration of circulatory arrest during deep hypothermia in dogs. *Can J Anaesth*. 1998;45(7):692-698.
65. Mitchell S, Pellett O, Gorman D. Cerebral protection by lidocaine during cardiac operations. *Ann Thorac Surg*. 1999;67:1117-1124.
66. Wang D, Wu X, Li J, et al. The effect of lidocaine on early postoperative cognitive dysfunction after coronary artery bypass surgery. *Anesth Analg*. 2002;95:1134-1141.
67. Shiga Y, Onodera H, Matsuo Y, et al. Cyclosporin A protects against ischemia-reperfusion injury in the brain. *Brain Res*. 1992;595:145-148.
68. Hagl C, Tatton N, Khaladj N, et al. Involvement of apoptosis in neurological injury after hypothermic circulatory arrest: a new target for therapeutic intervention? *Ann Thorac Surg*. 2001;72:1457-1464.
69. Strauch J, Spielvogel D, Haldenwang P, et al. Cooling to 100C and treatment with cyclosporine A improve cerebral recovery following prolonged hypothermic circulatory arrest in a chronic porcine model. *Eur J Cardiothorac Surg*. 2005; 27:74-80.
70. Tatton N, Hagl C, Nandor S, et al. Apoptotic cell death in the hippocampus due to prolonged hypothermic circulatory arrest: comparison of cyclosporine A and cycloheximide on neuron survival. *Eur J Cardiothorac Surg*. 2001;19: 746-755.
71. Redmond J, Gillinov A, Blue M, et al. The monosialoganglioside, GM_1, reduces neurologic injury associated with hypothermic circulatory arrest. *Surgery*. 1993;114: 324-333.
72. Sola A, Berrios M, Sheldon R, et al. Fructose-1, 6-bisphosphate after hypoxic ischemic injury is protective to the neonatal rat brain. *Brain Res*. 1996;741:294-299.
73. LeBlanc M, Farias L, Evans O, et al. Fructose-1, 6-bisphosphate, when given immediately before reoxygenation, or before injury, does not ameliorate hypoxic ischemic injury to the central nervous system in the newborn pig. *Crit Care Med*. 1991;19(1):75-83.
74. Romsi P, Kaakinen T, Kiviluoma K, et al. Fructose-1, 6-bisphosphate for improved outcome after hypothermic circulatory arrest in pigs. *J Thorac Cardiovasc Surg*. 2003;125: 686-698.
75. Quinn D, Pagano D, Bonser R, et al. Improved myocardial protection during cornary artery surgery with glucose-insulin-potassium: a randomized controlled trial. *J Thorac Cardiovasc Surg*. 2006;131:34-42.
76. Payne R, Tseng M, Schurr A. The glucose paradox of cerebral ischemia: evidence for corticosterone involvement. *Brain Res*. 2003;971:9-17.
77. Voll C, Auer R. Insulin attenuates ischemic brain damage independent of its hypoglycemic effect. *J Ceeb Blood Flow Metab*. 1991;11:1006-1014.
78. Auer R. Insulin, blood glucose levels, and ischemic brain damage. *Neurology*. 1998;51(Suppl 3):S39-S43.
79. Schipke J, Friebe R, Gams E. Forty years of glucose-insulin-potassium (GIK) in cardiac surgery: a review of randomized, controlled trials. *Eur J Cardiothorac Surg*. 2006;29: 479-485.
80. Young B, Ott L, Dempsey R, et al. Relationship between admission hyperglycemia and neurologic outcome of severely brain-injured patients. *Ann Surg*. 1989;210(4): 466-473.
81. Pulsinelli W, Levy D, Sigsbee B, et al. Increased damage after ischemic stroke in patients with hyperglycemia with or without established diabetes mellitus. *Am J Med*. 1983;74: 540-544.
82. den BG Van, Wouters P, Weekers F, et al. Intensive insulin therapy in critically ill patients. *N Engl J Med*. 2001;345: 1359-1367.
83. Vannucci R, Rossini A, Towfighi J. Effect of hyperglycemia on ischemic brain damage during hypothermic circulatory arrest in newborn dogs. *Pediatr Res*. 1996;40(2):177-184.
84. Ekroth R, Thompson R, Lincoln C, et al. Elective deep hypothermia with total circulatory arrest: changes in plasma creatine kinase BB, blood glucose, and clinical variables. *J Thorac Cardiovasc Surg*. 1989;97:30-35.
85. Steward D, Da Silva C, Flegel T. Elevated blood glucose levels may increase the danger of neurological deficit following profoundly hypothermic cardiac arrest. *Anesthesiology*. 1988;68:653.
86. Ceriana P, Barzaghi N, Locatelli A, et al. Aortic arch surgery: retrospective analysis of outcome and neuroprotective strategies. *J Cardiovasc Surg*. 1998;39:337-342.
87. De Ferranti S, Gauvreau K, Hickey P, et al. Intraoperative hyperglycemia during infant cardiac surgery is not

associated with adverse neurodevelopmental outcomes at 1, 4, and 8 years. *Anesthesiology*. 2004;100:1345-1352.
88. Ranasinghe A, Quinn D, Pagano D, et al. Glucose-insulin-potassium and tri-iodothyronine individually improve hemodynamic performance and are associated with reduced troponin I release after on-pump coronary artery bypass grafting. *Circulation*. 2006;114:I245-I250.
89. Akao M, Ohler A, O'Rourke B, et al. Mitochondrial ATP-sensitive potassium channels inhibit apoptosis induced by oxidative stress in cardiac cells. *Circ Res*. 2001;88:1267-1275.
90. Domoki F, Periaccante J, Veltkamp R, et al. Mitochondrial potassium channel opener diazoxide preserves neuronal-vascular function after cerebral ischemia in newborn pigs. *Stroke*. 1999;30:2713-2719.
91. Shake J, Peck E, Marban E, et al. Pharmacologically induced preconditioning with diazoxide: a novel approach to brain protection. *Ann Thorac Surg*. 2001;72:1849-1854.
92. Caparrelli D, Cattaneo S, Bethea B, et al. Pharmacological preconditioning ameliorates neurological injury in a model of spinal cord ischemia. *Ann Thorac Surg*. 2002;74:838-845.
93. Grilli M, Pizzi M, Memo M, et al. Neuroprotection by aspirin and sodium salicylate through blockade of NF-$_{\kappa}$B activation. *Science*. 1996;274:1383-1385.
94. Sawa Y, Morishita R, Suzuki K, et al. A Novel strategy for myocardial protection using in vivo transfection od cis element 'decoy' against nfkb binding site. *Circulation*. 1997;96(suppl II):II280-II285.
95. Ueno T, Sawa Y, Kitagawa-Sakakida S, et al. Nuclear factor-$_{\kappa}$B decoy attenuates neuronal damage after global brain ischemia: a future strategy for brain protection during circulatory arrest. *J Thorac Cardiovasc Surg*. 2001; 122(4): 720-727.
96. Calapai G, Marciano M, Corica F, et al. Erythropoietin protects against brain ichemic injury by inhibition of nitric oxide formation. *Eur J of Pharmacology*. 2000;401:349-356.
97. Sadamoto Y, Igase K, Sakanaka M, et al. Erythropoietin prevents place navigation disability and cortical infarction in rats with permanent occlusion of the middle cerebral artery. *Biochem Biophys Res Commun*. 1998;253:26-32.
98. Romsi P, Ronka E, Kiviluoma K, et al. Potential neuroprotective benefits of erythropoietin during experimental hypothermic circulatory arrest. *J Thorac Cardiovasc Surg*. 2002;124:714-723.
99. Givehchian M, Beschorner R, Ehmann C et al. Neuroprotective effects of erythropoietin during deep hypothermic circulatory arrest *Eur J Cardiothorac Surg*. 2010;37:662–668.

Off-Pump and On-Pump Coronary Artery Surgery and the Brain

16

R. Peter Alston

16.1 Introduction

Since its introduction into clinical practice in the early 1950s, cardiopulmonary bypass (CPB) has been the keystone that enabled many millions of patients to undergo heart surgery around the world.[1] However, brain damage has long been recognized as a complication of heart surgery with CPB.[2–4] By the 1970s, major neurological complications were frequently associated with heart surgery with an incidence of 19%.[5] In the intervening years, the incidences of major neurological complications have fallen to very low levels and, currently, less than two percent of patients undergoing coronary artery bypass grafting (CABG) surgery will develop strokes.[6–8] Nevertheless, with the burgeoning of CABG surgery in the 1980s, it became increasingly recognized that heart surgery was very commonly associated with another form of brain damage, cognitive decline, as almost 80% of patient had decrements in the early postoperative period following surgery.[9] Today, about 20–40% of patients undergoing CABG surgery will experience long-term cognitive decline, defined as 1 month or longer after surgery.[10–13] This form of brain damage is now so widely attributed to CPB that it is commonly referred to as "pump head," being a reference to the pump that is used to mechanically drive the blood around the body.[14] A news item in 2008 even cited the CPB used for his CABG surgery as the cause of former President Bill Clinton's uncharacteristic behavior when he was easily angered by hecklers and made factual mistakes and racial slurs while aggressively defending his wife, Hillary Clinton, and her campaign for presidency.[15]

Given that stroke and cognitive decline had been so firmly associated with the traditional use of CPB, a change from on- to off-pump CABG surgery has been widely advocated in recent years on the basis of preventing brain damage.[16] What evidence exists to support this contention? Remarkably, in a book on brain damage and heart surgery published in 2000, there was only one paragraph addressing off-pump CABG surgery and brain damage.[17] This paucity of information reflected the limited research available at that time comparing neurological and cognitive outcomes after off- and on-pump CABG surgery. In the intervening years, a rapidly increasing number of studies have compared the effects of off- and on-pump CABG surgery on the brain and there is now a large body of evidence relating to stroke and a moderate amount of information relating to cognition.

Initially, the results of published studies often supported the hypothesis that off-pump resulted in a lower incidence of stroke than on-pump CABG surgery.[18–21] Undertaken by pioneers who were likely enthusiasts for off-pump CABG surgery, these studies were extremely prone to selection bias, by the very nature of their observational and retrospective designs, and this greatly limited their interpretation. Subsequently, randomized controlled trials (RCTs), that greatly reduce selection bias, were undertaken examining cognitive outcomes as well as stroke, but the findings of these studies have been conflicting.[22–29] In addition, many of these RCTs had small populations and thus were underpowered and prone to Type II statistical error. To overcome these limitations, relevant RCTs have been subjected to systematic review and meta-analyses.[6–8,30–38]

R.P. Alston
Department of Anaesthesia, Critical Care and Pain Medicine, Royal Infirmary of Edinburgh, Edinburgh, Scotland, UK
e-mail: peter.alston@ed.ac.uk

R.S. Bonser et al. (eds.), *Brain Protection in Cardiac Surgery*,
DOI: 10.1007/978-1-84996-293-3_16, © Springer-Verlag London Limited 2011

The primary aim of this chapter is to review the published evidence base from these systematic reviews and meta-analyses to determine whether or not there are differences between off-pump and on-pump CABG surgery on neurological and cognitive outcomes. It will also review three RCTs examining cognitive outcome that were either published after the most recent meta-analyses or omitted from them.[29,39,40]

RCTs and meta-analyses were identified by searching MEDLINE, EMBASE, CINHAL, and the Cochrane databases using search algorithms, developed by the Scottish Intercollegiate Guideline Network (SIGN), including MESH terms for CABG and off-pump surgery.[41] Observational studies will only be considered in this chapter when seeking explanation for the findings of these meta-analyses and RCTs and to examine potential differences in pathophysiology. Before exploring the evidence on cerebral outcome, this chapter will first briefly review why there could be differences in adverse effects on the brain between off- and on-pump techniques.

16.2 Differences in Cerebral Pathophysiology Between Off- and On-Pump CABG Surgery

Over the years numerous mechanisms of injury have been associated with, or hypothesized as a cause of, brain damage following on-pump CABG surgery. As these have already been extensively reviewed in earlier chapters and elsewhere, this section will briefly review only cerebral hypoperfusion and emboli as the two major factors that may differ between off- and on-pump techniques[42] (Table 16.1).

Table 16.1 Putative differences in likelihood of mechanisms of brain injury during off- and on-pump coronary artery bypass grafting (CABG) surgery

Mechanism	On-pump CABG surgery	Off-pump CABG surgery
Dislocation of the heart	+	++
Non-pulsatile flow	++	–
Acid–base management	++	–
Hemodilution	++	–
Hyperthermia	++	–
CVP	+	–
Micro-emboli	++	–
Macro-emboli	++	+

unlikely, + likely, ++ very likely interval

16.2.1 *Cerebral Hypoperfusion*

Brain damage associated with CABG surgery has long been attributed to cerebral hypoperfusion during CPB. Cerebral hypoperfusion, as estimated by a jugular bulb oxyhemoglobin saturation < 50%, occurs frequently during on-pump CABG surgery.[10,12] However, this is not unique to on-pump techniques; not only does cerebral hypoperfusion also occur during off-pump CABG surgery but it occurs far more frequently than during on-pump CABG surgery.[43] There are a number of putative mechanisms that may be the cause of this cerebral hypoperfusion.

16.2.1.1 Dislocation of the Heart

The profound effects that off-pump CABG surgery has on heart function have been reviewed elsewhere.[44] Low cardiac output and hypotension during dislocation of the heart for grafting of the distal ends of the coronary anastomoses seem likely reasons why cerebral hypoperfusion is more common in off- than on-pump CABG surgery. Cerebral perfusion pressure depends on the difference between mean arterial and central venous pressures, so central venous hypertension can also cause cerebral hypoperfusion.[16] Venous return to the heart may become obstructed during off-pump manipulations causing central venous hypertension. However, this can sometimes also occur during on-pump CABG surgery as dislocation of the heart may be necessary to access the coronary arteries for grafting, particularly those on the posterior of the heart. So, dislocation of the heart may occur with both techniques causing cerebral hypoperfusion but is more likely during off- than on-pump CABG surgery.[43]

16.2.1.2 Cerebral Hyperthermia

Although a recent meta-analysis no longer supports the value of this technique, it was traditional to induce systemic hypothermia for organ protection, including the brain, during CPB.[45] As a consequence of induced hypothermia, the patient had to be rewarmed to normothermia or even mild hyperthermia, toward the end of CPB. However, too rapid rewarming from hypothermia has been associated with an adverse cognitive outcome.[46] The increased cerebral oxygen demand resulting from hyperthermia may outstrip oxygen delivery as it may be limited by a fixed cerebral blood flow. As a consequence, cerebral ischemia and resultant brain damage may occur. During off-pump CABG surgery normothermia is standard and rapid systemic rewarming should not occur, so cerebral hyperthermia is thus unlikely. As it is now recommended that rapid rewarming should be avoided to minimize the possibility of cerebral hyperthermia, this may no longer be a factor in on-pump CABG surgery but rewarming remains an important difference between the techniques when systemic hypothermia is used with CPB.[47]

16.2.1.3 Hemodilution

On commencement of CPB, the 2–3 L of crystalloid or colloid fluid that is used to prime the circuit mixes with the patient's circulating blood volume of approximately 5 L, causing marked dilution of the blood. This initial hemodilution is compounded by the addition of further crystalloid or colloid fluid during CPB to replace blood loss and maintain the circulating volume. The resultant hemodilution, by reducing the oxygen-carrying capacity of blood, may also be a cause of cerebral hypoperfusion. Indeed, Mathew and colleagues have found profound hemodilution during on-pump CABG surgery to be associated with adverse cognitive outcome in elderly patients.[48] By contrast, in a large observational study, hemodilution was not associated with stroke.[49] So what little evidence that exists regarding hemodilution is conflicting as far as cognition and stroke is concerned. However, hemodilution is a distinct difference between techniques as it is standard for on-pump and not used for off-pump CABG surgery and it has the potential to be a mechanism for cerebral hypoperfusion.

16.2.1.4 Character of Blood Flow

When bubble oxygenators were used, it was relatively easy to generate a pump flow during CPB that was pulsatile in character. Today, most CPB is conducted using membrane oxygenators and because of the complex technical difficulties required to achieve pulsatile flow, non-pulsatile flow is now standard.[50] Pulsatility, through a number of different mechanisms, may enhance blood flow in the cerebral microcirculation and so should improve cerebral outcome.[51–53] However, studies comparing the effects of pulsatile and non-pulsatile flow on neurological outcome have been reviewed and their results are conflicting.[42] In addition, one study indicates that pulsatile flow does not appear to influence cognitive outcome during on-pump CABG surgery.[54] However, non-pulsatile flow during on-pump CABG is yet another distinct physiological difference from off-pump CABG surgery when the heart is beating and, therefore, the blood flow is pulsatile. The lack of pulsatile flow during on-pump CABG surgery may cause cerebral hypoperfusion and, potentially, brain damage.

16.2.1.5 Acid–Base Management

In the past, two very different methods of acid–base management during hypothermic CPB existed. These were pH-stat and α-stat and their effects on cerebral blood flow are very different. In contrast to α-stat which preserves autoregulation, pH-stat acid–base management during hypothermia results in the loss of autoregulation and instead cerebral blood flow is pressure passive.[55] Moreover, compared to α-stat, pH-stat acid–base management has been found to have an adverse effect on cognitive outcome in elderly patients undergoing on-pump CABG surgery.[54] However, α-stat is now the recommended approach to acid–base management for on-pump CABG surgery.[47] During off-pump CABG surgery, there is no divergence of approach to acid–base management as patients are maintained normothermic and, therefore, acid–base management should not influence cerebral outcome. Currently, with the use of α(alpha)-stat during hypothermic CPB, it would seem unlikely that acid–base management is an important factor in differences in cerebral outcome between off- and on-pump CABG surgery.

16.2.2 Cerebral Embolization

Although cerebral hypoperfusion has been associated with brain damage following CABG surgery, cerebral embolization is an important alternative mechanism of injury or, even, an additional one.

16.2.2.1 Macro-Emboli

Strokes occurring during on-pump CABG surgery may be caused by cerebral macro-emboli dislodged from atheromatous plaques in the ascending aorta as a result of surgical manipulations such as cross-clamping, side-clamping and cannulation.[56] Aortic cross-clamping and cannulation are not required in off-pump CABG surgery and so there should be much less likelihood of dislodgement of atheromatous plaques and their embolization to the brain. However, during off-pump CABG surgery, side-clamping may still be used during the anastomoses of the proximal ends of vein or free arterial grafts so aortic manipulation may not be completely eliminated, unless the surgeon uses a total arterial grafting technique.[57,58] In addition, epi-aortic ultrasound scanning is increasingly being used to guide placement of the aortic cannula and clamps and this may reduce the incidence of macro-emboli and stroke during on-pump CABG surgery.[59] Nevertheless, manipulation and instrumentation of the ascending aorta will generally be far less with off-compared to on-pump CABG and this could have an important influence on cerebral outcome.

16.2.2.2 Micro-Emboli

In the past, high micro-emboli counts have been clearly associated with adverse cognitive outcome during on-pump CABG surgery.[60,61] Micro-embolization is a clear biological mechanism of injury and an important difference between the two techniques as the numbers of cerebral micro-emboli are exponentially greater during on-pump compared to off-pump CABG surgery.[20,29] Less surgical manipulation of the aorta, such as cross-clamping, along with the absence of the "sandblasting" effect of blood exiting the aortic cannula are likely explanations for this difference in the numbers of cerebral micro-emboli.[42,62,63] Theoretically, as with stroke, the use of epi-aortic scanning of the ascending aorta during on-pump CABG surgery to direct surgical manipulations should reduce disruption of atheromatous plaques and, thereby, reduce cerebral micro-embolization. Unfortunately, no reduction in the numbers of micro-emboli reaching the brain has been found using epi-aortic scanning and it is, consequently, unlikely to influence cognitive outcome.[64] Therefore, patients undergoing on-pump CABG surgery will continue to experience far greater numbers of cerebral micro-emboli and so should have more cerebral damage than those undergoing off-pump CABG surgery. Curiously, as will be discussed further in Sect 16.3.3.5, the association between cerebral micro-emboli and cognitive outcome after off- or on-pump CABG surgery is far less clear than this underlying hypothesis would suggest.

16.2.3 Summary of Differences in Cerebral Pathophysiology

Without doubt, there are a number of profound differences in the pathophysiological effects on the brain between off- and on-pump CABG surgery. While the relative importance of each of these factors is hard to estimate, the bulk of evidence indicates that on-pump causes far more physiological derangements to the brain than off-pump CABG surgery. On this basis, on-pump should be more liable to injure the brain, causing more strokes and cognitive decline than off-pump CABG surgery. However, the increased incidence of cerebral hypoperfusion associated with off-pump techniques gives concern that it may not be a completely benign procedure for the brain.

Although there are profound differences between off- and on-pump CABG surgery, one has to be very wary of simply translating these marked physiological differences into expected effects on patient outcomes from surgery. For example, COX-2 analgesics were initially highly promoted because they had a pharmacological profile that indicated they should have all the analgesic benefits of the nonspecific COX inhibitors with a far better safety profile. In reality, when the outcome of one, valdecoxib and its pro-drug parecoxib, were tested using RCTs in patients undergoing CABG surgery, the safety profile gave cause for concern and, in particular, it was associated with an increased incidence of thrombotic adverse events.[65,66]

16.3 Cerebral Outcomes: "T'ain't What You Do (It's the Way That You Do It)"

Comparison of the effects of off- and on-pump CABG surgery on the brain is not a simple question of black and white, as to focus only on CPB versus no CPB fails to take into account other important variations in surgical practice. Indeed, the day any two surgeons are found to apply exactly the same surgical techniques will be a notable one! Even with study protocols, surgical techniques vary greatly for both off- and on-pump CABG surgery and this increases variance within studies. This problem with internal validity can be overcome by small studies undertaken by a single surgeon.[24] Unfortunately, such studies have less external validity, as they are less generalizable to clinical practice. The variation in surgical technique creates even greater problems when considering and comparing results from different studies. For example, how the surgeon manipulates and clamps the ascending aorta, both for off- and on-pump CABG surgery, varies greatly and such differences in technique may have an important bearing on the amount of emboli that are generated and, thus, on cerebral damage.

As they have been reviewed elsewhere in this book, this chapter will not consider the influence of all the possible differences in surgical techniques as well as anesthesia and CPB that may affect cerebral outcome. However, the reader should be mindful when assessing the findings of RCTs and meta-analyses that additional, and potentially important, unidentified predictors of cerebral outcome may exist, other than simply the use of CPB or not. This limitation aside, RCTs and meta-analyses are our best source of information regarding the effects of CPB on cerebral outcome.

16.3.1 Methodology

Well-designed and conducted RCTs are the most reliable source of evidence as they limit the influence of bias on the results. There have been a large number of RCTs investigating CABG surgery and stroke. However, given the low incidence of stroke, none of the published studies have had the statistical power, in terms of sample size, required to determine this outcome.[34] By contrast, because the incidence of decrements is far higher than that of stroke, the studies that have examined cognitive outcome have largely been more appropriately powered. Nevertheless, probably because cognitive testing is far more resource intensive than simply recording the clinical outcome of stroke, there are only a few studies in this field (Table 16.2). The most recent meta-analysis could only identify a maximum of seven eligible studies while the earlier ones were based on three or fewer studies.[34,36,38] In addition, there is considerable variance in the incidence of cognitive decline between the studies due, at least in part, to the use of different definitions and timings of testing.[34]

Notwithstanding these limitations, the nine published systematic reviews and meta-analyses comparing outcome of stroke, or composite outcomes that include stroke, between off- and on-pump CABG surgery and the four comparing cognitive outcome were all examined for this review. The problems, outlined above, make their interpretation difficult and the role of methodological differences in explaining the conflicting findings will be discussed in more detail later in this chapter. This review also includes two RCTs comparing cognitive outcome, published since the most recent meta-analyses were undertaken, and one that was excluded because statistical analysis was continuous rather than categorical.[29,39,40]

16.3.2 Stroke

Cerebral vascular accidents after heart surgery may manifest in major ways that are clinically obvious including encephalopathy and visual, sensory and motor loss. For the purpose of this chapter, these major neurological outcomes will be grouped together under the general term of stroke, as this has been the approach taken by most papers. Formerly a more frequent complication, the incidence of stroke is now very low in patients undergoing isolated CABG surgery and recent RCTs report rates of about 2% or less.[6–8] Remarkably, many less obvious neurological changes are rarely documented as, with careful examination, new minor deficits, including motor and sensory loss, visual field defects, cerebellar signs and primitive reflexes, will be found in 50% or more of patients who undergo on-pump CABG surgery.[67,68] These subtle neurological deficits, although potentially important, have been infrequently investigated and no comparison of off- and on-pump CABG surgery has been undertaken. Moreover, although the incidence is very low, stroke greatly impairs quality of life and has a major impact on hospital resources as rehabilitation therapy and prolonged hospital stay are required (Chapt. 4). For these

Table 16.2 Meta-analyses comparing cognitive outcome between off- and on-pump coronary artery bypass grafting surgery

Year	Meta-analysis	Time period of cognitive testing after surgery									Comments
		Early			Medium			Late			
		n (*N*)	Actual TP	Estimate	*n* (*N*)	Actual TP	Estimate	*n* (*N*)	Actual TP	Estimate	
2005	Puskas et al.[36]	3 (335)	<2 week	OR 0.57 (0.21, 1.54)	3 (393)	2–6 mo	OR 0.56 (0.35, 0.89)	2 (334)	1 y	0.91 (0.57, 1.46)	Duplicate publication
2005	Cheng et al.[34]	3 (335)	<30 d	OR 0.57 (0.21, 1.54)	3 (393)	2–6 mo	OR 0.56 (0.35, 0.89)	2 (334)	1–2 y	OR 0.91 (0.57, 1.46)	Duplicate publication
2007	Takagi et al.[37]	5 (NP)	<2 week	RD–27% (–67%, 14%)	6 (NP)	1–3 mo	RD –9% (–16%, –2%)	4 (NP)	6–12 mo	RD –1% (–9%, 7%)	
2008	Marasco et al.[38]										
	Rey Auditory				5 (547)	<3 mo	WMD –0.16 (–1.83, 1.52)	4 (490)	>6 mo	WMD –1.03 (–2.84, 0.78)	
	Grooved pegboard				5 (547)	<3 mo	WMD –2.05 (–5.16, 1.06)	4 (490)	>6 mo	WMD –2.41 (–5.67, 0.84)	
	Trails A				6 (448)	<3 mo	WMD–2.62 (–4.79, –0.44)	5 (357)	>6 mo	WMD –4.96 (–7.35, –2.57)	
	Trails B				7 (696)	<3 mo	WMD –2.62 (–7.18, 1.94)	6 (617)	>6 mo	WMD 1.06 (–2.94, 5.06)	
	Digit Symbol				7 (614)	<3 mo	WMD 1.61 (–4.44, 1.22)	5 (559)	>6 mo	WMD –0.73 (–3.20, 1.73)	

n: number of trials, *N*: number of patients, Actual TP: Actual time period, NP: not presented, OR (): odds ratio (95% confidence interval), RD (): risk difference (95% confidence interval), WMD (): weighted mean difference (95% confidence interval), d: days, y: year, mo: months reasons this section will focus on stroke and will only review the differences in the incidence of stroke between off- and on-pump CABG surgery.

In recent years, nine systematic reviews and meta-analyses have compared the incidence of stroke between off- and on-pump CABG surgery and, although some have found significant differences in incidence, this is by no means the case for all (Table 16.2). Reston and colleagues undertook a systematic review and meta-analyses of a number of different outcomes including stroke.[30] Compared to on-pump, they found off-pump CABG surgery was associated with almost half the incidence of stroke (odds ratio [OR] 0.55, 95% confidence interval [95% CI] 0.43–0.69). A meta-analysis, undertaken for the International Society for Minimally Invasive Cardiothoracic Surgery (ISMICS) in 2004 by Puskas and colleagues, compared a number of outcomes from off- and on-pump CABG surgery and found that off-pump CABG surgery was associated with a reduction in the incidence of stroke of more than half (OR 0.45, 95% CI 0.34–0.60).[36] Athanasiou and colleagues restricted their meta-analysis to patients aged 70 years or older and found that off-pump CABG surgery was associated with a marked reduction, of more than 60%, in the incidence of stroke (OR 0.38, 95% CI 0.22–0.65).[32] Together, these three independent meta-analyses strongly indicate that off-pump is associated with a significant reduction in the incidence of stroke compared to on-pump CABG surgery.

In contrast, neither Parolari and colleagues[31] nor van der Heijden and colleagues[33] concurred as both meta-analyses, using a composite outcome that included stroke, found only a nonsignificant trend toward a lower incidence of stroke with off-pump CABG surgery.[31,33] A methodological difference, between these and the meta-analyses that found a statistically significant difference, relates to the inclusion or exclusion of observational studies. Wijeysundera and colleagues have argued that, in addition to economic considerations, observational research has important advantages over RCTs as all patients, including high risk, are included and the results are therefore more generalizable.[8] Nevertheless, problems with confounding and selection bias far outweigh these arguments as they often distort the findings from observational studies and their meta-analysis can provide very precise but spurious results.[69]

Table 16.2 Meta-analyses comparing the incidence of stroke between off- and on-pump coronary artery bypass grafting surgery

Year	Meta-analysis	Number of studies	Number of patients	Statistic	Study designs included	Comments
2003	Reston et al.[30]	38	34,126	OR 0.55 (0.43, 0.69)	Obs/RCTs	
2003	Parolari et al.[31]	9	1,090	OR 0.48 (0.21, 1.09)	RCTs	Composite outcome including stroke
2004	van der Heijden[33]	18	1,584	OR 0.66 (0.38, 1.15)	RCTs	Composite outcome including stroke
2005	Puskas et al.[36]	37	24,353	OR 0.45 (0.34, 0.60)	Obs/RCTs	
2005	Athanasiou et al.[32]	9	4475	OR 0.38 (0.22, 0.65)	Obs/RCTs	Over 70 years
2005	Wijeysundera et al. a)[8]	15	290,621	OR 0.61 (0.55–0.68)	Obs	Only high quality studies
	Wijeysundera et al. b)[8]	12	2,968	OR 0.69 (0.29,1.67)	RCTs	Only high quality studies
2005	Cheng et al.[34]	21	2,859	OR 0.68 (0.33, 1.40)	RCTs	Trials reporting no events included
2006	Sedrakyan et al.[6]	27	3,062	OR 0.50 (0.27,0.93)	RCTs	Trials reporting no events excluded
2007	Takagi et al. a)[7]	32	3,714	RR 0.50 (0.26, 0.98)	RCTs	Trials reporting no events included
	Takagi et al. b)[7]	18	2,607	RR 0.60 (0.34, 1.06)	RCTs	Trials reporting no events excluded

Year: year of publication, OR: odds ratio, RR: relative risk, (): (95% confidence

The danger of including observational studies in meta-analysis is exemplified by the two studies that were limited to RCTs and found no significant reduction in incidence of stroke associated with off-pump CABG surgery.[31,33] The effect of bias introduced by using observational studies is further emphasized by Wijeysundera and colleagues who undertook two meta-analyses, comparing off- and on-pump CABG surgery, using either only RCTs or only observational studies.[8] The meta-analysis of high-quality observational studies found that a reduced incidence of stroke was significantly associated with off-pump CABG surgery (OR 0.61, 95% CI 0.55–0.68). In contrast, when only RCTs were used, no significant difference was found (OR 0.69, 95% CI 0.29–1.67).[8]

Nonetheless, the controversy continued with the publication of two more meta-analyses looking at stroke, even though both only considered RCTs. Although Cheng and colleagues[34] reported no significant difference (OR 0.68, 95% CI 0.33–1.40), Sedrakyan and colleagues[6] reported a 50% reduction in the incidence of stroke in patients undergoing off-pump compared to on-pump CABG surgery (OR 0.50, 95% CI 0.27–0.93). The conflicting findings of these two meta-analyses are surprising as they analyzed papers from similar time periods and both applied seemingly robust methodology.

The most recently published meta-analysis by Takagi and colleagues, including literature up until March 2007, gives insight into why the findings of the meta-analyses by Sedrakyan and colleagues and Cheng and colleagues are conflicting.[7] Takagi and colleagues identified 32 trials containing a total of 3,714 patients. Pooled analysis of these results found the incidence of stroke was not significantly different in off-pump compared to on-pump CABG surgery (0.49% vs. 1.29%, relative risk [RR] 0.60, 95% CI 0.34–1.06). They found neither heterogeneity of trial results nor evidence of publication bias. When they re-analyzed the data using only studies that had at least one stroke in either the off- or on-pump CABG surgery groups, there remained 18 studies with only 2607 patients. Their re-analysis found that off-pump was associated with a 50% reduction in stroke rate compared to on-pump CABG surgery (0.69% vs. 1.85%, RR 0.50, 95% CI 0.26–0.98). So exclusion of 14 studies that reported no strokes and contained about 30% of the original patient population changed the results from being statistically nonsignificant into one that is clinically and statistically significant.

Thus, excluding studies that had no event rates inflated the statistical estimation and falsely increased the apparent risk of stroke. While Takagi and colleagues' meta-analysis has important limitations because the reporting of methodology is extremely limited, it offers a clear methodological explanation for the discrepancy in findings between the meta-analyses by Sedrakyan and colleagues and Cheng and colleagues as the former only assessed studies that had at least one stroke in either group and so found a significant effect whereas the latter included all studies and found no significant difference.[6,7,34]

Clearly this series of meta-analyses demonstrate that methodological rigor is paramount. Including observational studies of stroke associated with CABG surgery introduced bias and performing meta-analysis upon them produced precise but false results.[69] As in other areas of research in cardiothoracic anesthesia and surgery, clinically important differences tend to vanish like snow in spring when meta-analyses exclude observational studies and use only RCTs.[70] Even when only RCTs are used, the outcome of meta-analyses can be fundamentally different when a large amount of important data is omitted from analysis. In addition to the aspects already discussed, covert duplicate publication was a further methodological limitation that was identified by Cheng and colleagues in two of the meta-analyses as both Reston and colleagues and Parolari and colleagues included three duplicate reports of the same study populations.[30,31,34,71]

Where then does this leave our understanding about the differences between off- and on-pump CABG surgery on the incidence of stroke? Without an RCT with sufficient statistical power, we are unlikely to have a definitive answer and, given the impractically large patient sample that this would require, it is not anticipated that this will occur in the near future.[32,34] Until then, we will have to make do with meta-analyses of smaller trials and the current best evidence is that there is no significant difference in the incidence of stroke between off- and on-pump CABG surgery.

16.3.3 Cognition

While stroke is an infrequent adverse event after heart surgery, cognitive decrement is common. Decrements are, initially, extremely frequent and have been reported in the early postoperative period in up to 90% of patients undergoing CABG surgery.[11] Apart from surgery, there are many reasons why they might be so common in the first few postoperative weeks, including pain, analgesia, and sleep disturbances, and their importance in this time period is therefore limited. However, Newman and colleagues found that early decrements predict long-term cognitive outcome for up to 5 years after surgery.[13] While long-term cognitive decrements, defined as those present at 1 or more months after surgery occur much less frequently than early ones, they are estimated to affect about 20–40% of patients and are of far greater concern as they are believed to be permanent.[10,11,13]

In contrast to stroke, few RCTs have examined cognitive outcome and those that have often used different definitions of cognitive decline, which may have influenced their findings.[72] It is, therefore, unsurprising that there are only four published systematic reviews and meta-analyses examining cognitive outcome and, as two are duplicate publications, essentially there are only three (Table 16.3).[34,36–38] Cheng and colleagues and Puskas and colleagues report the same meta-analyses and, as the former is more fully reported than the later, it will be the only paper of the two that will be referenced henceforth.[34,36] Comparison of the three meta-analyses is difficult as the authors have taken different approaches to the selection of RCTs, to grouping the timings of cognitive testing and, very importantly, to the statistical analysis. In particular, Cheng and colleagues[34] and Takagi and colleagues[37] used incidences of dichotomized definitions of cognitive decline and Marasco and colleagues[38] used a continuous statistical approach.

16.3.3.1 Dichotomized Cognitive Outcomes

The meta-analyses that used categorical outcomes have three broad time periods of cognitive testing following surgery, early: less than 2 weeks or 1 month, medium: 1–6-months, and late: 6-months to 2-years. (Table 16.3) The reason why the studies used these time periods is unclear but probably reflects the underlying lack of a standardized approach to cognitive testing in the RCTs that were analyzed. Despite important inconsistencies in methodology, the two meta-analyses that used a dichotomized definition of cognitive decline have very similar findings.[34,37] In summary, they indicate that less than a month postoperatively there is no difference in the incidence of cognitive decline between off- and on-pump CABG surgery. Beyond a month and up to 6-months, off-pump surgery is associated with a significantly lower incidence of cognitive decline. After 6-months and up to about 2-years postoperatively, any differences have disappeared and there is no significant difference in incidence of cognitive decline between off- and on-pump CABG surgery.

16.3.3.2 Continuous Cognitive Outcomes

As difficult as these temporal differences in incidences are to explain, they would at least appear to be supported by two independent meta-analyses. However, their results become questionable once the third and most recent meta-analysis by Marasco and colleagues is examined.[38] Importantly, this meta-analysis uses a fundamentally different methodological approach from the previous two. Most studies have assessed cognition using a battery of tests that each result in a continuous measurement of outcome, for example, the time to undertake a specified task. Investigators have then dichotomized these continuous measures into impairment/no impairment using definitions such as one standard deviation. They then statistically compared the incidence of patients defined as having cognitive decrements between groups.

The author has heard David Stump state that a dichotomous approach to analysis of continuous data was originally taken to simplify grant applications for assessors in the early days of investigating heart surgery's effect on cognition. However, not only are the levels of these definitions completely arbitrary but such dichotomization of a continuous measurement has inherent statistical flaws and, in particular, when related to cognitive assessment produces spurious results.[73,74] For further information on this commonly repeated methodological flaw in cognitive assessment, readers are referred to the extensive review on the subject by MacCallum and colleagues.[73] Indeed, the methodology used in the meta-analysis by Takagi and colleagues has been criticized by Motallebzadeh and Jahangiri on the grounds that their use of dichotomized definitions is open to regression to the mean and increases variance because of the wide range of definitions of cognitive decrement between studies as well as the loss of important statistical information.[75] For these reasons, the most recent meta-analysis by Marasco and colleagues is of interest as it uses the continuous measurements of the cognitive tests rather than the incidences of cognitive impairment that have been defined by different arbitrary definitions.[38]

Marasco and colleagues were able to extract data to analyze five tests of cognition – four of which are recommended in a consensus statement – including Rey Auditory Learning, grooved pegboard, Trail Making A and B, and digit symbol.[38,76]

With the exception of Trail Making A, they could find no significant difference between off- and on-pump CABG surgery in any of the tests at any of the testing periods. In both time periods, Trail Making A was significantly better in patients having off- rather than on-pump CABG surgery. This is a curious finding because Trail Making B is an inherently harder test than Trail Making A and, therefore, is usually the more discriminating test (Ian Deary, personal e-mail communication). However, this meta-analysis also has limitations. The authors undertook multiple analyses of the individual cognitive tests and will thus have inflated the chance of a Type I statistical error and hence of finding a significant result. A more robust approach would have been to create a summary score of results to give a single overall measure of cognition.[10,29,77] Another difficulty with interpreting this study is that the authors have, without explanation, divided the time periods of cognitive testing into two, early (less than 3 months) and late (6 or more months) following surgery. This is different from the two categorical meta-analyses that used three time periods and seems just as arbitrary when presented without a scientific rationale. Notwithstanding these limitations, their approach to meta-analysis is far more highly powered statistically to detect very small differences between the groups than the two meta-analyses that used incidence of categorical definitions of cognitive decline.

When only the two meta-analyses that used a dichotomized definition of cognitive decline as the basis of their analyses are considered, it appears that the only difference in cognitive decrements occurs between 1 and 6 months postoperatively and that off-pump is associated with a lower incidence than on-pump CABG surgery.[34,37] At less than a month, or beyond 6 months postoperatively, there is no significant difference in cognition between off- and on-pump CABG surgery. Alternatively, if one considers only the meta-analysis by Marasco and colleagues, where continuous rather than dichotomized data were analyzed, there are no significant differences, with the exception of one test of cognition that is difficult to explain, regardless of the time after surgery.[38]

16.3.3.3 Randomized Controlled Trials

The meta-analysis by Takagi and colleagues did not include an RCT by Motallebzadeh and colleagues because data were analyzed as continua and incidences of cognitive decline were not reported.[29,37,78] Despite handling the data as continua, this RCT was also excluded from the meta-analysis by Marasco and colleagues because it reported only an overall summary score and did not provide the scores of the individual cognitive tests.[29,38] Importantly, using an overall summary measure of the cognitive tests and analyzing continuous data, Motallebzadeh and colleagues found that, although off-pump surgery was associated with better cognition at discharge from hospital, there were no significant differences between off- and on-pump CABG surgery at 6 weeks and 6 months postoperatively.[29]

Because the study by Hernandez and colleagues was not published until December 2007 and so beyond the final dates of their literature searches, it was not included in either the meta-analyses by Takagi and colleagues or Marasco and colleagues.[37–39] The authors found no significant differences between off- and on-pump CABG surgery in the incidence of cognitive decline at discharge from hospital (risk ratio [RR] 0.83, 95% CI 0.65–1.07) nor at 6 months after surgery (RR 0.94, 95% CI 0.70–1.28).

The third and most recent RCT by Tully and colleagues comparing cognitive outcome at 6 days and 6 months was published in August 2008 and so has not been included in any of the meta-analyses.[40] An accompanying editorial by Phillips-Bute and Mathew identifies a number of methodological limitations, the most important of which is the very small sample size ($n = 66$) that was based on the use of an unrealistic effect size in the power calculation, the use of a dichotomous definition of cognitive decline and multiple testing.[79] However, this study has several merits in that a control group who did not undergo CABG surgery was included and learning effects, measurement error and regression to the mean as well as differences in demographic characteristics were controlled statistically. While both groups experienced decrements, this study could find no difference in cognitive outcome at 6 days or 6 months between patients who had off- or on-pump CABG surgery.[40] While the cognitive outcome at hospital discharge differs, these three recent RCTs support the meta-analyses that have found no difference in cognitive deficits between off- and on-pump CABG surgery 6 months to a year post-operatively.[37,38,40]

16.3.3.4 Cognition More than 2 Years Postoperatively

A 5-year follow-up study by van Dijk and colleagues is the first to investigate any difference in cognitive outcome between off- and on-pump CABG surgery beyond 2 years postoperatively.[80] Using a dichotomized definition of 20% decline in performance in 20% of the cognitive test variables, they found no significant difference between off- and on-pump CABG surgery (absolute difference, 0% [95% CI 12.7–12.6%]). Interestingly, approximately 50% of patients in both groups had cognitive decrements and, as discussed further below, this points to a similar underlying cause. Therefore, although the only study comparing cognitive outcome at more than 2 years postoperatively found significant incidence of cognitive decline, the authors found no difference in outcomes between off- and on-pump CABG surgery.

16.3.3.5 Physiological Differences and Cognitive Outcome

Micro-emboli have long been believed to be the cause of cognitive deficits after on-pump CABG surgery. Indeed, landmark studies did find that the numbers of micro-emboli were associated to the incidence of cognitive deficits.[60,61] However, the techniques of CPB and surgery have changed and, for example, membrane rather than bubble oxygenators are now used and the numbers of micro-emboli generated are probably far less.[81,82] More importantly, while a recent RCT by Motallebzadeh and colleagues found that off-pump surgery resulted in significantly fewer cerebral micro-emboli than on-pump CABG surgery, the only significant association of micro-emboli counts with cognitive outcome was at discharge from hospital and there were no significant associations with cognition at 6 weeks or 6 months.[29] Thus the findings from Motallebzadeh and colleagues support the increasing body of evidence that there is no difference in long-term cognitive outcome between off- and on-pump CABG surgery and suggest a greatly diminished role for micro-emboli as an important cause of cognitive decrement.

16.3.3.6 CPB is Not a Cause of Cognitive Decrements

If there are no differences between off- and on-pump CABG surgery, what explanations are there for the long recognized association between cognitive outcome and CABG surgery? Newman and colleagues found that decline in cognition at 5 years after on-pump CABG surgery occurs in about 40% of patients.[13] Importantly, their study had no control group so it could not rule out the possibility that the cognitive decline was the result of underlying cardiovascular disease rather than CPB. Selnes and colleagues have recently reported a longitudinal observational study examining patients 6-years after CABG surgery that included a control group of patients with coronary artery disease, diagnosed by angiography, but who underwent only medical therapy.[83] They could find no significant difference in cognitive decline between patients who had on-pump CABG surgery and the medical control group after 6 years and concluded that long-term cognitive decline was not specific to the use of CPB. Currently, this would seem the most plausible explanation for the lack of any difference between off- and on-pump CABG surgery.

Indeed, as discussed earlier, the conclusion of the observational study by Selnes and colleagues is supported by the RCT by van Dijk and colleagues who found a 50% incidence of cognitive decline 5-years after surgery, whether performed off- or on-pump.[80] Furthermore, Wahrborg and colleagues, in an observational study comparing patients who were randomized to CABG surgery or percutaneous coronary intervention (PCI), found no significant difference in cognitive outcome between the groups at 6 and 12 months after the interventions.[84] Therefore, whatever the effect of surgical intervention for coronary artery disease, it is far outweighed by a more important determinant of long-term cognitive decline.

Cardiovascular disease may then seem the likely culprit for this cognitive decline as Aleman and colleagues have demonstrated that vascular risk factors predict performance on some cognitive tests.[85] However, it may not even be cardiovascular disease as van Dijk and colleagues have compared their combined off- and on- pump CABG surgery patients with a control group that had no cardiovascular disease and found no significant difference in the incidence of cognitive decline.[86] While the study has a number of important limitations, including lower baseline in the CABG surgery group and multiple confounding differences between groups that had to be statistically adjusted for, it is the largest study yet published and has a very low attrition rate. This study by van Dijk and colleagues indicates that a factor other than cardiovascular disease may determine cognitive decline. Whatever causes long-term cognitive decline, it appears not to be CABG surgery whether performed off- or on-pump.

16.4 Conclusions

This chapter has reviewed the evidence base from systematic reviews and meta-analyses as well as three recent RCTs to determine whether or not using CPB for CABG surgery affects cerebral outcome in the form of stroke and cognitive decrements. With regard to stroke, meta-analyses that included observational studies and so introduced selection bias found off-pump CABG surgery to have a lower incidence of stroke. When only RCTs were included, this effect disappeared unless the meta-analyses were methodologically flawed by their exclusion of large numbers of patients from studies that had no event rates. Where methodology was robust, meta-analyses have not found any difference in the incidence of stroke between off- and on-pump CABG surgery.

As far as the cognitive outcome is concerned, meta-analyses and RCTs indicate that while there may or may not be differences in the first 6 months, there is no difference in cognitive outcome from 6 months to 5 years after surgery whether performed off- or on-pump. Moreover, a recent RCT and two observational studies indicate that CPB is not the cause of the long-term cognitive decline that is associated with CABG surgery and it may be the progression of the underlying cardiovascular disease or even some other unidentified factor.

Therefore, attributing Bill Clinton's uncharacteristic behavior to "pump head" appears to be without adequate foundation. According to current evidence, it is probably an example of a "COX-2 paradox" by translating pathophysiological differences into expected outcomes and assuming that the former inevitably predicts the latter. It is probably more likely that Bill Clinton's atypical conduct was caused by something other than the CPB used to perform his CABG surgery or even the surgery itself. Finally, as the current evidence base does not support any significant influence from CPB, the decision whether or not to undertake CABG surgery off- or on-pump should be based on outcomes other than stroke or cognition.

Acknowledgments I wish to thank Linda Alston for her assistance in preparing and proofing this chapter.

References

1. Gibbon JH Jr. Application of a mechanical heart and lung apparatus to cardiac surgery. *Minn Med.* 1954;37:171-185.
2. Javid H, Tufo HM, Najafi H, Dye WS, Hunter JA, Julian OC. Neurological abnormalities following open-heart surgery. *J Thorac Cardiovasc Surg.* 1969;58:502-509.
3. Gilman S. Cerebral disorders after open-heart operations. *N Engl J Med.* 1965;272:489-498.
4. Aberg T. Effect of open heart surgery on intellectual function. *Scand J Thorac Cardiovasc Surg Suppl.* 1974;15:1-63.
5. Branthwaite MA. Neurological damage related to open-heart surgery. A clinical survey. *Thorax.* 1972;27:748-753.
6. Sedrakyan A, Wu AW, Parashar A, Bass EB, Treasure T. Off-pump surgery is associated with reduced occurrence of stroke and other morbidity as compared with traditional coronary artery bypass grafting: a meta-analysis of systematically reviewed trials. *Stroke.* 2006;37:2759-2769.
7. Takagi H, Tanabashi T, Kawai N, Umemoto T. Off-pump surgery does not reduce stroke, compared with results of on-pump coronary artery bypass grafting: a meta-analysis of randomized clinical trials. *J Thorac Cardiovasc Surg.* 2007; 134:1059-1060.
8. Wijeysundera DN, Beattie WS, Djaiani G, et al. Off-pump coronary artery surgery for reducing mortality and morbidity: meta-analysis of randomized and observational studies. *J Am Coll Cardiol.* 2005;46:872-882.
9. Shaw PJ, Bates D, Cartlidge NE, et al. Neurologic and neuropsychological morbidity following major surgery: comparison of coronary artery bypass and peripheral vascular surgery. *Stroke.* 1987;18:700-707.
10. Robson MJ, Alston RP, Deary IJ, Andrews PJ, Souter MJ, Yates S. Cognition after coronary artery surgery is not related to postoperative jugular bulb oxyhemoglobin desaturation. *Anesth Analg.* 2000;91:1317-1326.
11. Roach GW, Newman MF, Murkin JM, et al. Ineffectiveness of burst suppression therapy in mitigating perioperative cerebrovascular dysfunction. Multicenter Study of Perioperative

Ischemia (McSPI) Research Group. *Anesthesiol.* 1999;90: 1255-1264.
12. Croughwell ND, Newman MF, Blumenthal JA, et al. Jugular bulb saturation and cognitive dysfunction after cardiopulmonary bypass. *Ann Thorac Surg.* 1994;58:1702-1708.
13. Newman MF, Kirchner JL, Phillips-Bute B, et al. Longitudinal assessment of neurocognitive function after coronary-artery bypass surgery. *N Engl J Med.* 2001;344:395-402.
14. Alston RP. Pumphead - or not! Does avoiding cardiopulmonary bypass for coronary artery bypass surgery result in less brain damage? *Br J Anaesth.* 2005;94:699-701.
15. McDougall J. Bill Clinton's madness: a consequence of heart-bypass surgery brain damage. Available at: http://www.drmcdougall.com/misc/2008Other/080412clinton.htm. Accessed June 29, 2008.
16. Murkin JM, Boyd WD, Ganapathy S, Adams SJ, Peterson RC. Beating heart surgery: why expect less central nervous system morbidity? *Ann Thorac Surg.* 1999;68:1498-1501.
17. Newman SP, Harrison MJG, Stump DA, Smith P, Taylor K. *The brain and cardiac surgery: causes of neurological complications and their prevention.* Amsterdam: Harwood Academic; 2000.
18. Al-Ruzzeh S, Nakamura K, Athanasiou T, et al. Does off-pump coronary artery bypass (OPCAB) surgery improve the outcome in high-risk patients? A comparative study of 1398 high-risk patients. *Eur J Cardiothorac Surg.* 2003;23:50-55.
19. Patel NC, Deodhar AP, Grayson AD, et al. Neurological outcomes in coronary surgery: independent effect of avoiding cardiopulmonary bypass. *Ann Thorac Surg.* 2002;74: 400-405.
20. Bowles BJ, Lee JD, Dang CR, et al. Coronary artery bypass performed without the use of cardiopulmonary bypass is associated with reduced cerebral microemboli and improved clinical results. *Chest.* 2001;119:25-30.
21. Puskas JD, Thourani VH, Marshall JJ, et al. Clinical outcomes, angiographic patency, and resource utilization in 200 consecutive off-pump coronary bypass patients. *Ann Thorac Surg.* 2001;71:1477-1483.
22. van Dijk D, Jansen EW, Hijman R, et al. Cognitive outcome after off-pump and on-pump coronary artery bypass graft surgery: a randomized trial. *JAMA.* 2002;287:1405-1412.
23. Lee JD, Lee SJ, Tsushima WT, et al. Benefits of off-pump bypass on neurologic and clinical morbidity: a prospective randomized trial. *Ann Thorac Surg.* 2003;76:18-25.
24. Zamvar V, Williams D, Hall J, et al. Assessment of neurocognitive impairment after off-pump and on-pump techniques for coronary artery bypass graft surgery: prospective randomized controlled trial. *BMJ.* 2002;325:1268.
25. Lund C, Sundet K, Tennoe B, et al. Cerebral ischemic injury and cognitive impairment after off-pump and on-pump coronary artery bypass grafting surgery. *Ann Thorac Surg.* 2005; 80:2126-2131.
26. Ernest CS, Worcester MU, Tatoulis J, et al. Neurocognitive outcomes in off-pump versus on-pump bypass surgery: a randomized controlled trial. *Ann Thorac Surg.* 2006;81: 2105-2114.
27. Vedin J, Nyman H, Ericsson A, Hylander S, Vaage J. Cognitive function after on or off pump coronary artery bypass grafting. *Eur J Cardiothorac Surg.* 2006;30:305-310.
28. Al-Ruzzeh S, George S, Bustami M, et al. Effect of off-pump coronary artery bypass surgery on clinical, angiographic, neurocognitive, and quality of life outcomes: randomized controlled trial. *BMJ.* 2006;332:1365.
29. Motallebzadeh R, Bland JM, Markus HS, Kaski JC, Jahangiri M. Neurocognitive function and cerebral emboli: randomized study of on-pump versus off-pump coronary artery bypass surgery. *Ann Thorac Surg.* 2007;83:475-482.
30. Reston JT, Tregear SJ, Turkelson CM. Meta-analysis of short-term and mid-term outcomes following off-pump coronary artery bypass grafting. *Ann Thorac Surg.* 2003;76:1510-1515.
31. Parolari A, Alamanni F, Cannata A, et al. Off-pump versus on-pump coronary artery bypass: meta-analysis of currently available randomized trials. *Ann Thorac Surg.* 2003;76: 37-40.
32. Athanasiou T, Al-Ruzzeh S, Kumar P, et al. Off-pump myocardial revascularization is associated with less incidence of stroke in elderly patients. *Ann Thorac Surg.* 2004;77:745-753.
33. van der Heijden GJ, Nathoe HM, Jansen EW, Grobbee DE. Meta-analysis on the effect of off-pump coronary bypass surgery. *Eur J Cardiothorac Surg.* 2004;26:81-84.
34. Cheng DC, Bainbridge D, Martin JE, Novick RJ. Does off-pump coronary artery bypass reduce mortality, morbidity, and resource utilization when compared with conventional coronary artery bypass? A meta-analysis of randomized trials. *Anesthesiol.* 2005;102:188-203.
35. Parolari A, Alamanni F, Polvani G, et al. Meta-analysis of randomized trials comparing off-pump with on-pump coronary artery bypass graft patency. *Ann Thorac Surg.* 2005;80:2121-2125.
36. Puskas J, Cheng D, Knight J, et al. Off-pump versus conventional coronary artery bypass grafting: a meta-analysis and consensus statement from the 2004 ISMICS Consensus Conference. *Innovations.* 2005;1:3-27.
37. Takagi H, Tanabashi T, Kawai N, Umemoto T. Cognitive decline after off-pump versus on-pump coronary artery bypass graft surgery: meta-analysis of randomized controlled trials. *J Thorac Cardiovasc Surg.* 2007;134:512-513.
38. Marasco SF, Sharwood LN, Abramson MJ. No improvement in neurocognitive outcomes after off-pump versus on-pump coronary revascularisation: a meta-analysis. *Eur J Cardiothorac Surg.* 2008;33:961-970.
39. Hernandez F Jr, Brown JR, Likosky DS, et al. Neurocognitive outcomes of off-pump versus on-pump coronary artery bypass: a prospective randomized controlled trial. *Ann Thorac Surg.* 2007;84:1897-1903.
40. Tully PJ, Baker RA, Kneebone AC, Knight JL. Neuropsychologic and quality-of-life outcomes after coronary artery bypass surgery with and without cardiopulmonary bypass: a prospective randomized trial. *J Cardiothorac Vasc Anesth.* 2008;22:515-521.
41. SIGN. Search filters. Available at: http://www.sign.ac.uk/methodology/filters.html. Accessed June 15, 2008.
42. Hogue CW Jr, Palin CA, Arrowsmith JE. Cardiopulmonary bypass management and neurologic outcomes: an evidence-based appraisal of current practices. *Anesth Analg.* 2006;103:21-37.
43. Diephuis JC, Moons KG, Nierich AN, Bruens M, van Dijk D, Kalkman CJ. Jugular bulb desaturation during coronary artery surgery: a comparison of off-pump and on-pump procedures. *Br J Anaesth.* 2005;94:715-720.
44. Chassot PG, van der Linden P, Zaugg M, Mueller XM, Spahn DR. Off-pump coronary artery bypass surgery:

physiology and anaesthetic management. *Br J Anaesth.* 2004;92:400-413.

45. Rees K, Beranek-Stanley M, Burke M, Ebrahim S. Hypothermia to reduce neurological damage following coronary artery bypass surgery Cochrane Database of Systematic Reviews 2005; Issue 1. Art. No.: DOI: 10.1002/14651858. CD002138.
46. Grigore AM, Grocott HP, Mathew JP, et al. The rewarming rate and increased peak temperature alter neurocognitive outcome after cardiac surgery. *Anesth Analg.* 2002;94:4-10.
47. Shann KG, Likosky DS, Murkin JM, et al. An evidence-based review of the practice of cardiopulmonary bypass in adults: a focus on neurologic injury, glycemic control, hemodilution, and the inflammatory response. *J Thorac Cardiovasc Surg.* 2006;132:283-290.
48. Mathew JP, Mackensen GB, Phillips-Bute B, et al. Effects of extreme hemodilution during cardiac surgery on cognitive function in the elderly. *Anesthesiology.* 2007;107:577-584.
49. DeFoe GR, Ross CS, Olmstead EM, et al. Lowest hematocrit on bypass and adverse outcomes associated with coronary artery bypass grafting. Northern New England Cardiovascular Disease Study Group. *Ann Thorac Surg.* 2001;71:769-776.
50. Gourlay T, Taylor KM. Pulsatile flow and membrane oxygenators. *Perfusion.* 1994;9:189-196.
51. Watanabe T, Orita H, Kobayashi M, Washio M. Brain tissue pH, oxygen tension, and carbon dioxide tension in profoundly hypothermic cardiopulmonary bypass. Comparative study of circulatory arrest, nonpulsatile low-flow perfusion, and pulsatile low-flow perfusion. *J Thorac Cardiovasc Surg.* 1989;97:396-401.
52. Undar A, Masai T, Beyer EA, Goddard-Finegold J, McGarry MC, Fraser CD Jr. Pediatric physiologic pulsatile pump enhances cerebral and renal blood flow during and after cardiopulmonary bypass. *Artif Organs.* 2002;26:919-923.
53. Mutch WA, Warrian RK, Eschun GM, et al. Biologically variable pulsation improves jugular venous oxygen saturation during rewarming. *Ann Thorac Surg.* 2000;69:491-497.
54. Murkin JM, Martzke JS, Buchan AM, Bentley C, Wong CJ. A randomized study of the influence of perfusion technique and pH management strategy in 316 patients undergoing coronary artery bypass surgery: II. neurologic and cognitive outcomes. *J Thorac Cardiovasc Surg.* 1995;110:349-362.
55. Murkin JM, Farrar JK, Tweed WA, McKenzie FN, Guiraudon G. Cerebral autoregulation and flow/metabolism coupling during cardiopulmonary bypass: the influence of $PaCO_2$. *Anesth Analg.* 1987;66:825-832.
56. Goto T, Baba T, Matsuyama K, Honma K, Ura M, Koshiji T. Aortic atherosclerosis and postoperative neurological dysfunction in elderly coronary surgical patients. *Ann Thorac Surg.* 2003;75:1912-1918.
57. Mariani MA, D'Alfonso A, Grandjean JG. Total arterial off-pump coronary surgery: time to change our habits? *Ann Thorac Surg.* 2004;78:1591-1597.
58. Legare JF, Hassan A, Buth KJ, Sullivan JA. The effect of total arterial grafting on medium-term outcomes following coronary artery bypass grafting. *J Cardiothorac Surg.* 2007; 2:44.
59. Rosenberger P, Shernan SK, Loffler M, et al. The influence of epiaortic ultrasonography on intraoperative surgical management in 6051 cardiac surgical patients. *Ann Thorac Surg.* 2008;85:548-553.
60. Pugsley W, Klinger L, Paschalis C, Treasure T, Harrison M, Newman S. The impact of microemboli during cardiopulmonary bypass on neuropsychological functioning. *Stroke.* 1994;25:1393-1399.
61. Stump DA, Rogers AT, Hammon JW, Newman SP. Cerebral emboli and cognitive outcome after cardiac surgery. *J Cardiothorac Vasc Anesth.* 1996;10:113-118.
62. Scharfschwerdt M, Richter A, Boehmer K, Repenning D, Sievers HH. Improved hydrodynamics of a new aortic cannula with a novel tip design. *Perfusion.* 2004;19:193-197.
63. Muehrcke DD, Cornhill JF, Thomas JD, Cosgrove DM. Flow characteristics of aortic cannulae. *J Card Surg.* 1995; 10:514-519.
64. Djaiani G, Ali M, Borger MA, et al. Epiaortic scanning modifies planned intraoperative surgical management but not cerebral embolic load during coronary artery bypass surgery. *Anesth Analg.* 2008;106:1611-1618.
65. Ott E, Nussmeier NA, Duke PC, et al. Efficacy and safety of the cyclooxygenase 2 inhibitors parecoxib and valdecoxib in patients undergoing coronary artery bypass surgery. *J Thorac Cardiovasc Surg.* 2003;125:1481-1492.
66. Nussmeier NA, Whelton AA, Brown MT, et al. Complications of the COX-2 inhibitors parecoxib and valdecoxib after cardiac surgery. *N Engl J Med.* 2005;352:1081-1091.
67. Robson MJA, Alston RP, Deary IJ, Andrews PJD, Souter MJ. Jugular bulb oxyhemoglobin desaturation, S100β and neurologic and cognitive outcome after coronary artery surgery. *Anesth Analg.* 2001;93:839-845.
68. Shaw PJ, Bates D, Cartlidge NE, Heaviside D, Julian DG, Shaw DA. Early neurological complications of coronary artery bypass surgery. *BMJ.* 1985;291:1384-1387.
69. Egger M, Schneider M, Smith GD. Meta-analysis Spurious precision? Meta-analysis of observational studies. *BMJ.* 1998;316:140-144.
70. Alston RP. Cardiothoracic anesthesia and critical care. In: Moller A, Pederson T, eds. *Evidence-based anesthesia and intensive care.* Cambridge: Cambridge University Press; 2006.
71. Tramer MR, Reynolds DJM, Moore RA, McQuay HJ. Impact of covert duplicate publication on meta-analysis: a case study. *BMJ.* 1997;315:635-640.
72. Polunina AG. Selection of neurocognitive tests and outcomes of cardiac surgery trials. *Ann Thorac Surg.* 2008;85: 362.
73. MacCallum RC, Zhang S, Preacher KJ, Rucker DD. On the practice of dichotomization of quantitative variables. *Psychol Methods.* 2002;7:19-40.
74. Altman DG, Royston P. The cost of dichotomising continuous variables. *BMJ.* 2006;332:1080.
75. Motallebzadeh R, Jahangiri M. Meta-analysis of randomized controlled trials of cognitive decline after on-pump versus off-pump coronary artery bypass graft surgery. *J Thorac Cardiovasc Surg.* 2008;135:1400-1401.
76. Murkin JM, Newman SP, Stump DA, Blumenthal JA. Statement of consensus on assessment of neurobehavioral outcomes after cardiac surgery. *Ann Thorac Surg.* 1995; 59: 1289-1295.
77. Phillips-Bute B, Mathew JP, Blumenthal JA, et al. Association of neurocognitive function and quality of life 1 year after coronary artery bypass graft (CABG) surgery. *Psychosom Med.* 2006;68:369-375.

78. Takagi H, Kawai N, Umemoto T. Reply to the Editor. *J Thorac Cardiovasc Surg*. 2008;135:1400-1401.
79. Phillips-Bute B, Mathew JP. Cognitive outcomes analyses: two steps forward, one step back? *J Cardiothorac Vasc Anesth*. 2008;22:513-514.
80. van Dijk D, Spoor M, Hijman R, et al. Cognitive and cardiac outcomes 5 years after off-pump vs on-pump coronary artery bypass graft surgery. *JAMA*. 2007;297:701-708.
81. Gallagher EG, Pearson DT. Ultrasonic identification of sources of gaseous microemboli during open heart surgery. *Thorax*. 1973;28:295-305.
82. Deverall PB, Padayachee TS, Parsons S, Theobold R, Battistessa SA. Ultrasound detection of micro-emboli in the middle cerebral artery during cardiopulmonary bypass surgery. *Eur J Cardiothorac Surg*. 1988;2:256-260.
83. Selnes OA, Grega MA, Bailey MM, et al. Cognition 6 years after surgical or medical therapy for coronary artery disease. *Ann Neurol*. 2008;63:581-590.
84. Wahrborg P, Booth JE, Clayton T, et al. Neuropsychological outcome after percutaneous coronary intervention or coronary artery bypass grafting: results from the stent or surgery (SoS) trial. *Circulation*. 2004;110:3411-3417.
85. Aleman A, Muller M, de Haan EH, van der Schouw YT. Vascular risk factors and cognitive function in a sample of independently living men. *Neurobiol Aging*. 2005;26:485-490.
86. van Dijk D, Moons KG, Nathoe HM, et al. Cognitive outcomes five years after not undergoing coronary artery bypass graft surgery. *Ann Thorac Surg*. 2008;85:60-64.

17 Experimental Basis and Clinical Studies of Brain Protection in Pediatric Heart Surgery

Richard A. Jonas

17.1 Background: Improving Outcomes in Pediatric Cardiac Surgery

Over the last 20 years, there has been a steady and consistent reduction in mortality for pediatric cardiac surgery. This improvement has occurred in spite of an increase in complexity of cases undertaken as well as a shift to surgery in infants and neonates. At many major pediatric cardiac surgery centers such as Children's National Medical Center in Washington DC, approximately 30% of cardiac surgical patients today are neonates, 30% are infants between 1 month and 1 year of age, and the remaining are older. Even conditions such as hypoplastic left heart syndrome can now be palliated in the newborn period applying the Norwood procedure with a mortality as low as 10-15%.

The reasons behind the improvement in outlook for babies with congenital heart problems are many. They include improvements in ICU management, cardiac anesthesia, preoperative noninvasive diagnosis, interventional catheter techniques, and surgical techniques. Probably, the most important reason for the improvement in outcome, however, is related to improvements in cardiopulmonary bypass.

17.2 Improvements in Cardiopulmonary Bypass

Cardiopulmonary bypass for neonates and infants has improved in many areas.

R.A. Jonas
Children's National Medical Center, Washington, DC, USA
e-mail: rjonas@cnmc.org

17.2.1 Hardware

Twenty to 25 years ago, there were no oxygenators, filters, or cannulas designed specifically for neonates. Bubble oxygenators were used without arterial line filters until the late 1980s and were known to generate many gaseous microemboli which passed directly to the brain. In the late 1980s, with the introduction of the popular variable prime Cobe membrane lung (VPCML), the first flat sheet microporous membrane oxygenator was available for infants. In the early 1990s, various hollow fiber microporous membrane oxygenators designed specifically for neonates became available. Improvements in filters and cannulas have unquestionably improved cardiopulmonary bypass for neonates and infants (Figs. 17.1 and 17.2).

17.2.2 Hypothermia

Aggressive rapid cooling to deep hypothermia was a common strategy in the early to mid 1980s that was emphasized by Ebert.[1] Deep hypothermic circulatory arrest was widely employed at this time having been popularized by Barratt-Boyes in New Zealand and Castaneda in Boston.[2] Studies such as the Boston Circulatory Arrest study in the late 1980s began to cast doubt on the neuroprotective efficacy of deep hypothermic circulatory arrest.[3] The technique as applied at that time involved rapid cooling with severe hemodilution and an alkaline pH strategy. Furthermore, the technique at the time of the Boston study used no arterial line filter and a large prime volume flat sheet membrane oxygenator. Today various alternatives to hypothermic circulatory arrest such as antegrade regional cerebral

R.S. Bonser et al. (eds.), *Brain Protection in Cardiac Surgery*,
DOI: 10.1007/978-1-84996-293-3_17,

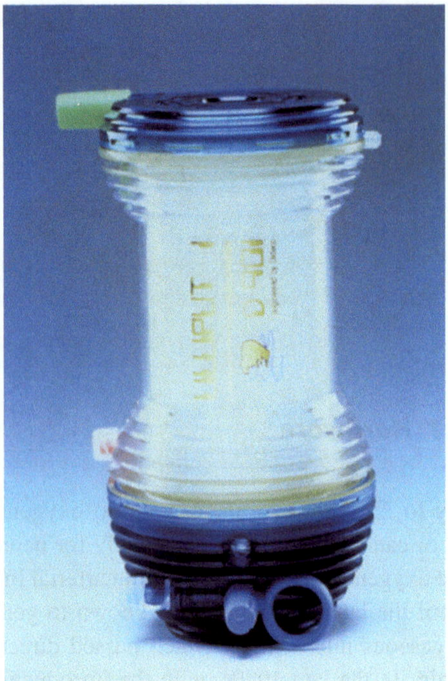

Fig. 17.1 Hollow-fiber microporous membrane oxygenators designed for neonates did not become available until the early 1990s

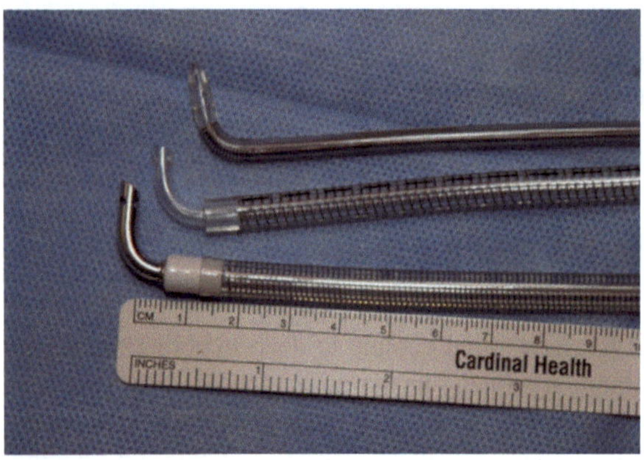

Fig. 17.2 New cannula designs have been helpful in improving cardiopulmonary bypass for neonates and premature neonates. Thin-walled all plastic cannulas (*top*) have replaced older models such as the traditional metal-tipped thick-walled "Pacifico" cannulas

perfusion[4] and retrograde cerebral perfusion[5] are being explored. Furthermore, cannulas designed for neonates have facilitated repair using standard cardiopulmonary bypass. An increasing number of centers use full-flow bypass at normothermia or with minimal cooling.[6]

17.2.3 Cardiopulmonary Bypass Prime

Refinements in the hardware of cardiopulmonary bypass have allowed a marked reduction in the cardiopulmonary bypass prime volume, thereby reducing exposure of the neonate or infant to the priming fluid. The question of optimal hematocrit for the prime is one that has been closely studied and is reviewed below.

17.2.4 Gas Strategy

The optimal oxygen and CO_2 strategy for pediatric cardiopulmonary bypass has been carefully studied and will be reviewed below.

17.2.5 Additives

Various additives such as steroids, vasodilators, and antifibrinolytics as well as anti-inflammatory agents such as aprotinin have been studied. The role of the anti-inflammatory and antifibrinolytic agent aprotinin is reviewed below.

17.3 pH Strategy and Hypothermic Bypass

17.3.1 pH Stat Strategy

The optimal pH strategy for hypothermic bypass has been strenuously debated for decades. In the early years of cardiopulmonary bypass the "pH stat" strategy was favored. Carbon dioxide is added to the gas mixture passing through the oxygenator so as to counteract the alkaline shift in the pH of neutrality that occurs during cooling. The pH stat strategy results in a pH of 7.40 and pCO_2 of 40 mm so long as the arterial blood gas is corrected to the patient's hypothermic body temperature. The blood gas result that is read directly from the blood gas machine (which routinely warms the blood sample to 37°C) should show an acidotic pH as low as 7.0–7.2 with a pCO_2 in the range of 60–100 mm according to the patient's temperature. The strategy requires the availability of carbon dioxide in the operating room.

17.3.2 Alpha Stat Strategy

The alternative alpha stat strategy was popularized in the early 1980s following theoretical discussion by animal physiologists.[7] The observation was made that cold blooded vertebrates which remain active at hypothermia follow the alpha stat strategy, that is, they allow their pH to shift in an alkaline direction and make no compensation for the natural alkaline shift. Interestingly, animals that hibernate are more likely to follow the pH stat strategy by hypoventilating and allowing their pCO_2 to increase. Unfortunately, few studies, either experimental or clinical, were undertaken before a widespread shift from the pH stat to the alpha stat strategy occurred in the mid-1980s.

17.3.3 An Epidemic of Choreoathetosis

Beginning in the mid-1980s coincident with the shift to the alpha stat strategy, a number of centers undertaking complex congenital cardiac surgery began to observe cases of choreoathetosis following cardiac surgery.[8] The risk appeared to be highest in toddler-age children, particularly those with pulmonary atresia with aortopulmonary collaterals. It was also more likely if deep hypothermic circulatory arrest was employed, particularly with shorter cooling time. Choreoathetosis had been seen in the early years of cardiac surgery but was exceedingly rare in the early 1980s. At Children's Hospital in Boston, there were no cases of choreoathetosis between 1982 and 1986. Between 1986 and 1990, there were 11 cases of severe choreoathetosis with four deaths.[8] This experience led to a retrospective review of cognitive development in 16 patients who underwent the Senning procedure for transposition of the great arteries between 1983 and 1988.[9] This time frame straddled the shift in pH strategy from the pH stat to the alpha stat strategy. A very strong correlation was found between pH strategy and developmental index with a p value of and 0.002. A more alkaline strategy, that is, the alpha stat strategy was associated with a worse outcome (Fig. 17.3).

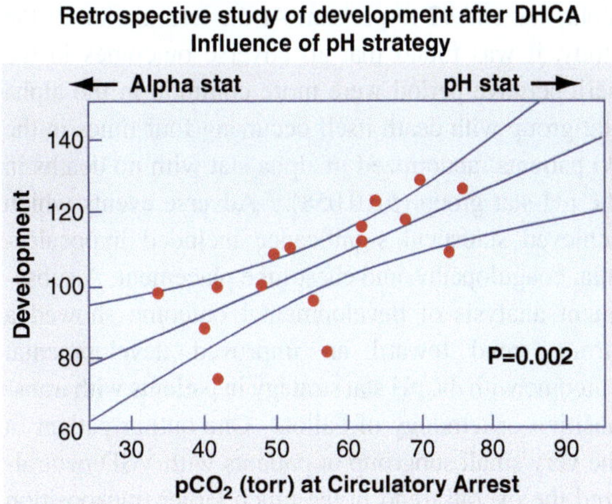

Fig. 17.3 A retrospective study of pH strategy documented a strong correlation between a more alkaline strategy, that is, the alpha stat strategy, and a worse developmental outcome. From Jonas RA et al.[9] Used with permission

17.3.4 Laboratory Study of pH Strategy

Two laboratory studies of pH strategy using piglets placed on cardiopulmonary bypass and studied with magnetic resonance spectroscopy demonstrated that preservation of cerebral high-energy phosphates was improved with application of the pH stat strategy relative to the alpha stat strategy.[10, 11] Based on the chronological coincidence of the choreoathetosis epidemic, the results of the retrospective pH study as well as the experimental data, a prospective randomized trial of pH strategy was funded by the NIH and undertaken at Children's Hospital Boston.

17.3.5 Randomized Prospective Trial of pH Strategy

The randomized trial of pH strategy for cardiopulmonary bypass in neonates and infants was undertaken between 1990 and 1994.[12, 13] One hundred and eighty two patients were enrolled with 90 being randomized to alpha stat and 92 to pH stat. At the termination of the study, it was found that all adverse outcomes in the perioperative period were more common in the alpha stat group with death itself occurring four times in the 90 patients randomized to alpha stat with no deaths in the pH stat group ($p=0.058$).[12] Adverse events which achieved statistical significance included hypocalcemia, coagulopathy, and chest tube placement. A subsequent analysis of developmental outcome showed a strong trend toward an improved developmental outcome with the pH stat strategy in patients with transposition or tetralogy of Fallot.[13] One outlier patient in the very small subgroup of patients with VSD neutralized the overall trend in the much larger transposition and tetralogy subgroups. Nevertheless, the perioperative outcome as well as the strong trends in the developmental outcomes together with our laboratory studies, retrospective clinical studies, and observational studies were sufficient to convince us and others that the pH stat strategy should be employed routinely for pediatric cardiac surgery. Subsequent reports from other groups have uniformly supported the advantages of the pH stat strategy, while there have been no reports demonstrating advantages of the alpha stat strategy for neonatal and infant bypass. These data have led the majority of pediatric centers to adopt the pH stat strategy.

17.4 Hemodilution and Cardiopulmonary Bypass

Hemodilution was introduced in 1960 during the early years of cardiopulmonary bypass as a means of reducing exposure of adult patients to large volumes of banked blood. This approach was necessary because of the extremely large priming volumes of early cardiopulmonary bypass circuits. The problem of autologous blood exposure was even more serious in infants and neonates in the early years of cardiopulmonary bypass because of the lack of circuits and oxygenators specifically designed for this patient population. Following the discovery of HIV and hepatitis C in the early 1980s hemodilution was practiced even more aggressively. Many centers recommended hemodilution to levels of 12–15%.[14] Interestingly, few clinical studies were undertaken to document the safety of this level of hemodilution, particularly the impact on developmental outcome in children.

17.4.1 Laboratory Study of Hemodilution

Two laboratory studies of hemodilution in piglets comparing hematocrits of 10%, 20%, and 30% documented both with magnetic resonance spectroscopy as well as near-infrared spectroscopy that cerebral oxygenation and preservation of high-energy phosphates were optimal with a hematocrit of 30%.[15, 16] In a survival study, the animals' behavioral scores and histological scores for brain injury were also optimal with minimal hemodilution to a hematocrit of 30%. The animals with severe hemodilution to a hematocrit of 10% suffered severe injury as seen on histological examination of the brain following sacrifice at 4 days postoperatively.

17.4.2 Retrospective Clinical Study of ASD Closure

A retrospective study of cognitive development was undertaken in children who had undergone ASD closure either by interventional catheter technique or surgery with cardiopulmonary bypass.[17] Surgery had been undertaken in an era when aggressive hemodilution was practiced. Patients who had surgical closure had worse outcomes. This remained true even when large ASDs were excluded. The only surgical variable which approached significance in a multivariable analysis of risk factors for worse developmental outcome was low hematocrit.

17.4.3 Randomized Clinical Trial of Hematocrit

A prospective randomized clinical trial of hemodilution was undertaken at Children's Hospital Boston between 1996 and 2000 comparing hematocrits of 20% and 30%.[18] The trial was shut down by the data and safety monitoring board because of an obvious improved outcome in motor skills with the higher hematocrit. The actual hematocrit difference between the two groups was only 6%, but nevertheless, the psychomotor development index assessed at 1 year of age was significantly better with a p value of.008 with the higher hematocrit. There was also a trend toward an improved mental development index. In the low hematocrit group, significantly more patients were developmentally delayed compared with the higher hematocrit group (Fig. 17.4).

A subsequent study between 2000 and 2004 compared outcomes following bypass with a lowest hematocrit of 25% versus 35%.[19,20] This study when analyzed in conjunction with the first randomized trial of hematocrit emphasized that a hematocrit of less than 20% was particularly dangerous. No clear advantage for a hematocrit of greater than 25% could be documented by analysis of the two hematocrits trials combined. Nevertheless, based on the overall information obtained from these two trials, it is our recommendation and current practice to maintain hematocrit at greater than 25% at all times and to aim, in general, for a hematocrit of between 25% and 30%. Interestingly, both trials documented that use of a higher hematocrit did not result in greater exposure to autologous blood products. The need for a greater amount of blood in the operating room was balanced by lesser need for blood products postoperatively, presumably secondary to reduced hemodilution of coagulation factors.

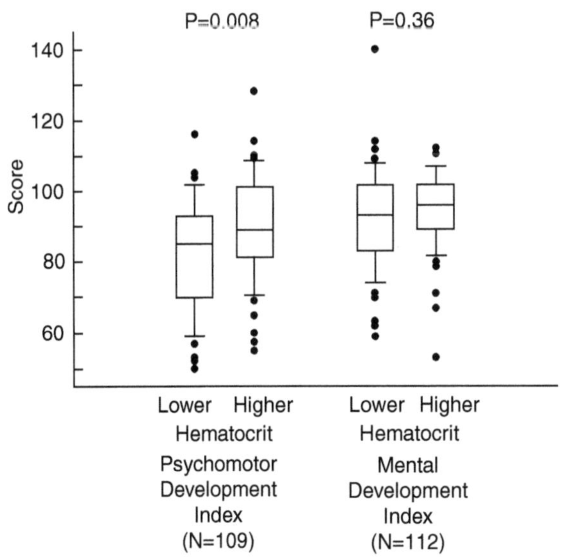

Fig. 17.4 A randomized prospective clinical trial of hematocrit strategy documented that a hematocrit of 28 was associated with a significantly improved score for motor skills (psychomotor development index) relative to hematocrit of 21.5

17.5 Interaction of Bypass Conditions to Determine Outcome after Circulatory Arrest or Low Flow Bypass

17.5.1 *Deep Hypothermic Circulatory Arrest*

An extensive laboratory study using piglets has documented that near-infrared spectroscopy is effective as a real-time monitor of the safe duration of hypothermic circulatory arrest.[21] Using behavioral outcome as well as histological outcome, these studies also documented that the safe duration of hypothermic circulatory arrest is influenced by not only temperature but also hematocrit level and pH.[22, 23] At lower temperatures, the pH strategy becomes increasingly important as documented in Fig. 17.5, which demonstrates the diverging lines for histological outcome. On the other hand, a greater degree of hemodilution becomes increasingly important at a higher temperature of circulatory arrest (Fig. 17.6). Thus a greater degree of hemodilution is increasingly dangerous if circulatory arrest is undertaken at 20°C rather than 15°C. As anticipated, both the temperature and duration of circulatory arrest also influence functional and structural outcomes. Table 17.1 documents

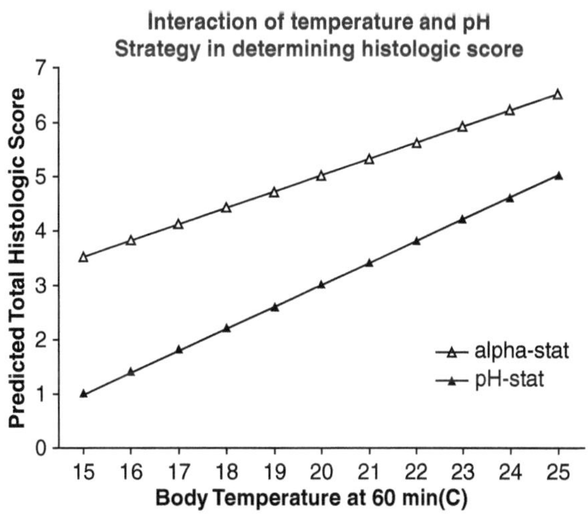

Fig. 17.5 At lower temperatures, pH strategy becomes increasingly important with improved cerebral histological outcome in laboratory animals with the pH stat strategy relative to the alpha stat strategy

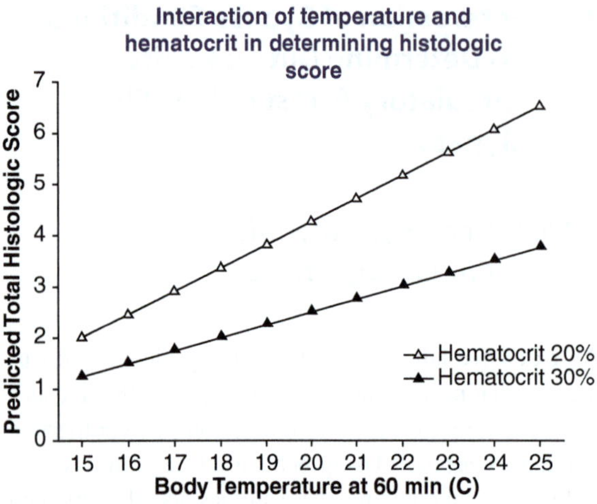

Fig. 17.6 At higher temperature, the degree of hemodilution becomes increasingly important with a worse outcome after hypothermic circulatory arrest

Table 17.1 Algorithm for predicting histologic score based on possible conditions

Multivariable predictor				
Temperature	pH strategy	Hematocrit (%)	HCA (Min)	Predicted total histologic score
15	pH	30	60	0.0
15	pH	20	60	0.5
15	Alpha	30	60	1.0
15	pH	30	80 or 100	1.5
15	Alpha	20	60	2.0
25	pH	30	60	2.5
15	Alpha	30	80 or 100	3.0
15	pH	20	80 or 100	3.0
25	pH	20	60	3.5
25	Alpha	30	60	4.0
15	Alpha	20	80 or 100	4.0
25	pH	30	80 or 100	4.5
25	Alpha	20	60	5.0
25	pH	20	80 or 100	6.0
25	Alpha	30	80 or 100	7.0
25	Alpha	20	80 or 100	8.0

the interaction of temperature, pH strategy, hematocrit, and circulatory arrest time. For example, circulatory arrest at 15°C using the pH stat strategy, a hematocrit of 30%, and a circulatory arrest time of 60 min is unlikely to result in any detectable histological injury. On the other hand, circulatory arrest at 15°C using the alpha stat strategy and a hematocrit of 20% with an arrest duration of 60 min results in a predicted total histological score of 2. A worst case scenario is the bottom row with a circulatory arrest temperature of 25°C in the setting of the alpha stat strategy, hemodilution to 20%, and an arrest duration of 80–100 min. This setting results in a predicted total histological score of 8 units.

17.5.2 Low Flow Bypass

Subsequent studies[24, 25] of reduced flow bypass using near-infrared spectroscopy as well as functional and structural outcomes in a piglet model have documented the utility of the tissue oxygenation index derived from near-infrared spectroscopy (Niro 300, Hammamatsu Corporation, Hammamatsu City, Japan) (Fig. 17.7). This new index is an absolute measure in contrast to the majority of near-infrared spectroscopy measures.[25] By employing three receiving optodes, it is possible to calculate the pathlength of the near-infrared beam of light

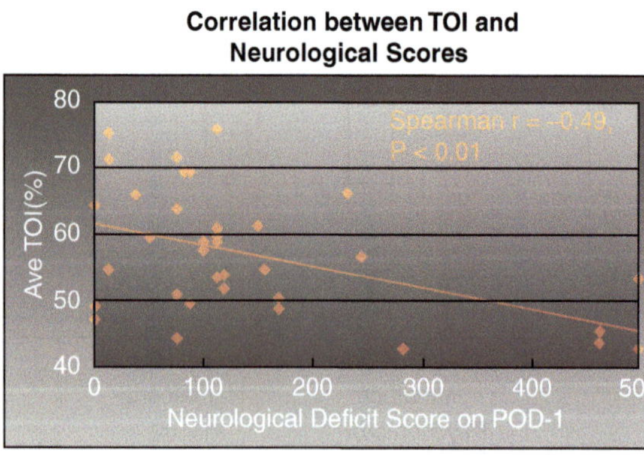

Fig. 17.7 The tissue oxygenation index derived from near-infrared spectroscopy is reliable in predicting functional and structural neurological outcome after reduced flow bypass. Near-infrared spectroscopy holds promise as a technique for monitoring adequacy of brain perfusion during repair of congenital anomalies

so that an absolute measure of tissue oxygenation can be obtained. Studies using piglets and near-infrared spectroscopy have confirmed that just as with the safe duration of circulatory arrest, the safe minimum flow rate is influenced by the cardiopulmonary bypass conditions including pH, hematocrit, and temperature. In general, a tissue oxygenation index of less than 55% throughout the low flow period or as a minimum value is highly predictive of important neurological injury. Intravital microscopy using a similar piglet model also documented that failure of the "functional capillary density" to return to baseline during rewarming also predicted worse functional and histological outcomes.[24] For example, at 15°C with the pH stat strategy and a hematocrit of 20% or 30% a flow rate as low as 10 mL/kg/min is safe for as long as 2 h. However, at 34°C under the same conditions, a flow rate of 10 mL/kg/min is very likely to be associated with neurological injury. The mechanism appears to involve preservation of endothelial function as determined by nitric oxide production.[26]

17.6 The Role of Serpins in Reducing Brain Injury During Cardiac Surgery

A number of pharmacological agents have been studied as helpful additives during cardiopulmonary bypass to reduce the probability of brain injury. Recent studies in our laboratory have highlighted the potential role of the serine protease inhibitor aprotinin in reducing brain injury during pediatric cardiac surgery.

17.6.1 *Background*

There are many serine protease inhibitors that play an important role in stabilizing various proteolytic cascades. For example, the plasminogen activator inhibitors PAI-1 and PAI-2 prevent excessive fibrinolysis.[27] Anti thrombin prevents excessive activation of the coagulation cascade, C-1 inhibitor modulates complement activation, and alpha 1 antitrypsin modulates connective tissue restructuring. Aprotinin is a serine protease inhibitor with a molecular weight of 6512 Da that is found in bovine lungs. It inhibits a wide range of proteases including kallikrein, trypsin, plasmin, complement activation, and plasmin neutrophil elastase. All of these proteolytic cascades are activated during cardiopulmonary bypass. Although some authors have suggested that aprotinin use in adults may be associated with an increased risk of stroke or encephalopathy,[28] an extensive meta analysis by Elefeteriades et al. in 2004 of 35 randomized trials including 3,887 patients suggested that aprotinin use is associated with a 47% reduction in the risk of stroke.[29] The recently published BART trial also documented no increased risk of stroke with aprotinin relative to the lysine analogues EACA and tranexamic acid.[30]

17.6.2 *Possible Mechanisms of Neuroprotection Afforded by Aprotinin*

17.6.2.1 Vascular and Anti-inflammatory

In a study by our group led by Aoki et al. and published in 1994,[31] we demonstrated that aprotinin has a role in preserving endothelial-dependent vasodilation after deep hypothermic circulatory arrest. Piglets treated with aprotinin showed greater in vivo cerebral and systemic endothelium-mediated vasodilation (acetylcholine response: cerebral $p<0.01$, systemic $p=0.04$) after reperfusion (Fig. 17.8). The response to endothelium-independent vasodilation (nitroglycerin) was the same in both groups. Aoki's study also documented that use of aprotinin was associated with accelerated recovery of cerebral high-energy phosphates measured by magnetic resonance spectroscopy. Brain water content postoperatively was 0.8077 in the aprotinin group and 0.8122 in control animals ($p = 0.06$).

17.6.2.2 Inhibition of NMDA Excitotoxicity by Aprotinin

In a study published in 2001, Nicole et al.[27] demonstrated that tissue plasminogen activator (TPA) can exaggerate NMDA excitotoxic brain injury. This observation is a possible explanation for the increase

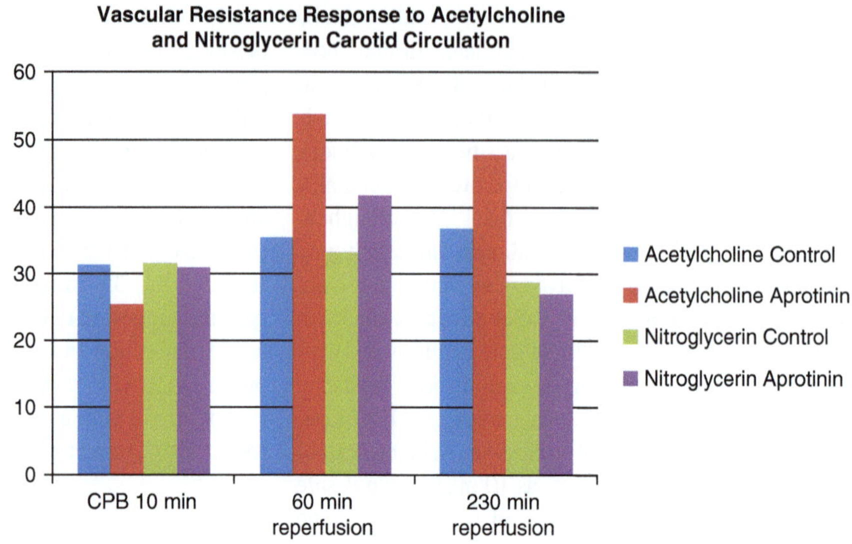

Fig. 17.8 The serine protease inhibitor aprotinin protects the vasculature from the deleterious effects of the systemic inflammatory response to cardiopulmonary bypass. Piglets treated with aprotinin show greater in vivo cerebral and systemic endothelium-mediated vasodilation (i.e., acetylcholine response relative to nitroglycerin response) relative to control animals not treated with aprotinin

in brain injury that is sometimes noted following the use of extrinsic TPA as a thrombolytic agent in patients suffering a cerebrovascular accident. An increase in neuronal injury and worsening clinical status is sometimes noted even in the absence of any hemorrhagic extension of the original stroke. Nicole and subsequently Labeurrier in 2004[32] demonstrated that inhibition of TPA by the serpins plasminogen activator inhibitor (PAI-1) and neuroserpin[33]reduced neuronal excitotoxic injury. We hypothesized that the broad-spectrum serine protease inhibitor aprotinin might also reduce excitotoxic neuronal injury.

17.6.2.3 Aprotinin and Excitotoxic Neuronal Injury in a Cell Culture Model

A cell culture study was undertaken similar to the original studies performed by Nicole and Labeurrier[27, 32] (Fig. 17.9). The efficacy of aprotinin in reducing NMDA excitotoxic cellular death both in a pure neuronal culture as well as a mixed neuronal and glial culture was studied. Cell culture plates were developed using fetal mouse brain. Exposure to a clinically relevant concentration of aprotinin between 100 and 200 KIU/mL resulted in a significant decrease in excitotoxic cellular death as documented by LDH release into the bathing medium. This was true both in pure and mixed cultures suggesting that the effect was directly mediated through neurons and was not dependent on interaction with glial cells.[34]

17.6.2.4 Laboratory Studies of Aprotinin in a Survival Porcine Model

Intravital Microscopy Study

Sixteen piglets at a mean weight of 13.6 kg underwent a severe neurological challenge with exposure to 2 h of deep hypothermic circulatory arrest at 15°C. Other animals underwent severely reduced low flow bypass at 25 mL/kg/min for 2 h at either 25°C or 34°C. Animals received either aprotinin or placebo. Endpoints included intravital microscopy. This study documented that the mean number of rolling leukocytes during rewarming was significantly less in all three subgroups when aprotinin was employed. In addition, the mean number of adherent leukocytes during rewarming was also significantly less. Recovery of functional capillary density was significantly inhibited during rewarming with hypothermic circulatory arrest in control animals, but not in animals that underwent circulatory arrest in the presence of aprotinin. The neurological damage score on postoperative day 1 was significantly less in aprotinin-treated animals in all three groups. There was a trend toward reduced histological injury which did not reach statistical significance.[35]

Near-Infrared Spectroscopy

In a follow-up study using near-infrared spectroscopy, 54 piglets were randomly assigned to one of three CPB

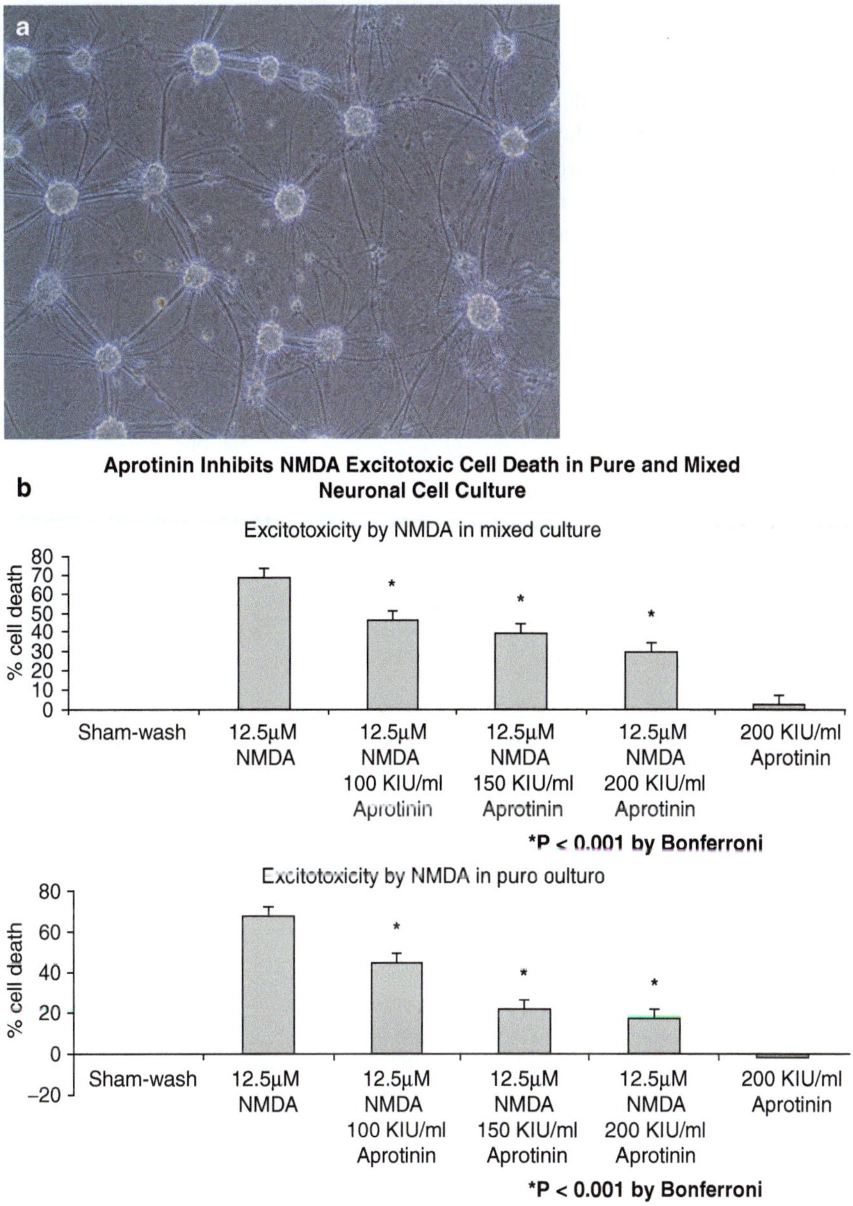

Fig. 17.9 (**a**) Neuronal cell culture studies have documented that serine protease inhibitors can reduce cell death following an excitotoxic insult such as that after ischemia. (**b**) Aprotinin, which is a serine protease inhibitor, has also been documented to be effective in reducing excitotoxic neuronal cell death in a cell culture model

groups designed to carry risk of postop cerebral and renal dysfunction.[36] Animals were randomized to: control (no aprotinin), low dose (30,000 KIU/kg into prime only), standard full dose (30,000 KIU/kg bolus IV into prime plus 10,000 KIU/kg infusion), and double full dose. Aprotinin significantly improved neurological scores on postoperative day 1 after ultralow flow bypass at 25°C or 34°C ($P<.01$). Linear regression indicated a strong dose–response relationship with higher aprotinin doses having the best neurological scores. During low flow, a higher TOI was correlated with a higher aprotinin dose ($P<.05$). Use of aprotinin and dose had no significant effect on creatinine or BUN on day 1. Low body weight was the only predictor of high BUN ($r = -0.39$, $P<.01$). We concluded from this study that aprotinin significantly improves neurologic recovery without compromising renal function in the young pig.

17.7 Conclusions

Both catastrophic and subtle neurological injuries are very much less frequent today than 20 to 30 years ago. Improvements in brain protection have paralleled improvements in overall mortality. Much of the improvement in outcome is attributed to improvement in cardiopulmonary bypass hardware and techniques. Further improvements in cardiopulmonary bypass are likely to be consequent to further developments in hardware design as well as adjunctive pharmacological agents such as serine protease inhibitors.

References

1. Turley K, Roizen M, Ebert PA. Deep hypothermia and total circulatory arrest: the effect of method of cooling on the catecholamine response to arrest. *J Surg Res*. 1981;30(4): 379-383.
2. Jonas RA, Newburger JW, Volpe JJ (eds) Brain Injury and Pediatric Cardiac Surgery. Butterworth-Heinemann, 1995
3. Newburger JW, Jonas RA, Wernovsky G, et al. A comparison of the perioperative neurologic effects of hypothermic circulatory arrest versus low flow cardiopulmonary bypass in infant heart surgery. *N Engl J Med*. 1993;329:1057-1064.
4. Goldberg CS, Bove EL, Devaney EJ, et al. A randomized clinical trial of regional cerebral perfusion versus deep hypothermic circulatory arrest: outcomes for infants with functional single ventricle. *J Thorac Cardiovasc Surg*. 2007; 133(4):880-887.
5. Duebener LF, Hagino I, Schmitt K, et al. Direct visualization of minimal cerebral capillary flow during retrograde cerebral perfusion: an intravital fluorescence microscopy study in pigs. *Ann Thorac Surg*. 2003;75(4):1288-1293.
6. McQuillen PS, Barkovich AJ, Hamrick SE, et al. Temporal and anatomic risk profile of brain injury with neonatal repair of congenital heart defects. *Stroke*. 2007;38(2 Suppl): 736-741.
7. Rahn H, Reeves RB, Howell BJ. Hydrogen ion regulation, temperature, and evolution. *Am Rev Respir Dis*. 1975;112(2): 165-172.
8. Wong PC, Barlow CF, Hickey PR, et al. Factors associated with choreoathetosis after cardiopulmonary bypass in children with congenital heart disease. *Circulation*. 1992;86(II):II–118-126.
9. Jonas RA, Bellinger DC, Rappaport LA, et al. Relation of pH strategy and developmental outcome after hypothermic circulatory arrest. *J Thorac Cardiovasc Surg*. 1993;106(2): 362-368.
10. Aoki M, Nomura F, Stromski ME, et al. Effects of pH on brain energetics after hypothermic circulatory arrest. *Ann Thorac Surg*. 1993;55(5):1093-1103.
11. Hiramatsu T, Miura T, Forbess JM, et al. pH strategies and cerebral energetics before and after circulatory arrest. *J Thorac Cardiovasc Surg*. 1995;109(5):948-957.
12. du Plessis AJ, Jonas RA, Wypij D, et al. Perioperative effects of alpha-stat versus pH-stat strategies for deep hypothermic cardiopulmonary bypass in infants. *J Thorac Cardiovasc Surg*. 1997;114(6):991-1000.
13. Bellinger DC, Wypij D, du Plessis AJ, et al. Developmental and neurologic effects of alpha-stat versus pH-stat strategies for deep hypothermic cardiopulmonary bypass in infants. *J Thorac Cardiovasc Surg*. 2001;121(2):374-383.
14. Cook DJ, Orszulak TA, Daly RC, MacVeigh I. Minimum hematocrit for normothermic cardiopulmonary bypass in dogs. *Circulation*. 1997;96((9):II–200-4.
15. Shin'oka T, Shum-Tim D, Jonas RA, et al. Higher hematocrit improves cerebral outcome after deep hypothermic circulatory arrest. *J Thorac Cardiovasc Surg*. 1996;112(6): 1610-1620.
16. Shin'oka T, Shum-Tim D, Laussen PC, et al. Effects of oncotic pressure and hematocrit on outcome after hypothermic circulatory arrest. *Ann Thorac Surg*. 1998;65(1): 155-164.
17. Visconti KJ, Bichell DP, Jonas RA, Newburger JW, Bellinger DC. Developmental outcome after surgical versus interventional closure of secundum atrial septal defect in children. *Circulation*. 1999;100(19):II145-50.
18. Jonas RA, Wypij D, Roth SJ, et al. The influence of hemodilution on outcome after hypothermic cardiopulmonary bypass: results of a randomized trial in infants. *J Thorac Cardiovasc Surg*. 2003;126(6):1765-1774.
19. Newburger JW, Jonas RA, Soul J, et al. Randomized trial of hematocrit 25% versus 35% during hypothermic cardiopulmonary bypass in infant heart surgery. *J Thorac Cardiovasc Surg*. 2008;135(2):347-354. 354.
20. Wypij D, Jonas RA, Bellinger DC, et al. The effect of hematocrit during hypothermic cardiopulmonary bypass in infant heart surgery: results from the combined Boston hematocrit trials. *J Thorac Cardiovasc Surg*. 2008;135(2):355-360.
21. Sakamoto T, Hatsuoka S, Stock UA, et al. Prediction of safe duration of hypothermic circulatory arrest by near-infrared spectroscopy. *J Thorac Cardiovasc Surg*. 2001;122(2): 339-350.
22. Sakamoto T, Zurakowski D, Duebener LF, et al. Interaction of temperature with hematocrit level and pH determines safe duration of hypothermic circulatory arrest. *J Thorac Cardiovasc Surg*. 2004;128(2):220-232.
23. Sakamoto T, Zurakowski D, Duebener LF, et al. Combination of alpha-stat strategy and hemodilution exacerbates neurologic injury in a survival piglet model with deep hypothermic circulatory arrest. *Ann Thorac Surg*. 2002;73(1):180-189.
24. Anttila V, Hagino I, Zurakowski D, et al. Specific bypass conditions determine safe minimum flow rate. *Ann Thorac Surg*. 2005;80(4):1460-1467.
25. Hagino I, Anttila V, Zurakowski D, Duebener LF, Lidov HG, Jonas RA. Tissue oxygenation index is a useful monitor of histologic and neurologic outcome after cardiopulmonary bypass in piglets. *J Thorac Cardiovasc Surg*. 2005;130(2): 384-392.
26. Anttila V, Christou H, Hagino I, et al. Cerebral endothelial nitric oxide synthase expression is reduced after very-low-flow bypass. *Ann Thorac Surg*. 2006 Jun;81(6):2202-2206.
27. Nicole O, Docagne F, Ali C, et al. The proteolytic activity of tissue-plasminogen activator enhances NMDA receptor-mediated signaling. *Nat Med*. 2001;7(1):59-64.

28. Mangano DT, Rieves RD, Weiss KD. Judging the safety of aprotinin. *N Engl J Med*. 2006;355(21):2261-2262.
29. Sedrakyan A, Treasure T, Elefteriades JA. Effect of aprotinin on clinical outcomes in coronary artery bypass graft surgery: a systematic review and meta-analysis of randomized clinical trials. *J Thorac Cardiovasc Surg*. 2004;128(3):442-448.
30. Fergusson DA, Hébert PC, Mazer CD, et al. the BART Investigators. A Comparison of Aprotinin and Lysine Analogues in High-Risk Cardiac Surgery. *N Engl J Med*. 2008;358:2319-2331.
31. Aoki M, Jonas RA, Nomura F, et al. Effects of aprotinin on acute recovery of cerebral metabolism in piglets after hypothermic circulatory arrest. *Ann Thorac Surg*. 1994;58(1): 146-153.
32. Lebeurrier N, Liot G, Lopez-Atalaya JP, et al. The brain-specific tissue-type plasminogen activator inhibitor, neuroserpin, protects neurons against excitotoxicity both in vitro and in vivo. *Mol Cell Neurosci*. 2005;30(4):552-558.
33. Cinelli P, Madani R, Tsuzuki N, et al. Neuroserpin, a neuroprotective factor in focal ischemic stroke. *Mol Cell Neurosci*. 2001;18:443-457.
34. Iwata Y, Nicole O, Okamura T, Zurakowski D, Jonas RA. Aprotinin confers neuroprotection by reducing excitotoxic cell death. *J Thorac Cardiovasc Surg*. 2008;135(3): 573-578.
35. Anttila V, Hagino I, Iwata Y, et al. Aprotinin improves cerebral protection: evidence from a survival porcine model. *J Thorac Cardiovasc Surg*. 2006;132(4):948-953.
36. Iwata Y, Okamura T, Ishibashi N, Zurakowski D, Lidov HGW, Jonas RA. Optimal dose of aprotinin for neuroprotection and renal function in a piglet survival model. *J Thorac Cardiovasc Surg*, submitted.

18 Experimental Basis and Clinical Studies of Brain Protection in Aortic Arch Surgery

Gabriele Di Luozzo and Randall B. Griepp

18.1 Introduction

The management of complex aortic arch disease has been and continues to be dependent upon reproducible neuronal protection strategies. Over the last 2 decades, numerous brain protection strategies have been investigated and employed in clinical practice. Since 1975, prolonged interruption of antegrade brain perfusion for the resection of aortic arch and ascending aortic aneurysms has relied principally on hypothermic circulatory arrest (HCA).[1] This method of brain protection has been embraced and still remains the primary brain protection strategy used by adult and pediatric cardiac surgeons worldwide. As surgical techniques have become more sophisticated, and our understanding of brain metabolism has improved, however, other strategies for brain protection have been introduced. Regardless of the methodology, the common denominator in almost all the strategies is hypothermia.

Laboratory research efforts dedicated to brain protection have produced a better understanding of brain physiology and neuronal injury, and have led to safer application of brain protection strategies in the clinical arena. The earliest investigations with regard to HCA examined cerebral metabolism as it is related to temperature, cerebral blood flow, and oxygen consumption.[2–4] We have investigated the neuroprotective effects and neurocognitive outcomes using various perfusion techniques in porcine and canine models as well as in clinical studies, and the results have had a significant influence in our current clinical practice.

G. Di Luozzo (✉)
Department of Cardiothoracic Surgery, Mount Sinai School of Medicine, New York, USA
e-mail: gabriele.diluozzo@mountsinai.org

We have focused this chapter on the efforts of research laboratories to understand brain protection during aortic arch surgery, and how the principles which emerge can be applied to clinical practice.

18.2 Hypothermic Circulatory Arrest

The replacement of the aortic arch was the paramount surgical challenge which initiated investigations focusing on protecting the human brain during periods of interrupting normal blood flow. As aortic surgery has evolved, more surgeons are utilizing HCA for the resection of ascending aortic aneurysms just proximal to the aortic arch and the proximal descending thoracic aorta just distal to the aortic arch. HCA offers the major benefits of simplicity and availability. It permits a dry operative field uncluttered by cannulae, and dramatic reduction in the manipulation of the aorta, reducing the likelihood of dislodging emboli. Moreover, any heart-lung machine with a heat exchanger can be used to provide hypothermia, and enable subsequent rewarming. The major disadvantage of HCA is its time limitation.

For many years, cardiac surgeons have been hoping not to exceed a duration of HCA which would allow them to complete their operation but still result in good neurologic outcomes. The initial experience with HCA for complex arch surgery, not uncommonly, required prolonged intervals of interrupted cerebral perfusion. Initially, neurologic recovery after 90 min of HCA at 18°C was thought to result in severe but reversible early impairment neurologically and behaviorally.[5] With clinical experience as well as on the basis of careful animal studies, however, it has become apparent that the safe interval of HCA is more limited. Because the brain requires oxygen for aerobic glycolysis at all

R.S. Bonser et al. (eds.), *Brain Protection in Cardiac Surgery*,
DOI: 10.1007/978-1-84996-293-3_18,

times, the measurement of cerebral metabolic rate of oxygen ($CMRO_2$) gives useful information on the metabolic state of the brain. Suppression of cerebral metabolic rate is achieved by means of thorough systemic, uniform cooling. The coefficient Q_{10}, a well-described physiological variable, describes the incremental decrease in cerebral metabolism with temperature. The Q_{10} estimates the oxygen requirement at a given hypothermic temperature, and can be used to assess the decrease in oxygen demand as a basis to estimate the safety of absent cerebral blood flow.[6] In the pig model, suppression of cerebral oxygen metabolism was found to be 50%, 19%, and 11% of baseline at 28°C, 18°C, and 8°C, respectively.[4] Quantitative electroencephalography showed no residual activity in the 8°C and 13°C groups, but significant slow wave activity was present at 18°C.[7] In the human model, the $CMRO_2$ is still 24% of baseline values at 20°C and 16% of baseline at 15°C.[3] After calculating the Q_{10} for a selected patient population and assuming that interrupting cerebral blood flow for 5 min at 37°C is safe, the duration of HCA for any blood temperature can be calculated (Table 18.1). Based on measurement of metabolic rates in dogs and pigs, and, in humans, on the frequency of temporary neurological dysfunction postoperatively and results of cognitive testing, an interval of 25–30 min represent the upper limits of absolutely safe duration of HCA at a nasopharyngeal temperature of 12–15°C.[5,8–10] Longer intervals of interrupted cerebral perfusion are sometimes inevitable, but should not be routinely accepted. Periods of HCA of 40 min or more result in an enhanced incidence of neurologic injury, and HCA intervals exceeding 65 min have been shown clinically to result in increased mortality.[11]

Table 18.1 Time intervals of safe HCA for a given nasopharyngeal temperature

Temperature (°C)	Cerebral metabolic rate(% of baseline)	Safe duration of HCA (min)
37	100	5
30	56 (52–60)	9 (8–10)
25	37 (33–42)	14 (12–15)
20	24 (21–29)	21 (17–24)
15	16 (13–20)	31 (25–38)
10	11 (8–14)	45 (36–62)

Calculations based on assumption that there is a 5-min tolerance for circulatory arrest at 37°C. Values in parenthesis are 95% confidence intervals. *HCA* hypothermic circulatory arrest

The technical details of establishing HCA are important. We believe that the patient should be cooled for least 30 min to allow for uniform cerebral cooling.[3,12] Some monitoring of cerebral metabolism using jugular venous saturations or near-infrared spectroscopy should assure that cerebral metabolic rates are adequately suppressed.[13,14] An upward drift in cerebral temperature occurs with intervals of HCA longer than 15–20 min, but can be prevented quite effectively by packing the head in ice. Careful deairing and removal of particulate debris prior to reestablishment of perfusion is important. Laboratory studies suggest that a brief period of cold perfusion at the end of HCA may decrease the incidence of cerebral edema and improve cerebral protection, and relatively slow warming preserves the balance of cerebral blood flow and metabolism. Reactive hyperemia – which often occurs with immediate rewarming after HCA – may pose its own luxury-perfusion-associated dangers (Fig. 18.1).[15] Slow rewarming, with a gradient of less than 10°C between the blood and the nasopharyngeal temperature, appears to be clinically important. Perhaps, most important is the prevention of overwarming: it is our belief that a blood temperature of greater than 36.5°C should never be used in patients who have undergone a period of cerebral hypoperfusion.

Hypothermia is the mainstay of all techniques of cerebral protection; its primary mechanism is reduction in cerebral metabolic demands. But regardless of the careful application of brain protection strategies and neuronal monitoring, a small number of patients will have a degree of temporary or permanent cognitive and behavioral dysfunction. Clinical and experimental models have shown that the exact mechanism of brain injury during aortic arch surgery is multifactorial. Surgical and perfusion techniques have been developed to deal with two major causes of brain injury during aortic arch surgery: stroke and global hypoperfusion. The first reflects particulate material embolization originating from the ostia of the cerebral vessels and aortic arch, especially during clamping and dissection (Fig. 18.2). The second is diffuse injury caused by lack of perfusion for an interval long enough to cause widespread neuronal damage or death within the central nervous system. It remains unclear whether most of the neuronal injury associated with a diffuse insult occurs during HCA itself or during reperfusion. A number of animal studies in our laboratory as well as some clinical measurements have

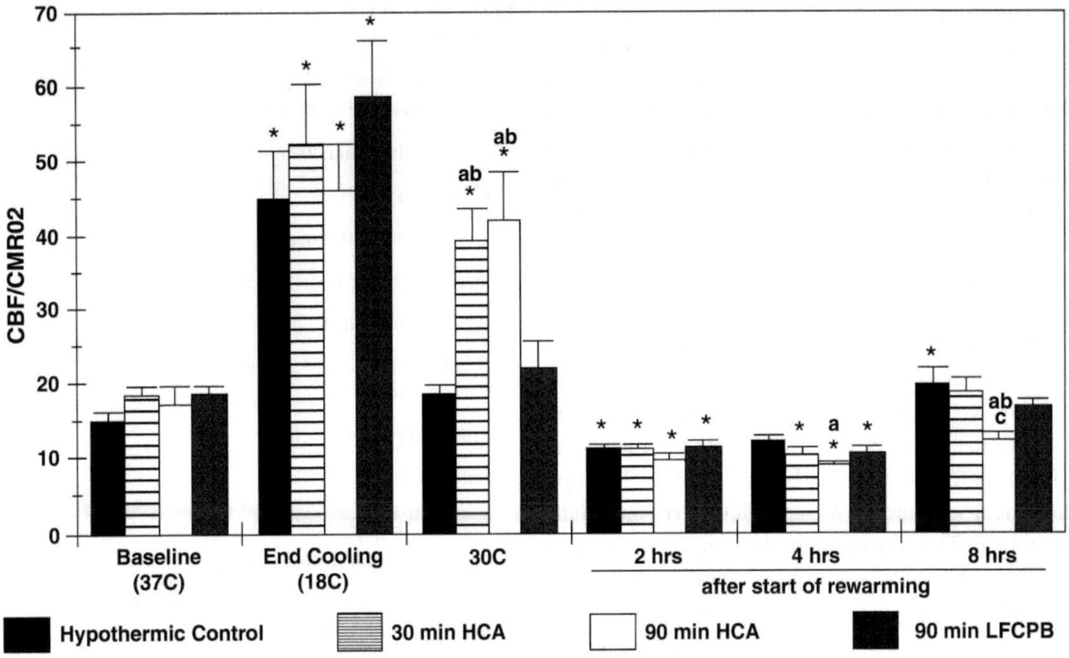

Fig. 18.1 Rate of cerebral blood flow (CBF) to cerebral metabolic rate of oxygen ($CMRO_2$), giving an estimate of appropriateness of cerebral blood flow. A ratio similar to what is seen at baseline, when cerebral autoregulation is intact, seems likely to represent an ideal value. By this standard, all groups had significant "luxury perfusion" by the end of cooling and only the HCA groups showed a marked hyperemia at 30°C. All groups show a lower-than-ideal ratio at 2 h, which persisted in all but the hypothermic control group at 4 h. By 8 h, the ratio of CBF/$CMRO_2$ had returned to values not significantly different from baseline in all groups, although the ratio was still significantly lower in the 90 min HCA group than in the other groups. *$P<0.05$ versus baseline (37°C); (*a*) $p<0.05$ versus control (18°C); (*b*) $p<0.05$ versus LFCPB (18°C); (*c*) $p<0.05$ versus 30 min HCA (18°C)

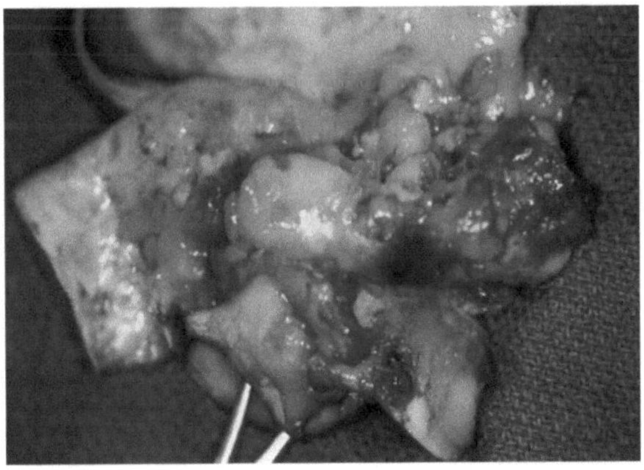

Fig. 18.2 Photograph of the resected aortic arch with evidence of atheromatous disease at the origin of the brachiocephalic vessels

suggested that in patients who have undergone HCA, a period of cerebral vasospasm may occur for as long as 8 h postoperatively (Fig. 18.1).[5] Adequate oxygen delivery (requiring stable hemodynamics, and a high hematocrit) is important during this vulnerable interval in order to avoid further injury and to allow recovery from whatever damage has already occurred. During this period of recovery from HCA, an equilibrium must be reestablished with respect to cerebral glucose metabolism, oxygen consumption, vascular resistance, and cerebral blood flow.

Contemporary outcomes for aortic arch surgery have improved dramatically, with only a 4% incidence of permanent neurologic impairment.[16] Technical advancements which have translated into better neurologic outcomes in aortic arch surgery have been achieved with axillary artery cannulation.[17,18] Focal embolic injury depends primarily on a surgical technique that avoids dislodgement of atheroemboli or clot into the cerebral circulation and removal of any debris from the cerebral vessels prior to reinstitution of perfusion. Dissection of diseased cerebral vessels can most safely be carried out during a period of hypothermic circulatory arrest, and anastomoses should be constructed beyond major atheromatous disease. Beyond focal neurologic injury, HCA durations exceeding 25 minutes have been shown to produce symptoms such as prolonged obtundation, disorientation, and Parkinson-like movements without localizing neurological signs, which were initially characterized by us as temporary neurologic dysfunction (TND), especially in elderly patients.[8] Our earlier findings showed a clear, almost linear relationship between circulatory arrest time and the development of TND, suggesting that TND reflects inadequate brain protection. But more quantitative neuropsychological evaluation has now shown that a duration of circulatory arrest exceeding 25 min is a predictor of long-term deficits in cognitive function.[19] Reich et al. showed that poor results on – or inability to undergo – early postoperative neuropsychological evaluation was predictive of poor late performance. The area of the brain which is thought to be affected the most is the hippocampus, which is responsible for acquisition of new information and memory; it is very sensitive to anoxia and ischemia due to the high metabolic rate. The prevalence of this injury in older patients, manifest as motor and memory dysfunction, may be related to slower recovery from injury due to an age-related reduction in brain reserve capacity. In consequence, we make a concerted effort to limit arrest duration, especially in older patients. In pursuing this strategy, we have primarily used antegrade selective cerebral perfusion during aortic arch surgery (Table 18.2).

Table 18.2 Mount Sinai protocol for HCA and selective cerebral perfusion

• Preoperative steroids (dexamethasone)
• Left jugular bulb catheter
• Right axillary cannulation
• Cooling to 15°C
• Cooling for approximately 30 min
• Hematocrit approximately 30%
• Ice packs to patient's head
• Jugular venous oxygen saturation >95% every 2 min once temperature is 15°C.
• Trendelenburg position
• Initiate DHCA
• Branched graft anastomosis
• Suction limbs of trifurcated graft
• Selective cerebral perfusion via right axillary artery with mean arterial pressure of 50mmHg or flow rate of 10 cc/kg/min
• Aortic reconstruction
• Dealring
• Rewarming with temperature gradient ≤ 10°C to a bladder temperature of 33°C
• Postoperative steroids if DHCA >30 min

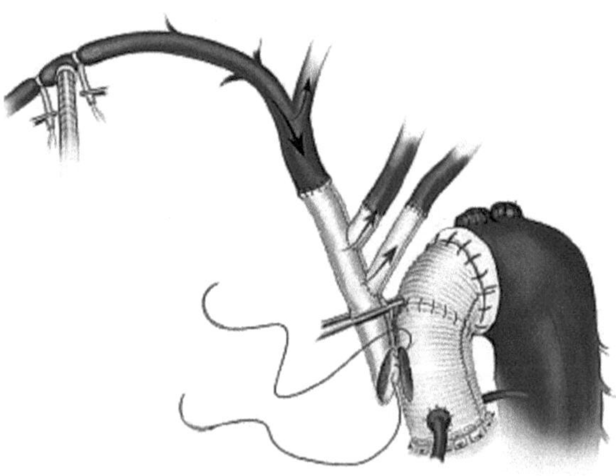

Fig. 18.3 The drawing demonstrates selective cerebral perfusion through the right axillary artery and into all three limbs of the trifurcated graft

18.3 Selective Antegrade Perfusion

Selective antegrade cerebral perfusion via some or all of the three arch vessels was used intermittently in the early days of cardiac surgery, but the complexity of cannulation and monitoring techniques, and the state of the art of bypass technology at that time resulted in only occasional success. As aortic surgery became more complex and the drawbacks of HCA became apparent, however, antegrade selective cerebral perfusion (SCP) was once again introduced into the clinical arena by Bachet in France and Kazui in Japan.[20,21] Currently, SCP is continuing to gain adherents as the preferred technique for brain protection during long periods of interruption of normal cerebral perfusion (Fig. 18.3). Moreover, some surgeons are advocating continuous SCP and using moderate HCA (22–25°C) with SCP in order to shorten cardiopulmonary bypass time.

All antegrade cerebral perfusion, however, is not identical, and a number of issues remain controversial. Direct balloon catheterization of cerebral vessels offers the advantage of being quick and minimizing the interval of HCA required for techniques which result in perfusion of the entire aortic arch. But these techniques require complex monitoring, inasmuch as catheters can be dislodged into the bifurcation of the innominate artery, and perfusion pressures may differ depending upon cannula size and resistance in the particular part of the brain perfused by each cannula.[22] In most series utilizing balloon catheter perfusion, only the innominate and the left carotid arteries are perfused. Kazui et al. reported on 472 patients undergoing total arch replacement with selective antegrade perfusion through the right axillary artery and either unilateral or bilateral cerebral perfusion, with a temporary and permanent neurologic dysfunction rate of 4.7% and 3.2%, respectively.[23] Advocates of this particular approach do not feel that the risk of embolization is elevated if the cerebral vessels are resected under HCA 1 cm beyond the diseased area, and the perfusing catheters are placed within an open vessel under direct vision. In addition, air embolism is not likely if patient is placed in the Trendelenburg position, and flow is begun before balloon inflation.

Monitoring of the adequacy of cerebral perfusion during antegrade SCP depends to some extent upon the technique utilized. If all cerebral vessels are connected to a common graft, only a single pressure needs to be monitored, but some monitoring of regional perfusion is also probably wise. Currently, the only readily available techniques for monitoring regional perfusion are near-infrared spectroscopy of the frontal lobes, and transcranial Doppler of the middle cerebral artery. The absence of a simple method for monitoring perfusion of the posterior cerebral circulation – coupled with a high incidence of variations in the circle of Willis – is a source of considerable reservation with regard to SCP strategies involving perfusion of fewer than three cerebral vessels. Approximately 2–3% of patients do not have a patent circle of Willis, and particularly the lack of a posterior communicating artery can give rise to a watershed infarct deep in white mater.[24] A dominant left vertebral artery or obstructed right vertebral artery can lead to vertebrobasilar ischemia if cerebral perfusion is approached exclusively through the innominate artery.

Hypoperfusion of the left cerebral hemisphere is a major concern with techniques perfusing fewer than all three head vessels. There are a several preoperative and intraoperative techniques used to assess whether cerebral circulation in the left hemisphere is appropriate. The following techniques are commonly employed: (1) preoperative angiography or magnetic resonance angiography to assess the circle of Willis and the posterior circulation; (2) a carotid occlusion test, using a cerebral balloon catheter to determine the adequacy of collateral blood flow; (3) intraoperative transcranial Doppler sonography to assess the left middle cerebral artery, and (4) assessment of the amount of backbleeding through the LCCA and LSA.[25] At present, we believe that rapid anastomosis of all three arch vessels to a trifurcation graft during HCA, followed by perfusion through an axillary artery, is the safest technique for SCP. We assess cerebral perfusion during SCP by left radial artery pressure and bi-hemispheric near-infrared spectroscopy.

In our quest to reduce the duration of DHCA, we have found selective antegrade cerebral perfusion for total arch replacement the most successful adjunct. Using this technique, the interruption of antegrade perfusion during aortic arch replacement can be limited to approximately 20–30 min, the time needed to complete three anastomoses with a trifurcated graft. Antegrade cerebral perfusion can be delivered via a side branch of a graft or the axillary artery once the reconstruction of the aortic arch is completed (Fig. 18.3). In an animal model, we reported similar results between continuous SCP and DHCA-SCP with regard to global cerebral protection and neurological recovery.[26] The short interval of DHCA did not significantly diminish the benefits of continuous SCP. Behavioral outcomes were not significantly worse after DHCA-SCP than with SCP alone.

If the total time necessary for aortic arch repair requiring arrest of the antegrade circulation is moderately long – between 40 and 80 min – the incidence of TND is lower with SCP than any other alternative cerebral protection strategy[10] (Fig. 18.4). If prolonged interruption of antegrade cerebral perfusion is anticipated, SCP is the technique of choice (Fig. 18.5). Nevertheless, we have shown, in a large series of patients, that SCP for more than 80 min is associated with a higher incidence of permanent stroke and death. Prolonged SCP alone may not be responsible, but may reflect more extensive operations involving the aortic arch in patients with severe atheromatous lesions.

Despite intense laboratory work and clinical studies, the optimal perfusion parameters for SCP need further delineation. In a series of experiments in the pig, we have demonstrated that a flow which generates pressures of 50–70 mmHg is safer than perfusion at higher pressures and that perfusion at 10°–15°C results in better cerebral recovery than at 20–25°C.[27]

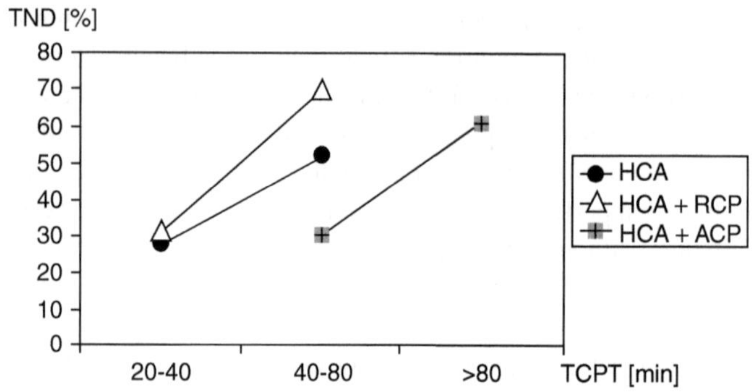

Fig. 18.4 Effect of increasing duration of cerebral protection (TCPT) on incidence of stroke, either transient or permanent, in all patients ($n=717$). In the HCA group TCPT corresponds to the interval of HCA, in the RCP group TCPT is equal to the sum of HCA and RCP times, and in the ACP group TCPT is the sum of the duration of HCA and selective ACP

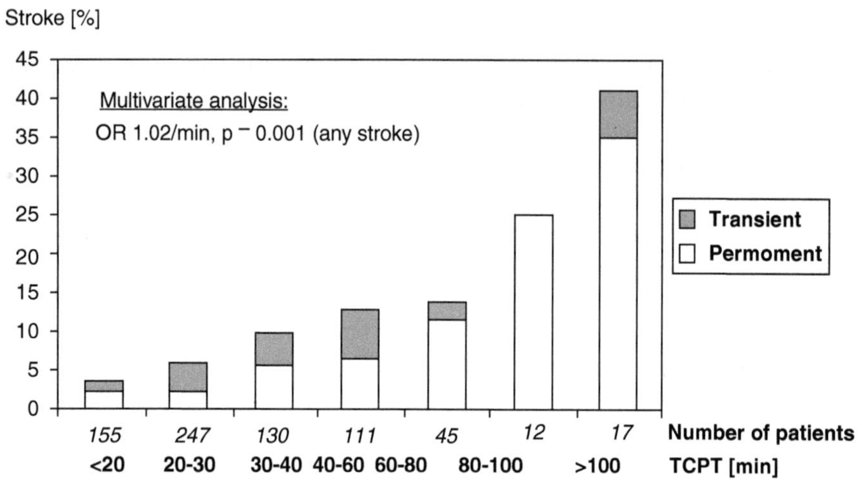

Fig. 18.5 Effect of increasing duration of cerebral protection on incidence of TND, as defined in the text, fractionated according to the cerebral protection method in all patients who survived operation without stroke since 1993 ($n=453$). In the HCA group TCPT corresponds to the interval of HCA, in the RCP group TCPT is equal to the sum of HCA and RCP times, and in the ACP group it is the sum of HCA and selective ACP. Although differences in patient selection require that comparisons between the groups undergoing different modes of cerebral protection be undertaken with caution, it is interesting to note that the incidence of TND with increasing TCPT appears to increase more sharply with RCP than with HCA alone, and that the levels of TND with ACP are comparatively low despite longer TCPT

We have confirmed observations by others suggesting that hemodilution during SCP results in a poorer neurological outcome, evident in our studies by significantly worse functional scores on early awakening and subsequent daily neurobehavioral analyses during recovery.[28] A hematocrit of 30% is preferable to one of 20%. Sakamoto et al. have elucidated better histological outcomes in piglets perfused with hematocrit of 30% versus 20%, especially in the hippocampus, an area known to be sensitive to ischemia.[29,30] In another porcine model, the reduced colloid oncotic pressure associated with low hematocrit levels has been shown to produce greater perioperative weight gain and cerebral edema.[31]

pH-stat acid–base management, although providing a higher cerebral blood flow, does not confer any benefit over perfusion using alpha-stat principles with regard to postoperative cerebral recovery in healthy pigs, but in dogs that have had an experimental cerebral infarct several weeks before SCP, there is some evidence that use of pH-stat perfusion may be preferable to use of alpha-stat strategy.[32] Given the equivalency of neurobehavioral outcome and the possible disadvantage of luxury perfusion in patients at risk of cerebral embolization, we utilize alpha-stat acid–base management in aortic arch surgery.

18.4 Retrograde Perfusion

In the early 1990s, reports of successful treatment of massive air embolism with retrograde cerebral perfusion (RCP) sparked an interest in this technique for cerebral protection in aortic surgery. There were a number of encouraging early laboratory and clinical reports, but in retrospect many of these relied on historical controls and relatively short intervals of interruption of normal antegrade cerebral perfusion. In a series of animal studies in our laboratory, we demonstrated that RCP was better than HCA alone, but no better than HCA combined with packing the head in ice.[33] Embolic material can be removed from the brain by RCP only with extremely high perfusion pressures brought about by clamping of both the superior and inferior vena cavae. Effective RCP is associated with a marked increase in fluid sequestration and elevated intracranial pressures postoperatively, and mild histological cerebral damage occurring as a consequence of the technique itself. Furthermore, in a study in pigs in which perfusion of brain capillaries was studied using fluorescent microspheres, it was shown that only a trivial amount – 0.01% of the blood injected into the superior vena cava –reaches cerebral capillaries.[34,35] In nonhuman primates, similar results have been reported.[36] Most of the blood during RCP is shunted into the inferior vena cava or passes through arteriovenous shunts. This information suggests that RCP does not provide any nutritive benefit during prolonged HCA, but may supplement the topical cooling provided by ice and thus provide an important benefit especially if cooling prior to HCA has been rapid.

In a series of clinical patients with cerebral protection times ranging between 40 and 80 min, we found that RCP was associated with a higher incidence of permanent stroke, and a much higher incidence of temporary neurological dysfunction than HCA or selective antegrade cerebral perfusion.[10] However, other authors have reported lower stroke rates and lower mortality with RCP in comparison to HCA alone.[37,38] Harrington et al. reported their results on the use of HCA ± RCP for aortic arch repairs, which showed normal neurologic outcomes despite significant changes on neuropsychometric testing.[39] RCP did not improve neurologic outcomes. In a small, randomized, prospective study comparing HCA alone, RCP and HCA and antegrade perfusion, there was no clinical benefit of any of the cerebral protection adjuncts over HCA alone.[40] The potential benefit of RCP in the hands of others may be secondary to continued cooling through veno-arterial and veno-venous anastomosis during HCA, but the updrift in temperature during prolonged HCA can be more safely prevented by thorough cooling and packing the head in ice. Currently, it is our belief that cold RCP may be an appropriate technique for treatment of massive intraoperative inadvertent air embolism, but otherwise, it is of historical importance only.

18.5 Axillary Artery Cannulation

The axillary artery is our preferred site of cannulation for proximal aortic and arch replacement surgery (Fig. 18.6). The incidence of stroke after replacement of the aortic arch and ascending aorta has been shown to be influenced by the site of cannulation and by perfusion technique. The preferred site of cannulation for CPB has traditionally been the ascending aorta, but sometimes, this poses an undesirable risk. When the ascending aorta is unsuitable for cannulation, the femoral artery has been the most common alternative. But retrograde flow in a severely atherosclerotic or dissected aorta poses major risks, including dislodgement of plaques, malperfusion, and aortic dissection, all of which may lead to cerebral and visceral organ malperfusion, as well as peripheral injury. Retrograde flow with blood destined for cerebral circulation through an atherosclerotic abdominal or thoracic aorta

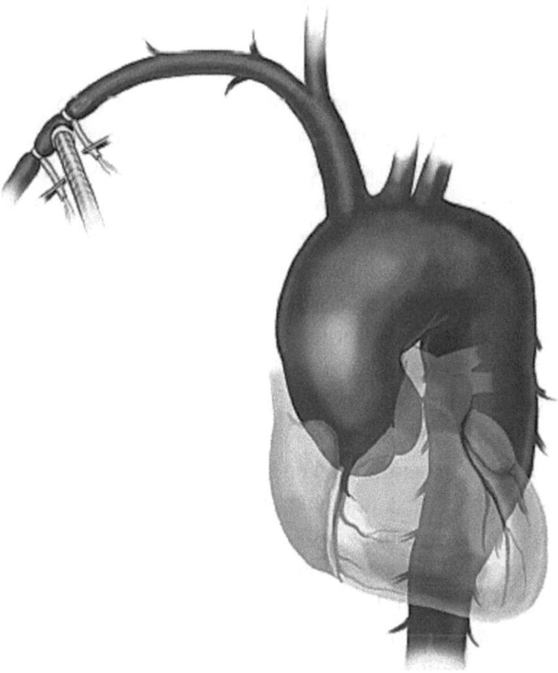

Fig. 18.6 A demonstration of direct axillary artery cannulation with an angled cannula in aortic arch surgery

unquestionably contributes to embolic load. For these reasons, cannulation of the axillary artery has become increasingly widespread.

Axillary artery cannulation preserves antegrade flow in the descending aorta while eliminating some of the risks associated with direct cannulation of the ascending aorta. It lowers the potential for embolization into right-sided cerebral vessels by perfusing them with flow which has not transversed the arch, and avoids the "sandblast" effect of turbulent flow from a catheter tip close to atherosclerotic lesions in the proximal aorta, and thus also reduces the risk of embolization into the left-sided cerebral vessels. Arterial inflow through the axillary artery increases the ease of using selective cerebral perfusion during the arch repair, which allows the surgeon to construct open proximal and distal anastomosis, while the lower body is kept hypothermic during circulatory arrest.

In 2004, we reported on 284 patients who had axillary artery cannulation for aortic arch and ascending aortic procedures. Our incidence of unsuccessful axillary artery cannulation was 2.1%, for reasons which included local dissection, small internal diameter, involvement in Type A dissection, or unusual location of the axillary artery. Brachial plexus injury occurred very infrequently in our series.[41] Axillary artery cannulation does not increase the risk of the procedure, and may be the optimal technique for reducing perfusion-related morbidity and adverse outcome in operations for acute dissection, atherosclerotic and degenerative aneurysmal disease. In a recent retrospective study, we reported on 451 patients who underwent proximal aortic or aortic arch surgery with axillary cannulation: patients with atherosclerotic aneurysms had better neurological outcomes and superior survival with axillary cannulation than with cannulation at other sites; the superiority of axillary cannulation for other etiologies of aortic aneurysms was less marked.[42] Our preference is for direct cannulation of the axillary artery, but another option is to suture a Hemashield graft end-to-side to the artery and then insert the cannula into the graft. If an end-to-side graft is utilized, it is probably wise to clamp the axillary artery distal to the graft, inasmuch as hyperperfusion of the right upper extremity and hypoperfusion of the remainder of the body may otherwise occur. If there are technical problems with the anastomosis or anatomical issues with the axillary artery, the cannula pressures may not be detected if the distal axillary artery is not clamped.

18.6 Trifurcated Graft Technique

The replacement of the aortic arch has notoriously been fraught with embolic strokes as a result of the burden of clot and atheroma in the aortic arch. A significant proportion of atheromatous disease is located at the ostia of the arch vessels. To reduce neurologic complications, we developed an aortic arch reconstruction technique in which a trifurcated graft is anastomosed to the individual brachiocephalic vessels distal to atheroma during DHCA, reducing the risk of embolization and minimizing cerebral ischemia (Fig. 18.7). Another advantage of this approach is bi-hemispheric antegrade cerebral perfusion through all three graft limbs as arch repair is completed. We have found that with this technique our circulatory arrest time is shorter, with a lower incidence of perioperative stroke and TND[16,18]. On average, we have found that the time of interruption of antegrade perfusion with the trifurcated graft technique has been approximately 30 min.

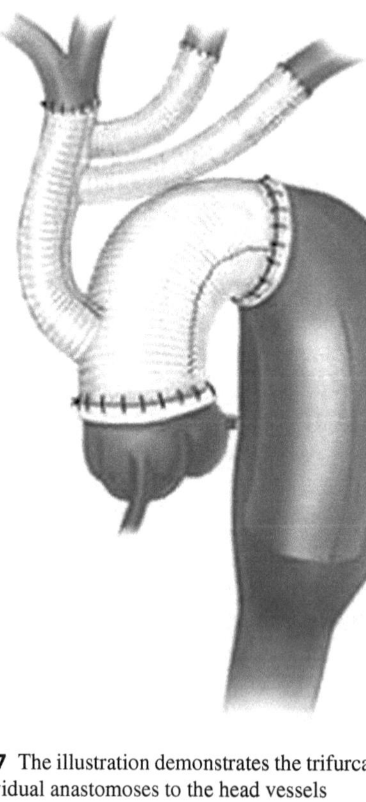

Fig. 18.7 The illustration demonstrates the trifurcated graft and the individual anastomoses to the head vessels

18.7 Summary

In summary, protection of the brain during aortic arch is reasonably satisfactory, resulting in mortality and stroke rates in the low single digits in contemporary series, but there is substantial room for further improvements. For short intervals of interruption of cerebral circulation, simple HCA is probably the preferable technique, although attention must be directed to its careful implementation. Appropriate cooling and rewarming protocols are mandatory for successful and reproducible neurologic outcomes. RCP may have a role in treatment of massive intraoperative air embolism, but in our view, it does not add substantially to cerebral protection and may actually cause cerebral edema. Antegrade cerebral perfusion will provide relatively safe periods of interruption of normal arch perfusion for up to 2–3 h, but the optimal techniques and perfusion parameters for its implementation are yet to be fully defined. As mentioned, implementing SCP exclusively through the innominate artery should be undertaken only with caution because it leaves the posterior circulation vulnerable to ischemia. Preoperative and intraoperative measures should be utilized to assure intracranial communication through the circle of Willis. Moreover, it is quite clear that longer periods of total cerebral protection do result in a higher incidence of transient neurological dysfunction, which may be associated with lasting albeit mild cognitive impairment. Clearly, factors other than those elucidated here, such as the rheology of cold blood and microembolization of air and fat, will require further study in the future if near-perfect cerebral protection is to be achieved.

References

1. Griepp RB, Stinson EB, Hollingsworth JF, Buehler D. Prosthetic replacement of the aortic arch. *J Thorac Cardiovasc Surg*. Dec 1975;70(6):1051-1063.
2. Ehrlich MP, McCullough JN, Zhang N, et al. Effect of hypothermia on cerebral blood flow and metabolism in the pig. *Ann Thorac Surg*. Jan 2002;73(1):191-197.
3. McCullough JN, Zhang N, Reich DL, et al. Cerebral metabolic suppression during hypothermic circulatory arrest in humans. *Ann Thorac Surg*. Jun 1999;67(6):1895-1899. discussion 1919-1821.
4. Mezrow CK, Midulla PS, Sadeghi AM, et al. Evaluation of cerebral metabolism and quantitative electroencephalography after hypothermic circulatory arrest and low-flow cardiopulmonary bypass at different temperatures. *J Thorac Cardiovasc Surg*. Apr 1994;107(4):1006-1019.
5. Mezrow CK, Gandsas A, Sadeghi AM, et al. Metabolic correlates of neurologic and behavioral injury after prolonged hypothermic circulatory arrest. *J Thorac Cardiovasc Surg*. May 1995;109(5):959-975.
6. Michenfelder JD, Milde JH. The relationship among canine brain temperature, metabolism, and function during hypothermia. *Anesthesiology*. Jul 1991;75(1):130-136.
7. Mezrow CK, Midulla PS, Sadeghi AM, et al. Quantitative electroencephalography: a method to assess cerebral injury after hypothermic circulatory arrest. *J Thorac Cardiovasc Surg*. May 1995;109(5):925-934.
8. Ergin MA, Galla JD, Lansman L, Quintana C, Bodian C, Griepp RB. Hypothermic circulatory arrest in operations on the thoracic aorta. Determinants of operative mortality and neurologic outcome. *J Thorac Cardiovasc Surg*. Mar 1994; 107(3):788-797. discussion 797-789.
9. Ergin MA, Uysal S, Reich DL, et al. Temporary neurological dysfunction after deep hypothermic circulatory arrest: a clinical marker of long-term functional deficit. *Ann Thorac Surg*. Jun 1999;67(6):1887-1890. discussion 1891-1884.
10. Hagl C, Ergin MA, Galla JD, et al. Neurologic outcome after ascending aorta-aortic arch operations: effect of brain protection technique in high-risk patients. *J Thorac Cardiovasc Surg*. Jun 2001;121(6):1107-1121.
11. Svensson LG, Crawford ES, Hess KR, et al. Deep hypothermia with circulatory arrest. Determinants of stroke and early mortality in 656 patients. *J Thorac Cardiovasc Surg*. Jul 1993;106(1):19-28. discussion 28-31.
12. Greeley WJ, Kern FH, Meliones JN, Ungerleider RM. Effect of deep hypothermia and circulatory arrest on cerebral blood flow and metabolism. *Ann Thorac Surg*. Dec 1993;56(6): 1464-1466.
13. Greeley WJ, Kern FH, Ungerleider RM, et al. The effect of hypothermic cardiopulmonary bypass and total circulatory arrest on cerebral metabolism in neonates, infants, and children. *J Thorac Cardiovasc Surg*. May 1991;101(5):783-794.
14. Griepp RB, Ergin MA, McCullough JN, et al. Use of hypothermic circulatory arrest for cerebral protection during aortic surgery. *J Card Surg*. 1997; Mar-Apr 12(2 Suppl): 312-321.
15. Ehrlich MP, McCullough J, Wolfe D, et al. Cerebral effects of cold reperfusion after hypothermic circulatory arrest. *J Thorac Cardiovasc Surg*. May 2001;121(5):923-931.
16. Spielvogel D, Etz CD, Silovitz D, Lansman SL, Griepp RB. Aortic arch replacement with a trifurcated graft. *Ann Thorac Surg*. Feb 2007;83(2):S791-795. discussion S824-731.
17. Strauch JT, Spielvogel D, Lauten A, et al. Technical advances in total aortic arch replacement. *Ann Thorac Surg*. Feb 2004;77(2):581-589. discussion 589-590.
18. Spielvogel D, Halstead JC, Meier M, et al. Aortic arch replacement using a trifurcated graft: simple, versatile, and safe. *Ann Thorac Surg*. Jul 2005;80(1):90-95. discussion 95.
19. Reich DL, Uysal S, Sliwinski M, et al. Neuropsychologic outcome after deep hypothermic circulatory arrest in adults. *J Thorac Cardiovasc Surg*. Jan 1999;117(1):156-163.
20. Kazui T, Kimura N, Yamada O, Komatsu S. Surgical outcome of aortic arch aneurysms using selective cerebral perfusion. *Ann Thorac Surg*. Apr 1994;57(4):904-911.

21. Bachet J, Guilmet D, Goudot B, et al. Cold cerebroplegia. A new technique of cerebral protection during operations on the transverse aortic arch. *J Thorac Cardiovasc Surg*. Jul 1991;102(1):85-93. discussion 93-84.
22. Kazui T, Yamashita K, Washiyama N, et al. Usefulness of antegrade selective cerebral perfusion during aortic arch operations. *Ann Thorac Surg*. Nov 2002;74(5):S1806-1809. discussion S1825-1832.
23. Kazui T, Yamashita K, Washiyama N, et al. Aortic arch replacement using selective cerebral perfusion. *Ann Thorac Surg*. Feb 2007;83(2):S796-798. discussion S824-731.
24. Schomer DF, Marks MP, Steinberg GK, et al. The anatomy of the posterior communicating artery as a risk factor for ischemic cerebral infarction. *N Engl J Med*. Jun 2 1994; 330(22):1565-1570.
25. Kazui T. Which is more appropriate as a cerebral protection method—unilateral or bilateral perfusion? *Eur J Cardiothorac Surg*. Jun 2006;29(6):1039-1040.
26. Strauch JT, Spielvogel D, Haldenwang PL, et al. Impact of hypothermic selective cerebral perfusion compared with hypothermic cardiopulmonary bypass on cerebral hemodynamics and metabolism. *Eur J Cardiothorac Surg*. Nov 2003;24(5):807-816.
27. Strauch JT, Spielvogel D, Lauten A, et al. Optimal temperature for selective cerebral perfusion. *J Thorac Cardiovasc Surg*. Jul 2005;130(1):74-82.
28. Halstead JC, Wurm M, Meier DM, et al. Avoidance of hemodilution during selective cerebral perfusion enhances neurobehavioral outcome in a survival porcine model. *Eur J Cardiothorac Surg*. Sep 2007;32(3):514-520.
29. Sakamoto T, Nollert GD, Zurakowski D, et al. Hemodilution elevates cerebral blood flow and oxygen metabolism during cardiopulmonary bypass in piglets. *Ann Thorac Surg*. May 2004;77(5):1656-1663. discussion 1663.
30. Sakamoto T, Zurakowski D, Duebener LF, et al. Combination of alpha-stat strategy and hemodilution exacerbates neurologic injury in a survival piglet model with deep hypothermic circulatory arrest. *Ann Thorac Surg*. Jan 2002;73(1): 180-189. discussion 189-190.
31. Shin'oka T, Shum-Tim D, Laussen PC, et al. Effects of oncotic pressure and hematocrit on outcome after hypothermic circulatory arrest. *Ann Thorac Surg*. Jan 1998;65(1): 155-164.
32. Halstead JC, Spielvogel D, Meier DM, et al. Optimal pH strategy for selective cerebral perfusion. *Eur J Cardiothorac Surg*. Aug 2005;28(2):266-273. discussion 273.
33. Midulla PS, Gandsas A, Sadeghi AM, et al. Comparison of retrograde cerebral perfusion to antegrade cerebral perfusion and hypothermic circulatory arrest in a chronic porcine model. *J Card Surg*. Sep 1994;9(5):560-574. discussion 575.
34. Yerlioglu ME, Wolfe D, Mezrow CK, et al. The effect of retrograde cerebral perfusion after particulate embolization to the brain. *J Thorac Cardiovasc Surg*. Nov 1995;110(5): 1470-1484. discussion 1484-1475.
35. Ehrlich MP, Hagl C, McCullough JN, et al. Retrograde cerebral perfusion provides negligible flow through brain capillaries in the pig. *J Thorac Cardiovasc Surg*. Aug 2001; 122(2):331-338.
36. Boeckxstaens CJ, Flameng WJ. Retrograde cerebral perfusion does not perfuse the brain in nonhuman primates. *Ann Thorac Surg*. Aug 1995;60(2):319-327. discussion 327-318.
37. Ueda Y, Okita Y, Aomi S, Koyanagi H, Takamoto S. Retrograde cerebral perfusion for aortic arch surgery: analysis of risk factors. *Ann Thorac Surg*. Jun 1999;67(6):1879-1882. discussion 1891-1874.
38. Ehrlich MP, Fang WC, Grabenwoger M, et al. Impact of retrograde cerebral perfusion on aortic arch aneurysm repair. *J Thorac Cardiovasc Surg*. Dec 1999;118(6):1026-1032.
39. Harrington DK, Bonser M, Moss A, Heafield MT, Riddoch MJ, Bonser RS. Neuropsychometric outcome following aortic arch surgery: a prospective randomized trial of retrograde cerebral perfusion. *J Thorac Cardiovasc Surg*. Sep 2003; 126(3):638-644.
40. Svensson LG, Nadolny EM, Penney DL, et al. Prospective randomized neurocognitive and S-100 study of hypothermic circulatory arrest, retrograde brain perfusion, and antegrade brain perfusion for aortic arch operations. *Ann Thorac Surg*. Jun 2001;71(6):1905-1912.
41. Strauch JT, Spielvogel D, Lauten A, et al. Axillary artery cannulation: routine use in ascending aorta and aortic arch replacement. *Ann Thorac Surg*. Jul 2004;78(1):103-108. discussion 103-108.
42. Etz CD, Plestis KA, Kari FA, et al. Axillary cannulation significantly improves survival and neurologic outcome after atherosclerotic aneurysm repair of the aortic root and ascending aorta. *Ann Thorac Surg*. Aug 2008;86(2):441-446. discussion 446-447.

The Future of Brain Protection in Cardiac Surgery

19

Min Lou and Magdy Selim

19.1 Introduction

Cerebral injury remains a continuing source of morbidity and mortality in patients undergoing cardiac surgery.[1] A variety of neurological disorders can occur after cardiac surgery, including stroke, cognitive dysfunction, and delirium.[2] The latter is mostly attributed to the use of anesthesia, and is often of short term. Attention is increasingly focused on the prevention and treatment of stroke and cognitive decline after cardiac surgery given their long-term morbidities and functional consequences. Strategies to optimize neurological outcomes in cardiac surgery patients continue to evolve. The purpose of this chapter is to briefly review the current strategies and to look into the future to suggest research priorities and approaches for brain protection in cardiac surgery. Our review is largely limited to clinical research with only modest examination of basic science and epidemiological studies.

19.2 Mechanisms of Brain Injury in Cardiac Surgery

A brief overview of the pathophysiology of cerebral injury in cardiac surgery, in particular coronary artery bypass grafting (CABG), is important to better understand the goals and targets of brain protection in patients undergoing heart surgery. The etiology of cerebral injury in cardiac surgery involves complex multifactorial mechanisms. Cerebral microembolization resulting from manipulations of an atheromatous aortic arch during clamping, the bypass machine, acquired coagulopathy, or peri-operative arrhythmias; hypoperfusion due to hemodynamic failure during surgery, postoperative pump failure or blood loss; inflammation (both cerebral as well as systemic); rapid rewarming after cardiopulmonary bypass, which may jeopardize sensitive brain tissue at risk for injury; as well as a genetic susceptibility to injury or genetic inability to repair following injury, have all been implicated.[3–5] Brain protection in cardiac surgery may be accomplished by impeding one or more of these etiologic factors and the resulting cascade of events leading to cerebral injury.

Strategies for brain protection in cardiac surgery can be considered in two stages, each utilizing pharmacological and nonpharmacological interventions. The first stage is prevention, which includes careful evaluation to identify high-risk patients, modifications of the surgical technique, and peri-operative monitoring to avoid the injury to brain before, during, and after surgery. The second is target-specific and directed towards preventing and treating secondary cerebral damage after surgery. Although numerous studies have focused on the latter solution, more success has been found with the former.[4] Similarly, more success has been found with nonpharmacological, as opposed to pharmacological, strategies.

19.3 Preoperative and Preventive Strategies

Several patient- and procedure-related factors are associated with increased risk of cerebral injury in

M. Lou (✉)
Assistant Professor, Department of Neurology,
The 2nd Affiliated Hospital of Zhejiang University, Hangzhou, Zhejiang, China
e-mail: loumingxc@vip.sina.com

R.S. Bonser et al. (eds.), *Brain Protection in Cardiac Surgery*,
DOI: 10.1007/978-1-84996-293-3_19,

cardiac surgery. An initial step in protecting the brain during cardiac surgery is to identify those patients at high risk for adverse neurological outcomes. Screening patients before they undergo surgery helps to optimize care, initiate appropriate treatment for co-existing morbidities, and allow the surgeon to modify the surgical technique, when possible, to minimize adverse outcomes while achieving the surgical goal.[6]

19.3.1 Clinical Risk Prediction

Multiple studies have defined the risk for cerebral injury in CABG patients on the basis of patient's clinical characteristics, and several risk-stratification models have been developed to predict a patient's risk, in particular for peri-operative stroke.[7,8] However, most of these studies were retrospective and lacked adequately designed and well-planned neurological and imaging assessments, thus limiting the utility of most risk-stratification models. Large-scale, prospective, clinical studies with appropriate controls and well-designed outcome assessment measures remain necessary to better identify how patient's characteristics contribute to neurological and cognitive impairment after cardiac surgery. This requires a coordinated effort between neurologists and cardiothoracic surgeons, increased involvement of the neurological community in the planning of these studies, and standardization of medical care management in cardiac surgery patients. The choice of centers for such studies is an important variable; expertise and ability to generalize results should be considered.

19.3.2 Genetic Identification

There is evidence that specific genetic polymorphisms and epistasis in biological pathways regulating inflammation, coagulation-thrombosis, cell matrix adhesion/interaction, lipid metabolism, and vascular reactivity may modulate the risk of neurological injury following cardiac surgery. In one study, patients with apolipoprotein ε4 allele had worse cognitive outcomes after CABG,[9] though subsequent studies did not replicate this finding.[10] Recent genetic studies in cardiac surgery patients found that carriers of minor alleles of C-reactive protein (CRP 1059G/C SNP) and P-selectin (SELP 1087A) had lower peri-operative serum CRP, less platelet activation, and less susceptibility to cognitive decline,[11] whereas polymorphism of the glycoprotein (GP) IIIa constituent of the platelet integrin receptor GP IIb/IIIa was associated with more severe neurocognitive decline after CABG.[12] Patients who develop neurocognitive decline after CABG seem to have significantly different gene-expression responses, involving inflammation, antigen presentation, and cellular adhesion among others, compared with that of patients without cognitive impairment.[13] Similarly, patients who have minor alleles for C-reactive protein (CRP 3'UTR 1846C/T) and interleukin(IL)-6 (-174G/C) may be at higher risk for stroke after CABG.[14] Most recently, carriers of the anti-oxidant response element dependent NAD(P)H:quinine oxidoreductase 1 (NQ01) gene, a regulatory element involved in the anti-inflammatory mechanism in the vasculature exposed to nonlaminar flow during cardiopulmonary bypass, were found to have higher serum levels of IL-6 during CABG than noncarriers.[15] These findings suggest that patients who undergo cerebral injury may have inherently different genetic responses to cardiopulmonary bypass compared with those of patients without adverse neurological outcomes; and that the genetic variations in inflammatory, cell adhesion, and apoptotic pathways could become a target for risk stratification and prevention of brain injury in cardiac surgery.

The promise that the genetic makeup of the individual can be used to identify patients at risks for cerebral injury after cardiac surgery is intriguing and represents a fertile area for the future research. Identifying specific single nucleotide peptides associated with neurological injury and the specific mechanisms whereby a genetic polymorphism mediates its effects is important to identify molecular and genetic targets for future therapies aiming to improve neurological outcome in patients undergoing cardiac surgery. Furthermore, a patient's genetic makeup may be useful to determine his/her response to a particular therapy. The ability to identify surgical patients with genetic susceptibility to cerebral injury pre-operatively could have important utility when new neuroprotective strategies become available by facilitating rational allocation of these likely high-cost therapies to the highest risk patients.

19.3.3 Biochemical Markers

Few preliminary studies have investigated the association between biochemical markers of brain injury and the inflammatory response and neurological outcomes after CABG. Most of these studies have focused on S-100β (beta), neuron-specific enolase (NSE), and Tau proteins. In one study, serum levels of NSE and Tau were better associated with post-operative cognitive decline and less influenced by cardiotomy suction compared with S-100β (beta).[16] A recent study showed that patients with a positive pre-operative serum N-Methyl-D-Aspartate (NMDA) receptor subunit NR2 antibodies test (≥2.0 ng/mL) were nearly 18 times more likely to experience an adverse post-operative neurological event than patients with a negative test.[17] Future studies are needed to optimize the measurement of biomarkers of brain injury, and to better define and assess their potential role in the prediction of neurological outcome after cardiac surgery.

19.3.4 Pharmacological Preventive Strategies

Peri-operative administration of a variety of drugs to CABG patients may decrease the incidence of stroke and cognitive decline after surgery. Although studies provide conflicting results, there is convincing evidence to support the use of statins and β-blockers peri-operatively, including the pre-operative period.[18–20] In a retrospective cohort study, preoperative statin treatment was associated with reduced post-operative mortality and morbidity in patients undergoing cardiac surgery.[19] In another prospective observational study, taking statins, at least 4 weeks prior to surgery, was independently associated with lower risk of peri-operative cerebrovascular events.[20] The neuroprotective effects of statins seem to be multifactorial. Statins exert multiple pleiotropic properties, independent of their effects on low-density lipoprotein cholesterol, which result in direct anti-atherosclerotic, anti-thrombotic, anti-oxidative, and anti-inflammatory effects.[21–24] Statins may also be protective against postoperative atrial fibrillation, possibly due to alterations in the extracellular matrix and remodeling after CABG.[25, 26] A recent prospective study of 22 patients undergoing CABG who were randomized to a combination of statins and angiotensin-converting enzyme inhibitors (ACE-inhibitors) found that early treatment with high doses (ramipril 10 mg or enalapril 20 mg and simvastatin 80 mg or atorvastatin 40 mg), but not standard doses (ramipril 2.5 mg and simvastatin 20 mg or atorvastatin 10 mg), drastically attenuated plasma levels of IL-6, tumor necrosis factor-α (alpha), E-selectin, and sVCAM-1 after surgery.[27] This suggests that statins/ACE-inhibitor mediated modulation of CABG-associated inflammatory response may be dose-dependent.

Observational studies also suggest that the use of β(beta)-adrenergic antagonists during the peri-operative period in patients undergoing cardiac surgery is associated with a substantial reduction in the incidence of post-operative neurological complications, including stroke and transient ischemic attacks.[28] This neuroprotective effect of β-blockers may be related to reduced incidence of myocardial ischemia and post-operative arrhythmias; modulating both cerebrovascular tone and CABG-related inflammatory events; and anti-oxidant and anti-apoptosis properties.[29–31]

The use of statins, β(beta)-blockers, and ACE-inhibitors has increased among patients with coronary artery disease during the past few years. It is thus an appealing concept to use these drugs for peri-operative prophylaxis against cerebral injury after CABG. Prospective, large, randomized, controlled trials investigating the effects of peri-operative use of statins, ACE-inhibitors, angiotensin receptor blockers, and β(beta)-blockers among CABG patients are needed to confirm the above findings. The doses, duration of therapy, and possible synergistic effects of various combinations also warrant further investigations.

19.4 Intraoperative Strategies

Cerebral microembolism is the leading cause of brain injury in cardiac surgery.[32] Several studies have demonstrated that embolization during CABG is predominantly related to manipulations of the aortic arch and dislodging of atheromatous plaques during application and removal of cross-clamps.[33] Therefore, developing strategies to minimize aortic manipulations during surgery and to prevent the travel of the generated microemboli to the brain represents the main cornerstone of brain protection during the peri-operative period in cardiac surgery. Improved monitoring for cerebral embolization during surgery is also important, as it could allow for instantaneous modification of the surgical technique to minimize further embolism and subsequent brain injury.

19.4.1 Minimizing Emboli Generation

Many approaches have been used to minimize emboli generation during cardiac surgery. Small studies have shown that the use of heparin-bonded circuits and cell saver,[34,35] which minimizes the amount of particulate and lipid-laden material in the blood prior to returning it to the venous reservoir, could be beneficial. A multicenter, randomized trial in 1,289 patients showed that the use of an intra-aortic filter during cardiac surgery is safe and effective, as demonstrated by an emboli capture rate of 97%, and might reduce the incidence of postoperative neurological complications in high-risk patients.[36,37] Changes in the surgical techniques may also reduce emboli generation. Avoiding manipulation of the aorta by using only a single clamp application was demonstrated to reduce postoperative cognitive impairment.[38] There is some evidence, albeit inconclusive, that off-pump CABG in patient with severe aortic atherosclerosis may decrease cerebral microembolization.[39,40] A recent systematic review assessing the quality of published reports of randomized controlled trials comparing off- vs. on-pump CABG techniques found that the overall quality of reporting was poor and insufficient compared with the Consolidated Standards for Reporting Trials (CONSORT) statement.[41] Future, well-designed, well-reported, large-scale, randomized, controlled trials are needed to clarify the role of these various surgical techniques in patients at high risk for cerebral injury after cardiac surgery. Patient stratification based on the degree and extent of aortic atherosclerosis should be addressed in these trials, and the use of pre-operative techniques, such as magnetic resonance angiography and transesophageal echocardiography, for screening high-risk patients and guiding the choice of the surgical technique warrant investigations. In addition, innovative technologies aiming to reduce atheromatous plaque dislodgement and embolization, such as the use of sutureless and clampless aortic anastomotic devices, need to be developed and studied in the clinical setting.

19.4.2 Brain Monitoring

Improved monitoring for evidence of cerebral embolization or ischemia during surgery can play an important role in brain protection during CABG. Rapid detection of an evidence of cerebral compromise can prompt immediate surgical and therapeutic interventions to minimize the risk of permanent cerebral injury. Transcranial Doppler provides a noninvasive measure of blood flow velocity and allows the detection of high-intensity transient signals (HITS), which may signify that cerebral embolism electroencephalography (EEG) and near-infrared spectroscopy (NIRS) can provide a measure of brain activity, perfusion, and oxygenation status. The utilization of these various neurological monitoring techniques in cardiac surgery is currently limited. Intraoperative neurological monitoring holds a great promise in detecting and reducing neurological abnormalities during cardiac surgery in the future.[42] Observational studies are needed to collect hemodynamic data, and to synchronize these data with those from TCD, EEG, and NIRS to identify the association between various clinical strategies and the development of precursors of neurological injury during CABG. Studies are also needed to assess the role of on-line TCD, EEG, and NIRS in the assessment and refinement of current surgical techniques, and the development of new techniques and therapies.

19.4.3 Temperature Control

A great deal of investigation has focused on the influence of intra-operative temperature on neurological outcome after cardiac surgery. Animal studies have demonstrated a protective effect of mild hypothermia (2–5 C decrease in brain temperature) in the setting of global cerebral ischemia followed by reperfusion.[43,44] Multimodal effects of hypothermia were suggested, in addition to its measurable effect on suppressing cerebral metabolism.[45] However, clinical trials have yielded conflicting results regarding the neuroprotective effects of hypothermia. A meta-analysis only showed a trend toward a reduction in the rate of peri-operative stroke when the patient's core body temperature during CABG was 31.4–33.1 C, as compared with a temperature of more than 33.2 C.[46] A recent randomized, double-blind study demonstrated that mild intra-operative hypothermia did not decrease the incidence of neurocognitive deficits in patients undergoing cardiac surgery.[47] Although the limitations to the existing data preclude definitive conclusions about the neuroprotective effect of intra-operative hypothermia, there is emerging evidence that rapid post-operative rewarming and hyperthermia during the first 48 h after CABG have harmful neurological effects.[48,49] Grocott et al. found an association between peak body temperature within 24 h of CABG and cognitive decline postoperatively.[48] Grigore et al.[50] demonstrated that, when compared to conventional faster rewarming, slower rewarming results in a lower incidence of neurocognitive dysfunction 6 weeks after cardiac surgery. Similarly, Nathan et al.[51,52] reported that rewarming from mild hypothermia to 34 C was associated with fewer cognitive deficits after CABG surgery compared with rewarming to a body temperature of 37 C, suggesting that mild postoperative hypothermia may be beneficial. Given these results, it appears that some degree of the neuroprotection afforded by intra-operative hypothermia may be negated by the postoperative change in temperature after cardiac surgery. The efficacy of reducing inadvertent postoperative hyperthermia, controlling the rewarming process and possibly extending mild hypothermia into the period after cardiac surgery to reduce subsequent neurological complications merit further future investigations.

19.5 Postoperative Interventions

At present, there are no proven interventions that can be recommended for prophylactic neuroprotection in the postoperative period aside from the good clinical practice of acid-base management and blood glucose control. There are promising data on the potential benefits of some drugs that attenuate blood loss, activation of hemostatic system, inflammation, and excitatory amino acids signaling pathways. However, future investigations are still needed before any of these agents can be recommended for brain protection in cardiac surgery patients.

19.5.1 Strategies for Blood Conservation

Excessive blood loss after cardiac surgery is an important cause of morbidity and can contribute to cerebral hypoperfusion and secondary neurological injury. Factors contributing to blood loss include hemodilution, consumption of clotting factors, platelet-consumption dysfunction, activation of the inflammatory cascade, and fibrinolysis. Various strategies to decrease blood loss have been investigated with different results. Several studies showed that aprotonin, a nonspecific serine protease inhibitor, significantly reduces the need for blood transfusions and the number of units of blood transfused in cardiac surgery patients.[53] Treatment with high-dose aprotinin was shown to reduce the incidence of cognitive deficits, stroke, and atrial fibrillation after CABG.[54, 55] Nevertheless, animal investigations failed to show any direct benefit of aprotonin on either functional or neurohistologic outcome following cerebral ischemia,[56] suggesting that aprotinin may have had its beneficial effects independent of any direct neuroprotective effect through an indirect effect of modulating cerebral embolization.[4] Most recently, however, a retrospective study that used propensity scoring to adjust for the higher overall risk in CABG patients receiving aprotinin reported an increase in stroke rate with aprotinin use.[57] In recent years, there has been a rising interest in using recombinant activated factor VII (rFVIIa) in cardiac surgery patients,[58] and a multicenter trial is currently underway. Future studies are needed to confirm the safety of these pro-coagulant factors in cardiac patients and to ascertain their effects and other blood-conserving strategies on CABG-related neurological injury.

19.5.2 N-Methyl-D-Aspartate (NMDA) Blocker

Excitotoxicity, modulated through the NMDA receptor-mediated pathways, has received much attention in the field of neuroprotection. To date, only preliminary reports of studies of NMDA antagonists in cardiac surgery have appeared in the literature. In one study, peri-operative treatment with remacemide, a noncompetitive NMDA antagonist, was shown to improve the neuropsychiatric performance in patients undergoing CABG.[59] Xenon gas, an NMDA receptor antagonist, was also found to attenuate cardiopulmonary bypass-induced neurological and neurocognitive dysfunction in the rat.[60] Although there are concerns that xenon's disposition to expand gaseous bubbles destined to become cerebral air emboli during CABG could abolish its beneficial effect or even worsen cerebral outcome,[61] a recent open-label phase-I study in 16 patients undergoing CABG showed that treatment with Xenon was safe and did not result in increased cerebral embolization on TCD.[62] These results suggest that neuroprotective drugs that operate through the excitotoxic pathway may be beneficial in cardiac surgery. The neuroprotective potential of NMDA antagonists, in particular xenon, merits further investigations in large placebo-controlled, randomized clinical trials. The timing of NMDA blockade and the status of NMDA receptor after cardiac surgery, as assessed by serum assays, should be considered in the planning of these trials.

19.5.3 Magnesium

Magnesium is another potential candidate for brain protection in cardiac surgery. It blocks voltage-gated calcium influx and NMDA receptor-operated calcium channels, thereby attenuating neuronal excitotoxicity. Magnesium also reduces the incidence of postoperative atrial fibrillation.[63] In addition, magnesium affects other pathways potentially involving inflammatory processes.[64] In patients undergoing CABG, changes in serum S-100β(beta) concentrations correlate with those in serum total magnesium concentrations, where a decrease in serum magnesium results in an elevation in serum S-100β(beta).[65] A recent preliminary study found that magnesium administration improves neurological function after cardiac surgery, particularly in preserving short-term memory and cortical control over brainstem functions.[66] Future studies to delineate the optimal duration and timing of magnesium therapy and targeted serum concentrations are needed to further investigate the potential benefits of magnesium in brain protection after cardiac surgery.

19.5.4 Deferoxamine

Cardiopulmonary bypass and the superimposed period of ischemia-reperfusion are situations in cardiac surgery that promote free radical generation and subsequent lipid peroxidation. Ferric iron, derived from hemolysis and cardioplegia solutions during CABG, catalyzes these reactions. Diminishing the production of free radicals by reducing ferric iron in cardiac surgery could be beneficial. Several studies have shown that the addition of the iron chelator deferoxamine to the cardioplegia solution prevents the generation of oxygen free radicals and decreases the incidence of arrhythmias.[67] A small number of clinical trials have shown that cardioplegia with deferoxamine can reduce oxygen free radical activity and lipid peroxidation and attenuate apoptotic cell death after CABG.[68] More recently, deferoxamine infusion for 8 h prior to CABG was reported to ameliorate oxygen free radical production, protect the myocardium against reperfusion injury, and improve postoperative cardiac recovery and function.[69] The benefits of deferoxamine were particularly evident in patients with a lower pre-operative left ventricular ejection fraction. Furthermore, treatment with deferoxamine significantly increased cerebral perfusion and improved neurological deficit scores in rat models of cardiac arrest and resuscitation.[70] These observations have not been translated into large-scale, randomized, controlled trials to examine the impact of treatment with deferoxamine on patients' neurological outcomes after CABG. They merit future investigations.

19.5.5 Complement Inhibitors

Activation of complement during CABG is a major contributor to CABG-associated systemic inflammatory response. A few preliminary studies have examined the impact of complement inhibitors on neurological outcomes after CABG. In one study, a C5 inhibitor was shown to attenuate cognitive decline after cardiac surgery.[71] In another study, the use of pexelizumab (a complement C5 inhibitor) 24 h peri-operatively ameliorated the decline in visuo-spatial function at hospital discharge, but had no significant effect on overall cognition.[72] Further investigations are required to delineate the role of complement inhibition in brain protection after CABG.

In conclusion, brain protection in cardiac surgery needs to be considered from several perspectives. Although rigorous research is still needed, our lessons from the past and the rapid pace of accumulating knowledge regarding the pathophysiological, molecular, and biochemical changes leading to brain injury after cardiac surgery encourage optimism that more effective brain protective strategies will become available in the future. We anticipate that new approaches will be pursued, including: novel surgical and technical strategies to minimize the risk of cerebral microembolization during surgery; agents that are tailored to ameliorate the postoperative cascade of events associated with cerebral injury; and the development of genetic and biochemical markers to facilitate identification of high-risk patients to whom potential neuroprotective therapies should be administered. The use of multitherapy, as opposed to monotherapy, and combining pharmacological with nonpharmacological protective strategies are likely to be more effective. Although most efforts will remain focused on preventing brain injury in cardiac surgery in the near future, the concept of brain protection is likely to expand to include strategies to restore function and facilitate recovery from neurological injury. Much has been learnt about how to plan, conduct, and report large-scale, multicenter, clinical studies in this area, and much more will be learnt over the coming years to maximize ongoing efforts in this therapeutic endeavor.

References

1. Ferguson TB Jr, Hammill BG, Peterson ED, et al. A decade of change-risk profiles and outcomes for isolated coronary artery bypass grafting procedures, 1990-1999: a report from the STS National Database Committee and the Duke Clinical Research Institute. *Ann Thorac Surg*. 2002;73:480-489.
2. Roach GW, Kanchuger M, Mangano CM, et al. Adverse cerebral outcomes after coronary bypass surgery. *N Engl J Med*. 1996;335:1857-1864.
3. Newman MF, Mathew JP, Grocott HP, et al. Central nervous system injury associated with cardiac surgery. *Lancet*. 2006;368:694-703.
4. Grocott HP, Yoshitani K. Neuroprotection during cardiac surgery. *J Anesth*. 2007;21:367-377.
5. McKhann GM, Grega MA, Borowicz LM Jr, et al. Stroke and encephalopathy after cardiac surgery: an update. *Stroke*. 2006;37:562-571.
6. Selim M. Perioperative stroke. *N Engl J Med*. 2007;356: 706-713.
7. Newman MF, Wolman R, Kanchuger M, et al. Multicenter preoperative stroke risk index for patients undergoing coronary artery bypass graft surgery. *Circulation*. 1996;94:II74-80.
8. Charlesworth DC, Likosky DS, Marrin CA, et al. Development and validation of a prediction model for strokes after coronary artery bypass grafting. *Ann Thorac Surg*. 2003;76:436-443.
9. Tardiff BE, Newman MF, Saunders AM, et al. Preliminary report of a genetic basis for cognitive decline after cardiac operations. *Ann Thorac Surg*. 1997;64:715-720.
10. Steed L, Kong R, Stygall J, et al. The role of apolipoprotein E in cognitive decline after cardiac operation. *Ann Thorac Surg*. 2001;71:823-826.
11. Mathew JP, Podgoreanu MV, Grocott HP, et al. Genetic variants in P-selectin and C-reactive protein influence susceptibility to cognitive decline after cardiac surgery. *J Am Coll Cardiol*. 2007;49:1934-1942.
12. Mathew JP, Rinder CS, Howe JG, et al. Platelet PlA2 polymorphism enhances the risk of neurocognitive decline after cardiopulmonary bypass. *Ann Thorac Surg*. 2001;71: 663-666.
13. Ramlawi B, Otu H, Rudolph JL, et al. Genomic expression pathways associated with brain injury after cardiopulmonary bypass. *J Thorac Cardiovasc Surg*. 2007;134:996-1005.
14. Grocott HP, White W, Morris RW, et al. Genetic Polymorphisms and the risk of stroke after cardiac surgery. *Stroke*. 2005;36:1854-1858.
15. Isbir CS, Ergen A, Tekeli A, et al. The effect of NQ01 polymorphism on the inflammatory response in cardiopulmonary bypass. *Cell Biochem Funct*. Dec 2007;20.
16. Ramlawi B, Rudolph JL, Mieno S, et al. Serologic markers of brain injury and cognitive function after cardiopulmonary bypass. *Ann Surg*. 2006;244:593-601.
17. Bokesch PM, Izykenova GA, Justice JB, et al. NMDA receptor antibodies predict adverse neurological outcome after cardiac surgery in high-risk patients. *Stroke*. 2006;37: 1432-1436.
18. Ali IS, Buth KJ. Preoperative statin use and outcomes following cardiac surgery. *Int J Cardiol*. 2005;103:12-18.
19. Clark LL, Ikonomidis JS, Crawford FA Jr, et al. Preoperative statin treatment is associated with reduced postoperative mortality and morbidity in patients undergoing cardiac surgery: an 8-year retrospective cohort study. *J Thorac Cardiovasc Surg*. 2006;131:679-685.
20. Aboyans V, Labrousse L, Lacroix P, et al. Predictive factors of stroke in patients undergoing coronary bypass grafting: statins are protective. *Eur J Cardiothorac Surg*. 2006;30: 300-304.
21. Kinlay S, Schwartz GG, Olsson AG, et al. High-dose atorvastatin enhances the decline in inflammatory markers in patients with acute coronary syndromes in the MIRACL study. *Circulation*. 2003;108:1560-1566.
22. Shishehbor MH, Brennan ML, Aviles RJ, et al. Statins promote potent systemic antioxidant effects through specific inflammatory pathways. *Circulation*. 2003;108:426-431.
23. Cipollone F, Fazia M, Iezzi A, et al. Suppression of the functionally coupled cyclooxygenase-2/prostaglandin E synthase as a basis of simvastatin- dependent plaque stabilization in humans. *Circulation*. 2003;107:1479-1485.
24. Saito S, Fujiwara T, Matsunaga T, et al. Increased adiponectin synthesis in the visceral adipose tissue in men with coronary artery disease treated with pravastatin: A role of the attenuation of oxidative stress. *Atherosclerosis*. Dec 2007;26.
25. Blanchard L, Collard CD. Non-antiarrhythmic agents for prevention of postoperative atrial fibrillation: role of statins. *Curr Opin Anaesthesiol*. 2007;20:53-56.
26. Marín F, Pascual DA, Roldán V, et al. Statins and postoperative risk of atrial fibrillation following coronary artery bypass grafting. *Am J Cardiol*. 2006;97:55-60.
27. Radaelli A, Loardi C, Cazzaniga M, et al. Inflammatory activation during coronary artery surgery and its dose-dependent modulation by statin/ACE-inhibitor combination. *Arterioscler Thromb Vasc Biol*. 2007;27:2750-2755.
28. Amory DW, Grigore A, Amory JK, et al. Neuroprotection is associated with beta-adrenergic receptor antagonists during cardiac surgery: evidence from 2575 patients. *J Cardiothorac Vasc Anesth*. 2002;16:270-277.

29. Andrews TC, Reimold SC, Berlin JA, et al. Prevention of supraventricular arrhythmias after coronary artery bypass surgery: A meta-analysis of randomized control trials. *Circulation.* 1991;84:III236-244.
30. Wallace A, Layug B, Tateo I, et al. Prophylactic atenolol reduces postoperative myocardial ischemia. *Anesthesiology.* 1998;88:7-17.
31. Savitz SI, Erhardt JA, Anthony JV, et al. The novel beta-blocker, carvedilol, provides neuroprotection in transient focal stroke. *J Cereb Blood Flow Metab.* 2000;20:1197-1204.
32. Likosky DS, Marrin CA, Caplan LR, et al. Determination of etiologic mechanisms of strokes secondary to coronary artery bypass graft surgery. *Stroke.* 2003;34:2830-2834.
33. Bergman P, Hadjinikolaou L, Van Der Linden J. Aortic atheroma is related to number of particulates captured by intra-aortic filtration in CABG. *Eur J Cardiothorac Surg.* 2002;22:539-544.
34. Aldea GS, Soltow LO, Chandler WL, et al. Limitation of thrombin generation, platelet activation, and inflammation by elimination of cardiotomy suction in patients undergoing coronary artery bypass grafting treated with heparin-bonded circuits. *J Thorac Cardiovasc Surg.* 2002;123:742-755.
35. Jewell AE, Akowuah EF, Suvarna SK, et al. A prospective randomised comparison of cardiotomy suction and cell saver for recycling shed blood during cardiac surgery. *Eur J Cardiothorac Surg.* 2003;23:633-636.
36. Wimmer-Greinecker G. International Council of Emboli Management Study Group. Reduction of neurologic complications by intra-aortic filtration in patients undergoing combined intracardiac and CABG procedures. *Eur J Cardiothorac Surg.* 2003;23:159-164.
37. Banbury MK, Kouchoukos NT, Allen KB, et al. Emboli capture using the Embol-X intraaortic filter in cardiac surgery: A multicenter randomized trial of 1289 patients. *Ann Thorac Surg.* 2003;76:508-515.
38. Hammon JW, Stump DA, Butterworth JF, et al. Single cross-clamp improves 6-month cognitive outcome in high-risk coronary bypass patients: the effect of reduced aortic manipulation. *J Thorac Cardiovasc Surg.* 2006;131:114-121.
39. Sedrakyan A, Wu AW, Parashar A, et al. Off-pump surgery is associated with reduced occurrence of stroke and other morbidity as compared with traditional coronary artery bypass grafting: a meta-analysis of systematically reviewed trials. *Stroke.* 2006;37:2759-2769.
40. Légaré JF, Hirsch G. Off-pump coronary artery bypass graft surgery is standard of care: where do you stand? *Can J Cardiol.* 2006;22:1107-1110.
41. Farrokhyar F, Chu R, Whitlock R, et al. A systematic review of the quality of publications reporting coronary artery bypass grafting trials. *Can J Surg.* 2007;50:266-277.
42. Andropoulos DB, Stayer SA, Diaz LK, et al. Neurological monitoring for congenital heart surgery. *Anesth Analg.* 2004;99:1365-1375.
43. Fukuda S, Warner DS. Cerebral protection. *Br J Anaesth.* 2007;99:10-17.
44. Hoesch RE, Geocadin RG. Therapeutic hypothermia for global and focal ischemic brain injury—a cool way to improve neurologic outcomes. *Neurologist.* 2007;13:331-342.
45. Erecinska M, Thoresen M, Silver IA. Effects of hypothermia on energy metabolism in Mammalian central nervous system. *J Cereb Blood Flow Metab.* 2003;23:513-530.
46. Rees K, Beranek-Stanley M, Burke M, et al. Hypothermia to reduce neurological damage following coronary artery bypass surgery. *Cochrane Database Syst Rev.* 2001; CD002138.
47. Boodhwani M, Rubens F, Wozny D, et al. Effects of sustained mild hypothermia on neurocognitive function after coronary artery bypass surgery: a randomized, double-blind study. *J Thorac Cardiovasc Surg.* 2007;134:1443-1450.
48. Grocott HP, Mackensen B, Grigore AM, et al. Postoperative hyperthermia is associated with cognitive dysfunction after coronary artery bypass graft surgery. *Stroke.* 2002;33: 537-541.
49. Thong WY, Strickler AG, Li S, et al. Hyperthermia in the forty-eight hours after cardiopulmonary bypass. *Anesth Analg.* 2002;95:1489-1495.
50. Grigore AM, Grocott HP, Mathew JP, et al. The rewarming rate and increased peak temperature alter neurocognitive outcome after cardiac surgery. *Anesth Analg.* 2002;94: 4-10.
51. Nathan HJ, Wells GA, Munson JL, et al. Neuroprotective effect of mild hypothermia in patients undergoing coronary artery surgery with cardiopulmonary bypass: a randomized trial. *Circulation.* 2001;104:I85-91.
52. Nathan HJ, Parlea L, Dupuis JY, et al. Safety of deliberate intraoperative and postoperative hypothermia for patients undergoing coronary artery surgery: a randomized trial. *J Thorac Cardiovasc Surg.* 2004;127:1270-1275.
53. Kristeller JL, Stahl RF, Roslund BP, et al. Aprotinin use in cardiac surgery patients at low risk for requiring blood transfusion. *Pharmacotherapy.* 2007;27:988-994.
54. Harmon DC, Ghori KG, Eustace NP, et al. Aprotinin decreases the incidence of cognitive deficit following CABG and cardiopulmonary bypass: a pilot randomized controlled study. *Can J Anaesth.* 2004;51:1002-1009.
55. Frumento RJ, O'Malley CM, Bennett-Guerrero E. Stroke after cardiac surgery: a retrospective analysis of the effect of aprotinin dosing regimens. *Ann Thorac Surg.* 2003;75: 479-483.
56. Grocott HP, Sheng H, Miura Y, et al. The effects of aprotinin on outcome from cerebral ischemia in the rat. *Anesth Analg.* 1999;88:1-7.
57. Mangano DT, Tudor IC, Dietzel C. The risk associated with aprotinin in cardiac surgery. *N Engl J Med.* 2006;354:353-365.
58. Romagnoli S, Bevilacqua S, Gelsomino S, et al. Small-dose recombinant activated factor VII (NovoSeven) in cardiac surgery. *Anesth Analg.* 2006;102:1320-1326.
59. Arrowsmith JE, Harrison MJG, Newman SP, et al. Neuroprotection of the brain during cardiopulmonary bypass. A randomized trial of remacemide during coronary artery bypass in 171 patients. *Stroke.* 1998;29:2357-2362.
60. Ma D, Yang H, Lynch J, et al. Xenon attenuates cardiopulmonary bypass-induced neurologic and neurocognitive dysfunction in the rat. *Anesthesiology.* 2003;98:690-698.
61. Jungwirth B, Gordan ML, Blobner M, et al. Xenon impairs neurocognitive and histologic outcome after cardiopulmonary bypass combined with cerebral air embolism in rats. *Anesthesiology.* 2006;104:770-776.
62. Lockwood GG, Franks NP, Downie NA, et al. Feasibility and safety of delivering xenon to patients undergoing coronary artery bypass graft surgery while on cardiopulmonary bypass: phase I study. *Anesthesiology.* 2006;104:458-446.

63. Miller S, Crystal E, Garfinkle M, et al. Effects of magnesium on atrial fibrillation after cardiac surgery: a meta-analysis. *Heart*. 2005;91:618-623.
64. Baker WL, White CM. Post-cardiothoracic surgery atrial fibrillation: a review of preventive strategies. *Ann Pharmacother*. 2007;41:587-598.
65. Dabrowski W. Do changes in S100beta protein correlate with serum magnesium concentrations in patients undergoing extracorporeal circulation? *Magnes Res*. 2007;20:168-176.
66. Bhudia SK, Cosgrove DM, Naugle RI, et al. Magnesium as a neuroprotectant in cardiac surgery: a randomized clinical trial. *J Thorac Cardiovasc Surg*. 2006;131:853-861.
67. Euler DE. Role of oxygen-derived free radicals in canine reperfusion arrhythmias. *Am J Physiol*. 1995;268:H295-300.
68. Menasché P, Antebi H, Alcindor LG, et al. Iron chelation by deferoxamine inhibits lipid peroxidation during cardiopulmonary bypass in humans. *Circulation*. 1990;82:IV390-396.
69. Paraskevaidis IA, Iliodromitis EK, Vlahakos D, et al. Deferoxamine infusion during coronary artery bypass grafting ameliorates lipid peroxidation and protects the myocardium against reperfusion injury: immediate and long-term significance. *Eur Heart J*. 2005;26:263-270.
70. Liachenko S, Tang P, Xu Y. Deferoxamine improves early postresuscitation reperfusion after prolonged cardiac arrest in rats. *J Cereb Blood Flow Metab*. 2003;23:574-581.
71. Fitch JC, Rollins S, Matis L, et al. Pharmacology and biological efficacy of a recombinant, humanized, single-chain antibody C5 complement inhibitor in patients undergoing coronary artery bypass graft surgery with cardiopulmonary bypass. *Circulation*. 1999;100:2499-2506.
72. Mathew JP, Shernan SK, White WD, et al. Preliminary report of the effects of complement suppression with pexelizumab on neurocognitive decline after coronary artery bypass graft surgery. *Stroke*. 2004;35:2335-2339.

Index

R.S. Bonser et al. (eds.), *Brain Protection in Cardiac Surgery*,
DOI: 10.1007/978-1-84996-293-3, © Springer-Verlag London Limited 2011

MIX
Papier aus verantwortungsvollen Quellen
Paper from responsible sources
FSC® C105338

If you have any concerns about our products,
you can contact us on
ProductSafety@springernature.com

In case Publisher is established outside the EU,
the EU authorized representative is:
Springer Nature Customer Service Center GmbH
Europaplatz 3, 69115 Heidelberg, Germany

Printed by Libri Plureos GmbH
in Hamburg, Germany